Fibromyalgia Syndrome

For Churchill Livingstone

Commissioning Editor: Mary Law
Project Development Manager: Valerie Dearing
Project Manager: Ewan Halley
Page Make-up: Gerard Heyburn

Fibromyalgia Syndrome

A Practitioner's Guide to Treatment

Leon Chaitow ND DO
Practitioner and Senior Lecturer, Centre for Community Care and Primary Health,
University of Westminster, London, UK

With contributions by
Peter Baldry MB FRCP

Regina P. Gilliland MD

Gina Honeyman-Lowe BLS DC

John C. Lowe MA DC

Mark Pellegrino MD

Paul J. Watson BSc(Hons) MCSP

Foreword by
Dr Sue Morrison
General Practitioner, Marylebone Health Centre, London and
Associate Dean, Postgraduate General Practice, North Thames (West), UK

Illustrated by
Graeme Chambers BA(Hons)
Medical Artist

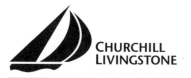
CHURCHILL
LIVINGSTONE

EDINBURGH LONDON NEW YORK PHILADELPHIA ST LOUIS SYDNEY TORONTO 2000

CHURCHILL LIVINGSTONE
An imprint of Harcourt Publishers Limited

© Harcourt Publishers Limited 2000

⚓ is a registered trade mark of Harcourt Publishers
Limited

First published 2000
  Reprinted 2000

ISBN 0 443 06227 7

British Library Cataloguing in Publication Data
A catalogue record for this book is available from the British
Library.

Library of Congress Cataloging in Publication Data
A catalog record for this book is available from the Library of
Congress.

Note
Medical knowledge is constantly changing. As new information becomes available, changes in treatment, procedures,
equipment and the use of drugs become necessary.
The editors, contributors and the publishers have, as far as it
is possible, taken care to ensure that the information given in
this text is accurate and up to date. However, readers are
strongly advised to confirm that the information, especially
with regard to drug usage, complies with current legislation
and standards of practice.

Printed in China

Contents

Contributors

Peter Baldry MB FRCP
Emeritus Consultant Physician, Ashford
Hospital, North-West London, UK; Private
Practice, Fladbury, Pershore, Worcester, UK
6. Acupuncture treatment of fibromyalgia and myofascial pain

Regina P. Gilliland MD
Private Practitioner, Birmingham, Alabama, USA
8. A medical perspective on fibromyalgia

Gina Honeyman-Lowe BLS DC
Adviser in Metabolic Therapy, Fibromyalgia
Research Foundation, Tulsa, Oklahoma, USA
10. The metabolic rehabilitation of fibromyalgia patients

John C. Lowe MA DC
Director of Research, Fibromyalgia Research
Foundation, Tulsa, Oklahoma, USA
10. The metabolic rehabilitation of fibromyalgia patients

Mark Pelligrino MD
Private Practitioner, Ohio Rehab Center Inc.,
Canton, Ohio, USA
9. Physical medicine and a rehabilitation approach to treating fibromyalgia

Paul J. Watson BSc(Hons) MSc MCSP
Research Fellow, Rheumatic Diseases Centre,
Hope Hospital, Salford, UK
7. Interdisciplinary pain management in fibromyalgia

Foreword

Chronic pain and 'unwellness' are the bread and butter of primary health care: our patients come to see us because they don't feel well. This is expressed in all manner of ways, often dictated by cultural habit, but most practitioners are familiar with the complaints of 'I feel tired all the time' or 'I ache all over' or 'My body condition is not good'. This may be what a patient with fibromyalgia syndrome tells us, but the condition is unlikely to be diagnosed, and the patient may be called a 'somatiser', or 'depressed'.

These presentations make the hearts and minds of many mainstream medical practitioners sink, as they search their memory for any skills learned in medical training appropriate to help relieve these symptoms. This mismatch between a still largely reductionist cure-seeking approach taught in medical schools, and a case-load comprising approximately 80% 'psychosocial' distress in the primary health care setting, is daunting.

However, a steadily growing mutual awareness between traditional and complementary therapies and approaches has begun to address this gap. Many physicians have now heard of fibromyalgia, and are delighted to be able to make sense of a cluster of symptoms that are commonly presented, especially in the primary care setting. While most practitioners would be wary of rigid labelling of conditions, being able to use the shorthand for this syndrome and associated conditions facilitates our communication with our colleagues and patients.

This is true integrated medicine, where understanding each other's therapeutic worlds allows us to progress from multiprofessional to interprofessional learning and working.

Leon Chaitow's exploration of the main aetiological hypotheses for fibromyalgia syndrome makes very intelligent reading, avoiding the temptation to condense theory into fact. Readers will be able to distil their own management approach from clinical experience which they can now underpin with current thinking and practice. The sizeable contributions in the text from several therapeutic disciplines view fibromyalgia syndrome through the lenses of different clinical perspectives and promote understanding between complementary and traditional orientations.

The author has provided us not only with an excellent opportunity to explore the complexities and satisfactory management of a common and challenging condition, but also with a framework for formulating truly integrated protocols and guidelines. This model can be usefully extended to other areas of practice, and will serve as a learning tool for the multiprofessional practice team who are wishing to develop integrated medical practice.

The layout of the text and tables makes the information easily accessible to busy practitioners, who may wish to dip in and out of it to refer to both general themes (e.g. health and disease influences on the human condition) and to more specific topics (e.g. exclusion diets, stress, and the gut). The self-help material will be of great interest to patients.

Our learning as adults is driven by the need to know particular information; primary care practitioners who are struggling on a daily basis with how to deal with the conditions described in this book will be relieved to be able to formulate new ways to understand and work with patients who have some of these chronic conditions (for example, see Chapter 12: irritable bowel syndrome, depression, premenstrual syndrome, sleep disorder, allergy).

Leon Chaitow has written a pivotal book here: his readable style, underpinned by a critical evidence base, makes this text invaluable to primary health care practitioners, traditional or complementary, who are genuinely interested in the pursuit and maintenance of health, and not merely freedom from illness. This book should be a welcome addition to any clinical practitioner's individual library or primary health care learning facility and will significantly develop the collaborative agenda between traditional and complementary medicine.

London, 1999   Sue Morrison

Preface

Fibromyalgia syndrome (FMS) has much in common with chronic fatigue syndrome (CFS) and also superficially resembles aspects of myofascial pain syndrome (MPS). How is it possible to make sense of the complex aetiology of FMS and CFS which seems often to involve a cocktail of biochemical, biomechanical and psychosocial factors ? It becomes increasingly obvious that these umbrella terms, FMS and CFS, incorporate conditions in which, although symptoms may be very similar, aetiological factors are often quite different. In some instances an obvious trauma, whiplash for example, can be shown to have triggered FMS. In others a biochemical (endocrine imbalance, toxicity etc) scenario is demonstrable, while in yet others severe emotional distress seems to have been the precipitating factor.

Research into these often debilitating conditions continues at an explosive rate, breeding a variety of hypotheses and treatment approaches. What this book attempts is a review of what is currently agreed as well as what is conceptualized and hotly debated about FMS. It also summarizes what is being done therapeutically in various contexts. To assist in this process of review a selection of practitioners from an eclectic range of professional backgrounds, both orthodox and unconventional, have provided their own particular insights, and in some instances protocols.

Following the broad overview and debate, and the individual chapters which represent different viewpoints, a practical guide is offered incorporating osteopathic and naturopathic therapeutic approaches. These are the methods which the principle author has found to be effective over the past 15 years of treating CFS and FMS, both privately and in an NHS setting. As far as is possible research evidence is presented to support these.

It is worth emphasising that although FMS manifests primarily as musculoskeletal pain, this is not where the problem arises. The 'bodywork' protocols are therefore offered as a means of providing symptomatic relief, assisting in rehabilitation, but not as a 'cure'. Out of the wide range of choices discussed, and in some instances described in detail, it should be possible to make choices, based on the individual patient's needs as well as the belief system and training of the practitioner or therapist. As reported in chapter 2, the most important and valuable contribution to recovery or control of their condition, as specified by the majority of FMS patients, is derived from gaining an understanding of their condition. I hope that the information in this book will allow for a greater degree of understanding in what is, by any standards, a little understood, major health problem.

Corfu, Greece, May 1999   Leon Chaitow

Acknowledgements

My deep and sincere thanks go to Peter Baldry, Regina Gilliland, Gina Honeyman-Lowe, John Lowe, Mark Pellegrino and Paul Watson for their collaborative contributions to this book. In addition I want to offer thanks to Melvyn Werbach, who provided me with so much research evidence regarding nutritional influences on fibromyalgia. I strongly believe that it is only by seeing this confusing condition from a variety of perspectives that some understanding is possible of its complex nature. Out of these differing viewpoints emerges a strong message which suggests that by means of integrated therapeutic endeavours, recovery becomes more likely. The value of integrated practice is one which has been brought into reality in my experience for the past 7 years, at that pioneering National Health Service practice, Marylebone Health Centre, London. I wish to acknowledge my enormous professional debt to all those with whom I have had the privilege of working at Marylebone, in particular the person who invited me to join it, Patrick Pietroni, to whom I dedicate this book, with affection and thanks.

Publisher's Acknowledgements

Figs 1.1, 1.4, 6.3, 6.4, 6.5, 13.14, 13.15, 13.16, 13.17A&B, 13.18, 13.19A&B, 13.20A&B, 13.21A&B from Chaitow (1996) Modern Neuromuscular Technique, reproduced with permission of Harcourt Publishers Ltd.

Figs 13.1, 13.2, 13.6, 13.8, 13.9, 13.10A&B, 13.11A&B, 13.12A&B, 13.13A&B, 13.22, 13.23, 13.24, 13.25, 13.26, 13.27A-C from Chaitow (1996) Muscle Energy Techniques, reproduced with permission of Harcourt Publishers Ltd.

Figs 13.3, 13.4, 13.5 from Chaitow (1996) Palpation Skills (1998), reproduced with permission of Harcourt Publishers Ltd.

Figs 13.7, 13.28, 13.29, 13.30A-C, 13.31, 14.1, 14.2, 14.3, 14.5 from Chaitow (1996) Positional Release Techniques, reproduced with permission of Harcourt Publishers Ltd.

Figs 6.1, 6.2 from Baldry (1993) Acupuncture, Trigger Points and Musculoskeletal Pain (Second edition), reproduced with permission of Harcourt Publishers Ltd.

1

The history and definition of fibromyalgia

HISTORY

Historically, fibromyalgia – or conditions very like it – have been reported for hundreds of years, under many names, including the most unsatisfactory 'fibrositis'. The fascinating history of what are now known as fibromyalgia syndrome (FMS) and myofascial pain syndrome (MPS) has been catalogued by several modern clinicians working in the sphere of chronic muscle pain, from whose work the material summarised in Box 1.1 has been compiled. Thanks are due to these individuals (Peter Baldry, David Simons and Richard van Why in particular) for revealing so much about past studies into the phenomenon of chronic muscle pain. What we can learn from this information is just how long ago (well over 150 years) particular features were recognised, such as pain referral patterns and characteristics such as taut bands and 'nodules', as well as insights from many astute researchers and clinicians into the pathophysiology of these conditions.

AMERICAN COLLEGE OF RHEUMATOLOGY DEFINITION

It was not until the 1980s that a redefining of what was by then a confused and confusing picture of a common condition took place. In 1987 fibromyalgia was recognised as a distinct syndrome by the American Medical Association (Starlanyl & Copeland 1996), although at that time detailed knowledge of what it comprised was not as clear as the current, generally accepted, American College of Rheumatology (ACR) definition, which was produced in 1990 (see Box 1.2 and Fig. 1.1).

1

Box 1.1 Historical (pre-1990) research into chronic muscle pain (Baldry 1993, Simons 1988, van Why 1994)

Guillaume de Baillou (late 16th century) *Liber de Rheumatismo* (published in 1736, over 100 years after death of de Baillou).
Used term **rheumatism** to describe muscular pain as well as acute rheumatic fever.

Thomas Sydenham (1676) *Observationes Medicae*.
Confused the use of word **rheumatism** by using it to describe symptoms of acute rheumatic fever.

William Balfour (1815) 'Observations on the Pathology and Cure of Rheumatism.' *Edinburgh Medical and Surgical Journal* 11:168-187
Suggested that an inflammatory process in connective tissue was responsible for the pain of what was then called **muscular rheumatism.**

C. Scudamore (1827) *A Treatise on the Nature and Cure of Rheumatism*. Longman, London
Supported the concepts promoted by Balfour.

F. Valleix (1841) *Treatise on Neuralgia*. Paris
Noted that when certain painful points were palpated they produced shooting pain to other regions (**neuralgia**). He also reported that diet was a precipitating factor in the development of the painful aching symptoms of the back and cervical region.

Johan Mezger (mid-19th century) (W. Haberling *Johan Georg Mezger of Amsterdam. Founder of Modern Scientific Massage*. Medical Life, 1932)
Dutch physician, developed massage techniques for treating 'nodules' and taut cord-like bands associated with this condition.

T. Inman (1858) 'Remarks on Myalgia or Muscular Pain.' *British Medical Journal*: 407–408, 866–868
Was able clearly to state that radiating pain in these conditions (**myalgia**) was independent of nerve routes.

Uno Helleday (1876) *Nordiskt Medecinkst Arkiv* 6 & 8 (8)
Swedish physician described nodules as part of '**chronic myitis**'.

H. Strauss (1898) Über die sogenaunte 'rheumatische muskelschwiele'. *Klinische Wochenschrift* 35: 89–91
German physician distinguished between palpable nodules and 'bands'.

A. Cornelius (1903) 'Narben und Nerven.' *Deutsche Militartzlische Zeitschrift* 32: 657–673
German physician who demonstrated the pain influencing features of tender points and nodules, insisting that the radiating pathway was not determined by the course of nerves. He also showed that external influences, including climatic, emotional or physical exertion, could exacerbate the already hyper-reactive neural structures associated with these conditions. Cornelius also discussed these pain phenomena as being due to **reflex mechanisms**.

Sir William Gowers (1904) 'Lumbago: Its Lessons and Analogues.' *British Medical Journal* 1: 117–121
Suggested that the word **fibrositis** be used – believing erroneously that inflammation was a key feature of 'muscular rheumatism'.
(Lecture, National Hospital of Nervous Diseases, London)

Ralph Stockman (1904) 'Causes, Pathology and Treatment of Chronic Rheumatism.' *Edinburgh Medical Journal* 15: 107–116, 223–225
Offered support for Gowers's suggestion by reporting finding evidence of inflammation in connective tissue in such cases (never substantiated), and suggested that pain sensations emanating from nodules could be due to nerve pressure (now discounted).

Sir William Osler (1909) *Principles and Practice of Medicine*. Appleton, New York
Considered the painful aspects of muscular rheumatism (**myalgia**) to involve '**neuralgia of the sensory nerves** of the muscles'.

W. Telling (1911) 'Nodular Fibromyositis – an Everyday Affliction and its Identity with so-called Muscular Rheumatism.' *The Lancet* 1: 154–158
Called the condition '**nodular fibromyositis**'.

A. Muller (1912) 'Untersuchbefund am Rheumatish Erkranten Musckel.' *Zeitschrift Klinische Medizine* 74: 34–73
German physician who noted that to identify nodules and bands required refined palpation skills – aided, he suggested, by lubricating the skin.

L. Llewellyn (1915) *Fibrositis*. Rebman, New York
Broadened the use of the word **fibrositis** to include other conditions, including gout.

F. Albee (1927) 'Myofascitis – a Pathological Explanation of any Apparently Dissimilar Conditions.' *American Journal of Surgery* 3: 523–533
Called the condition '**myofascitis**'.

G. Murray (1929) 'Myofibrositis as Simulator of other Maladies.' *The Lancet* 1: 113–116
Called the condition '**myofibrositis**'.

E. Clayton (1930) 'Fibrositis.' *The Lancet* 1: 1420–1423
Called the condition '**neuro-fibrositis**'.

A. H. Rowe (1930) 'Allergic Toxemia and Migraine due to Food Allergy.' *California West Medical Journal* 33: 785
Demonstrated that muscular pains associated with fatigue, nausea, gastrointestinal symptoms, weakness, headaches, drowsiness, mental confusion and slowness of thought, as well as irritability, despondency and widespread bodily aching, often had an allergic aetiology which he termed '**allergic toxaemia**'.

Box 1.1 (Contd.)   Historical (pre-1990) research into chronic muscle pain (Baldry 1993, Simons 1988, van Why 1994)

C. Hunter (1933) 'Myalgia of the Abdominal Wall.'
Canadian Medical Association Journal 28: 157–161
Described referred pain (**myalgia**) resulting from tender points situated in the abdominal musculature.

F. Gudzent (1935) 'Testunt und Heilbehandlung von Rheumatismus und Gicht mid Specifischen Allergen.'
Deutsche Medizinsche Wochenschrift 61: 901
German physician noted that chronic '**muscular rheumatism**' may at times be allergic in origin and that removal of certain foods from the diet resulted in clinical improvement.

J. Edeiken, C. Wolferth (1936) 'Persistent Pain in the Shoulder Region Following Myocardial Infarction.' *American Journal of Medical Science* 191: 201–210
Showed that pressure applied to tender points in scapula region muscles could reproduce shoulder pain already being experienced. This work influenced Janet Travell (see below).

Sir Thomas Lewis (1938) 'Suggestions Relating to the Study of Somatic Pain.' *British Medical Journal* 1: 321–325
A major researcher into the phenomenon of pain in general, he charted several patterns of pain referral and suggested that Kellgren (see below), who assisted him in these studies, continue the research.

J. Kellgren (1938) 'Observations on Referred Pain Arising from Muscle.' *Clinical Science* 3: 175–190
Identified (in patients with '**fibrositis**'/'**myalgia**') many of the features of our current understanding of the trigger point phenomenon, including consistent patterns of pain referral – to distant muscles and other structures (teeth, bone, etc.) from pain points ('spots') in muscle, ligament, tendon, joint and periosteal tissue – which could be obliterated by use of novocaine injections.

A. Reichart (1938) 'Reflexschmerzen auf Grund von Myoglosen.' *Deutsche Medizinische Wochenschrift* 64: 823–824
Czech physician who identified and charted patterns of distribution of **reflex pain** from tender points (nodules) in particular muscles.

M. Gutstein (1938) 'Diagnosis and Treatment of Muscular Rheumatism.' *British Journal of Physical Medicine* 1: 302–321
Refugee Polish physician working in Britain who identified that in treating **muscular rheumatism,** manual pressure applied to tender (later trigger) points produced both local and referred symptoms, and that these referral patterns were consistent in everyone, if the original point was in the same location. He deactivated these by means of injection.

A. Steindler (1940) 'The Interpretation of Sciatic Radiation and the Syndrome of Low Back Pain.' *Journal of Bone and Joint Surgery* 22: 28–34
American orthopaedic surgeon who demonstrated that novocaine injections into tender points located in the low back and gluteal regions could relieve sciatic pain. He called these points 'trigger points'. Janet Travell (see below) was influenced by his work and popularised the term 'trigger points'.

M. Gutstein-Good (1940) (same person as M. Gutstein above) 'Idiopathic Myalgia Simulating Visceral and other Diseases.' *The Lancet* 2: 326–328
Called the condition '**idiopathic myalgia**'.

M. Good (1941) (same person as M. Gutstein and M. Gutstein-Good above) 'Rheumatic Myalgias.' *The Practitioner* 146: 167–174
Called the condition '**rheumatic myalgia**'.

James Cyriax (1948) 'Fibrositis.' *British Medical Journal* 2: 251–255
Believed that chronic muscle pain derived from nerve impingement due to disc degeneration. 'It [pressure on dura mater] has misled clinicians for decades and has given rise to endless misdiagnosis; for these areas of "**fibrositis**", "trigger points", or "myalgic spots", have been regarded as the primary lesion – not the result of pressure on the dura mater' (J. Cyriax, 1962 *Text-Book of Orthopaedic Medicine* , 4th edn. Cassell, London, vol. 1).

P. Ellman, D. Shaw (1950) 'The Chronic "Rheumatic" and his Pains. Psychosomatic Aspects of Chronic Non-articular Rheumatism.' *Annals of Rheumatic Disease* 9: 341–357
Suggested that because there were few physical manifestations to support the pain claimed by patients with chronic muscle pain, their condition was essentially psychosomatic (**psychogenic rheumatism**): 'the patient aches in his limbs because he aches in his mind'.

Theron Randolph (1951) 'Allergic Myalgia.' *Journal of Michigan State Medical Society* 50: 487
This leading American clinical ecologist described the condition as '**allergic myalgia**' and demonstrated that widespread and severe muscle pain (particularly of the neck region) could be reproduced 'at will under experimental circumstances' following trial ingestion of allergenic foods or inhalation of house dust extract or particular hydrocarbons – with relief of symptoms often being achieved by avoidance of allergens. Randolph reported that several of his patients who achieved relief by these means had previously been diagnosed as having '**psychosomatic rheumatism**'.

James Mennell (1952) *The Science and Art of Joint Manipulation*. Churchill, London, vol. 1.
British physician described 'sensitive areas' which referred pain. Recommended treatment was a choice between manipulation, heat, pressure and deep friction. He also emphasised the importance of diet, fluid intake, rest and the possible use of cold and procaine injections, as well as suggesting cupping, skin rolling, massage and stretching in normalisation of '**fibrositic deposits**'.

Box 1.1 (Contd.)   Historical (pre-1990) research into chronic muscle pain (Baldry 1993, Simons 1988, van Why 1994)

Janet Travell, S. Rinzler (1952) 'The Myofascial Genesis of Pain.' *Postgraduate Medicine* 11: 425–434
Building on previous research, and following her own detailed studies of the tissues involved, Travell coined the word 'myofascial', adding it to Steindler's term to produce 'myofascial trigger points', and finally '**myofascial pain syndrome**'.

I. Neufeld (1952) 'Pathogenetic Concepts of "Fibrositis" – Fibropathic Syndromes.' *Archives of Physical Medicine* 33: 363–369
Suggested that the pain of '**fibrositis–fibropathic syndromes**' was due to the brain misinterpreting sensations.

F. Speer (1954) 'The Allergic–Tension–Fatigue Syndrome.' *Pediatric Clinician of North America* 1: 1029
Called the condition the '**allergic–tension–fatigue syndrome**' and added to the pain, fatigue and general symptoms previously recognised (see Randolph above) the observation that oedema was a feature – especially involving the eyes.

R. Gutstein (1955) 'Review Of Myodysneuria (Fibrositis).' *American Practitioner* 6: 570–577
Called the condition '**myodysneuria**'.

M. Kelly (1962) 'Local Injections For Rheumatism.' *Medical Journal of Australia* 1: 45–50
Australian physician who carried on Kellgren's concepts from the early 1940s, diagnosing and treating pain (**rheumatism**) by means of identification of pain points and deactivating these using injections.

H. Moldofsky, P. Scarisbrick, R. England, H. Smythe 1975 'Musculoskeletal Symptoms and Non-Rem Sleep Disturbance in Patients with Fibrositis Syndrome and Healthy Subjects.' *Psychosomatic Medicine* 371: 341–351
Canadian physician who, together with co-workers, identified sleep disturbance as a key feature of chronic muscle pain (**fibrositis**).

M. Yunus, A. Masi, J. Calabro, K. Miller, S. Feigenbaum (1981) 'Primary Fibromyalgia (Fibrositis) Clinical Study of 50 Patients with Matched Controls.' *Seminars in Arthritis and Rheumatism* 11: 151–171
First popularised the word **fibromyalgia.**

Janet Travell, David Simons (1983) *Myofascial Pain and Dysfunction: the Trigger Point Manual.* Williams and Wilkins, Baltimore, vol. 1. (Revised 1998)

The definitive work (with volume 2, 1992) on the subject of **myofascial pain syndrome** (MPS).

David Simons (1986) 'Fibrositis/Fibromyalgia: a Form of Myofascial Trigger Points?' *American Journal of Medicine* 81(S3A): 93–98
American physician who collaborated with Travell in joint study of MPS and who also conducted his own studies into the connection between **myofascial pain syndrome** and **fibromyalgia syndrome**, finding a good deal of overlap.

D. Goldenberg, D. Felson, H. Dinerman et al (1986) 'Randomized Controlled Trial of Amitriptyline and Naproxen in Treatment of Patients with FMS.' *Arthritis and Rheumatism* 29: 1371–1377
Demonstrated that low dose tricyclic antidepressant medication improved sleep quality, reduced morning stiffness, and alleviated pain in **fibromyalgia** (see Ch. 11).

G. McCain, R. Scudds (1988) 'The Concept of Primary Fibromyalgia (Fibrositis) Clinical Value, Relation and Significance to other Chronic Musculoskeletal Pain Syndromes.' *Pain* 33: 273–287
Showed that there was some benefit to **fibromyalgia** symptoms from cardiovascular fitness training ('aerobics') (see Ch. 11).

M. Margoles (1989) 'The Concept of Fibromyalgia.' *Pain* 36: 391
States that most patients with **fibromyalgia** demonstrate numerous active myofascial trigger points.

R. Bennett (1990) 'Myofascial Pain Syndromes and the Fibromyalgia Syndrome'. In: R. Fricton, E. Awad. (eds) *Advances in Pain Research and Therapy*. Raven Press, New York
Showed that many 'tender points' in **fibromyalgia** are in reality latent trigger points. He believes that MPS and FMS are distinctive syndromes but are 'closely related'. States that many people with MPS progress to develop fibromyalgia.

American College of Rheumatology (1990) 'Criteria for the Classification of **Fibromyalgia**.' *Arthritis and Rheumatism* 33: 160–172
Official definition for FMS syndrome. Subsequently expanded in 1992 by the Copenhagen Declaration: Consensus Document on Fibromyalgia (Consensus Document 1992; see also p. 6).

What can be said with certainty about fibromyalgia syndrome is that:

- It is a nondeforming rheumatic condition and, indeed, one of the commonest such conditions

- It is an ancient condition, newly defined as a disease complex or syndrome
- There is no single cause, or cure, for its widespread and persistent symptoms

Box 1.2   ACR definition of fibromyalgia syndrome

The definition of fibromyalgia syndrome (FMS) as stated by the American College of Rheumatologists (ACR 1990) is as follows:

1. A history of widespread pain for at least 3 months. Pain is considered widespread when all of the following are present: pain in the left side of the body, the right side of the body, below the waist and above the waist. In addition there should be axial pain (cervical spine or anterior chest or thoracic spine or low back).

2. Pain (with the patient reporting 'pain' and not just 'tenderness') in 11 of 18 tender point sites on digital pressure involving 4K of pressure. The sites are all bilateral and are situated:

- At the suboccipital muscle insertions (close to where rectus capitis posterior minor inserts)

- At the anterior aspects of the inter-transverse spaces between C5 and C7
- At the midpoint of the upper border of upper trapezius muscle
- At the origins of supraspinatus muscle above the scapula spines
- At the second costochondral junctions, on the upper surface, just lateral to the junctions
- 2 centimetres distal to the lateral epicondyles of the elbows
- In the upper outer quadrants of the buttocks in the anterior fold of gluteus medius
- Posterior to the prominence of the greater trochanter (piriformis insertion)
- On the medial aspect of the knees, on the fatty pad, proximal to the joint line.

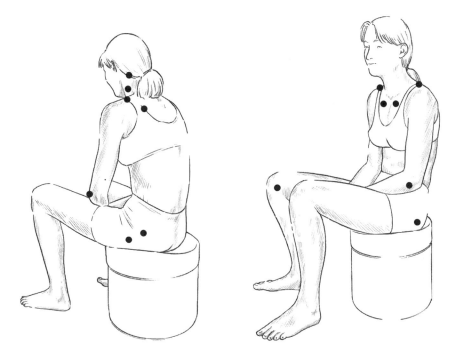

Figure 1.1   The sites of the 18 fibromyalgia tender points as defined by the American College of Rheumatologists.

- Its complex causation seems to require more than one essential aetiological factor to be operating, and there are numerous theories as to what these might be (see Ch. 4)
- There has been an explosion of research into the subject over the past decade (one data search on the internet revealed over 20 000 papers which mention fibromyalgia as a key word).

Despite its earlier medical meaning which suggested involvement of both articular and nonarticular structures, the word *rheumatic* has, through common usage, come to mean 'a painful but nondeforming soft tissue musculoskeletal condition', as distinct from the word *arthritic* which suggests articular and/or deforming features (Block 1993).

Problems arising from the ACR definition

There are distinct and obvious problems with a definition as precise as that offered by the ACR:

- If pressure varies only slightly, so that on a 'good day', a patient may report sensitivity and tenderness rather than 'pain' when tender points are being tested, the patient may therefore not 'qualify' for a definition which could have very real insurance benefit implications, as well as leaving a distressed individual still seeking a diagnosis which might help them understand their suffering.
- If all other criteria are present, and fewer than 11 of the 18 possible sites are reported as 'painful' (say only 9 or 10), what diagnosis is appropriate?
- If there are 11 painful sites but the 'widespread' nature of the pain is missing (as per the definition above), what diagnosis is appropriate?

Clearly, what is being observed in people with widespread pain, who also demonstrate at least 11 of the 18 test points as being painful, is a situation which represents the distant end of a spectrum of dysfunction. Others who do not quite meet the required (for a diagnosis of FMS) number of tender points may well be progressing towards that unhappy state.

It is reported that approximately 2% of the population meet all the ACR criteria (Wolfe et al 1993). A great many more people, however, are advancing in that direction, according to both British and American research which shows that about 20% of the population suffer 'widespread' pain which matches the ACR definition, with almost the same number, *but not necessarily the same people*, demonstrating 11 of the specified 18 tender points as being painful on appropriate testing, also in accordance with the ACR definition. Some people have the widespread pain and not enough painful 'points', others have the

points but their generalised pain distribution is not sufficiently widespread.

What condition do they have if it is not FMS (Croft et al 1992)?

If all the criteria are not fully met, and people with, say, 9 or 10 points, rather than the 11 needed, are offered a diagnosis of FMS (and therefore become eligible for insurance reimbursement or disability benefits, or suitable for inclusion in research projects), what of the person with only 8 painful points who meets all the other criteria?

In human terms this is all far from an academic exercise, for pain of this degree is distressing and possibly disabling, whether or not 11 (or more) points are painful.

Clinically such patients should receive the same attention, wherever they happen to be in the spectrum of disability, and whatever the tender point score, if their pain is sufficient to require professional attention.

SYMPTOMS OTHER THAN PAIN

In 1992 a consensus document on fibromyalgia was produced at the Second World Congress on Myofascial Pain and Fibromyalgia in Copenhagen, and later published in *The Lancet* (Consensus document on FMS 1992). This declaration accepted the ACR fibromyalgia definition as the basis for a diagnosis, and added a number of symptoms to that definition (apart from widespread pain and multiple tender points), including persistent fatigue, generalised morning stiffness and non-refreshing sleep.

This declaration recognised that people with FMS may indeed at times present with fewer that 11 painful points – which is clearly important if most of the other criteria for the diagnosis are met. In such a case a diagnosis of 'possible FMS' is thought appropriate, with a follow-up assessment suggested to reassess the condition.

There are practical implications for a cut-off point (of symptoms or tender point numbers for example) in making such a diagnosis: these relate directly to insurance reimbursement and/or disability benefits, as well as, possibly, to differential diagnosis.

The Copenhagen document adds that FMS is seen to be a part of a larger complex which includes symptoms such as headache, irritable bladder, dysmenorrhoea, extreme sensitivity to cold, restless legs, odd patterns of numbness and tingling, intolerance to exercise and others.

MIND ISSUES

The addition, the Copenhagen Declaration of the symptoms associated with FMS (over and above pain, which is clearly the defining feature) also addresses the psychological patterns often related to FMS – anxiety and/or depression.

The possible psychological component in FMS is an area of study fraught with entrenched beliefs and defensive responses. A large body of medical opinion assigns the entire FMS – and chronic fatigue syndrome (CFS) – phenomenon to the arena of psychosomatic/psychosocial illness, while an equally well-defined position exists, occupied by many health care professionals (as well as most patients), which holds that anxiety and depression symptoms are more commonly a result, rather than a cause, of the pain and disability being experienced in FMS (McIntyre 1993).

A 1994 review paper analysed all British medical publications on the topic of CFS from 1980 onwards and found that 49% favoured a nonorganic cause while only 31% favoured an organic cause. When the popular press was examined in the same way, between 70% (newspapers) and 80% (women's magazines) favoured an organic explanation (McClean & Wesseley 1994).

Many leading researchers into FMS who hold to an organic – biochemical – neurological explanation for the main symptoms are dismissive of psychological explanations for the condition. Dr Jay Goldstein, whose detailed and important research and clinical insights into the care of patients with CFS and FMS will be outlined later in this book, uses the term 'neurosomatic' to describe what he sees as a disorder of central information processing. He makes clear his position regarding the nonorganic, psychosocial school of thought (Goldstein 1996):

Many of the illnesses [CFS, FMS] treated using this model [neurosomatic] are still termed 'psychosomatic' by the medical community and are treated psychodynamically by psychiatrists, neurologists and general physicians. Social anthropologists also have their theories describing CFS as the 'neurasthenia' of the 1990s, and a 'culture bound syndrome' that displaces the repressed conflicts of patients unable to express their emotions ('alexithymics') into a culturally acceptable viral illness or immune dysfunction. Cognitive–behavioural therapy is perhaps more appropriate, since coping with the vicissitudes of their illnesses, which wax and wane unpredictably, is a major problem for most of those afflicted. Few investigators in psychosomatic illness (except those researching panic disorders) have concerned themselves about the pathophysiology of the patients they study, seeming content to define this population in psychosocial phenomenological terms. This position becomes increasingly untenable as the mind–body duality disappears. (Goldstein 1996)

Goldstein says that he only refers patients for psychotherapy if they are suicidally depressed. He emphasises the normalisation (using a variety of medications) of the biochemical basis for neural network dysfunction, which he has satisfied himself is the underlying cause of these (and many other) conditions.

WHEN IS A CAUSE NOT A CAUSE?

Goldstein's methods will be examined in later chapters; however, it might prove useful at this stage to make a slight diversion in order to clarify the importance of looking beyond apparent causes to attempt to uncover their origins.

As we progress through the saga which is FMS (and CFS) we will come across a number of well-defined positions which maintain that the dominant cause is X or Y – or a more usually a combination of X and Y (and possibly others). The truth is that in some important instances these 'causes' themselves have underlying causes which might usefully be therapeutically addressed.

An example – which will emerge in more detail later – is the suggestion that many of the problems associated with FMS (and CFS) are allergy related (Tuncer 1997). This may well be so in the sense that particular foods or substances can be shown, in given cases, to provoke or exacerbate symptoms of pain and fatigue. But what produces this increased reactivity/ sensitivity? Is there an identifiable cause of the (usually food) intolerance itself?

In some cases this can be shown to result from malabsorption of large molecules through the intestinal wall, possibly due to damage to the mucosal surfaces of the gut (Tagesson 1983). In some cases the mucosal damage itself can be shown to have resulted from abnormal yeast or bacterial overgrowth, resulting from prior (possibly inappropriate) use of antibiotics and consequent disturbance of the normal flora, and their control over opportunistic organisms (Crissinger 1990).

The layers of the onion can be peeled away, one by one, revealing causes which lie ever further from the obvious. The pain is aggravated by allergy, which results from bowel mucosa damage, which results from yeast overgrowth, which results from . . . and so on. The allergy in this example is not a cause per se but an exacerbating factor, a link in a chain, and while treating it might satisfactorily reduce symptoms, it would not necessarily deal with causes. Neither would treating the bacterial or yeast overgrowth, although this too might well assist in reducing overall symptom distress.

Where does the cause lie in this particular individual's FMS? Probably in a complex array of interlocking features which may be impossible to untangle. Therefore, approaches such as those which direct themselves at the allergy or at the bowel flora status, while possibly (in this instance) valid and helpful, are not necessarily dealing with fundamental causes.

Does this matter? In Goldstein's model of FMS and CFS aetiology we are faced with a neural network which is dysfunctional. He acknowledges that the evolution of such a state requires several interacting elements:

- A basic susceptibility which is probably genetically induced
- Some developmental factors in childhood (abuse for example)
- Probably a degree of viral encephalopathy (influenced by 'situational perturbations of the immune response')

- Increased susceptibility to environmental stressors resulting from reduction in neural plasticity.

The 'causes' within this model can be seen to be widely spread. Goldstein's (apparently successful) interventions deal with what is happening at the end of this complex sweep of events when the neural network has, as a result, become dysfunctional. By manipulating the biochemistry of that end-state many (Goldstein says most) of his patients' symptoms apparently improve dramatically and rapidly.

Such improvement does not necessarily indicate that underlying causes have been addressed; if these are still operating, future health problems may yet be expected to eventually emerge. The schematic representation of a 'stairway to ill-health' (see Fig. 1.2) indicates some of the possible features ongoing in complicated dysfunctional patterns such as FMS, where adaptive resources have been stretched to their limits, and the 'stage of exhaustion' in Selye's general adaptation syndrome has been reached (Selye 1952).

Dysfunctional patterns such as chronic fatigue syndrome and FMS seem to have three overlapping aetiological features interacting with the unique inborn and subsequently acquired characteristics of individuals to determine their particular degree of vulnerability and susceptibility (Fig. 1.3):

1. Biochemical factors. These can include toxicity, deficiency, infectious, endocrine, allergic and other characteristics
2. Biomechanical factors. These can include:
   a. structural (congenital – i.e. short leg or hypermobility features – postural or traumatically induced characteristics)
   b. functional (overuse patterns, hyperventilation stresses on respiratory mechanisms, etc.)
3. Psychosocial factors. These can include depression and/or anxiety traits, poor stress coping abilities, etc.

Let us briefly consider Dr Goldstein's model of dysfunction, which suggests neural network dysfunction as the 'cause' of FMS, itself being a result of a combination of features as outlined above (Goldstein 1996).

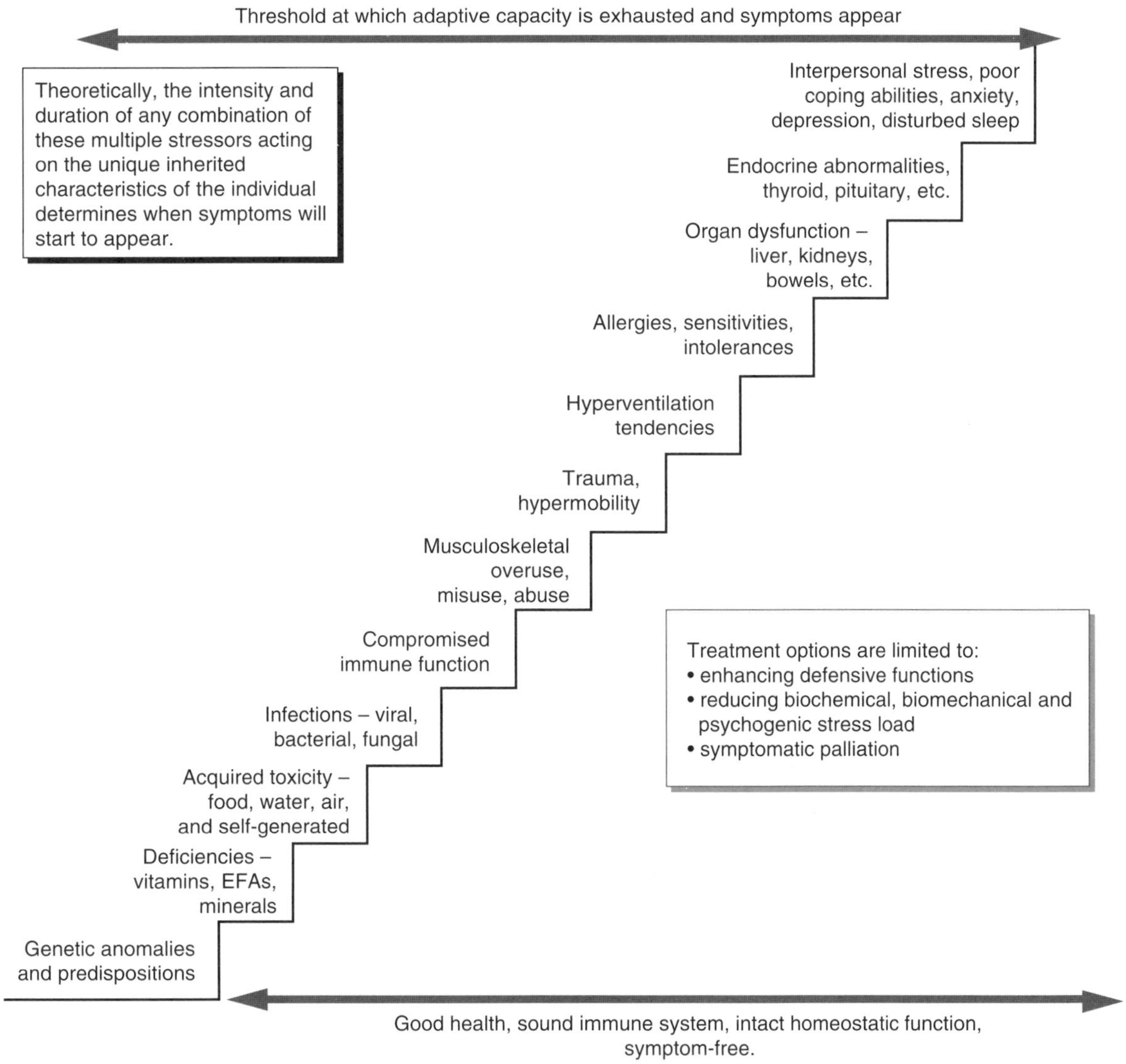

Threshold at which adaptive capacity is exhausted and symptoms appear

Interpersonal stress, poor
coping abilities, anxiety,
depression, disturbed sleep

Endocrine abnormalities,
thyroid, pituitary, etc.

Organ dysfunction –
liver, kidneys,
bowels, etc.

Allergies, sensitivities,
intolerances

Hyperventilation
tendencies

Trauma,
hypermobility

Musculoskeletal
overuse,
misuse, abuse

Compromised
immune function

Infections – viral,
bacterial, fungal

Acquired toxicity –
food, water, air,
and self-generated

Deficiencies –
vitamins, EFAs,
minerals

Genetic anomalies
and predispositions

Theoretically, the intensity and
duration of any combination of
these multiple stressors acting
on the unique inherited
characteristics of the individual
determines when symptoms will
start to appear.

Treatment options are limited to:
• enhancing defensive functions
• reducing biochemical, biomechanical and
  psychogenic stress load
• symptomatic palliation

Good health, sound immune system, intact homeostatic function,
symptom-free.

According to Selye's General Adaptation Syndrome the cumulative effects
of multiple stressors, each demanding adaptation on the part of the
immune, defence and repair systems, eventually reaches a point where
finite defence and repair resources become exhausted, at which time
frank disease becomes inevitable.
  The primary task of the holistic physician or therapist is to minimise the
'load' which is being carried as well as enhancing the body's defence
capabilities – there are few other choices apart from offering palliative
and symptom oriented attention.
  Healing is the prerogative of the body itself – and this occurs when
homeostasis is operating efficiently. When defence and repair functions
are impaired heterostatic influences are needed – i.e. appropriate
treatment – which ideally cause no further harm.

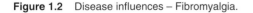

Figure 1.2   Disease influences – Fibromyalgia.

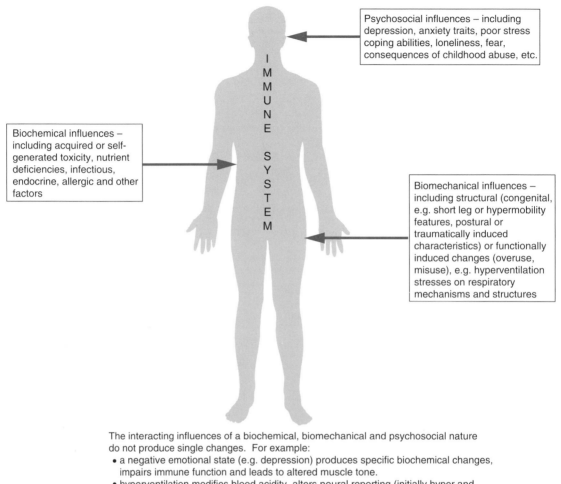

Psychosocial influences – including depression, anxiety traits, poor stress coping abilities, loneliness, fear, consequences of childhood abuse, etc.

Biochemical influences – including acquired or self-generated toxicity, nutrient deficiencies, infectious, endocrine, allergic and other factors

Biomechanical influences – including structural (congenital, e.g. short leg or hypermobility features, postural or traumatically induced characteristics) or functionally induced changes (overuse, misuse), e.g. hyperventilation stresses on respiratory mechanisms and structures

The interacting influences of a biochemical, biomechanical and psychosocial nature do not produce single changes. For example:
- a negative emotional state (e.g. depression) produces specific biochemical changes, impairs immune function and leads to altered muscle tone.
- hyperventilation modifies blood acidity, alters neural reporting (initially hyper and then hypo), creates feelings of anxiety/apprehension and directly impacts on the structural components of the thoracic and cervical region – muscles and joints.
- altered chemistry affects mood; altered mood changes blood chemistry; altered structure (posture for example) modifies function and therefore impacts on chemistry (e.g. liver function) and potentially on mood.

Within these categories – biochemical, biomechanical and psychosocial – are to be found most major influences on health.

Figure 1.3 Major categories of health influence.

If we utilise the clinical options suggested in Figure 1.2, we can see that it is possible to attempt to:

1. Reduce the biochemical, biomechanical or psychogenic 'stress' burden to which the person is responding
2. Enhance the defence, repair, immune functions of the person so that they can handle these stressors more effectively

3. Palliate the symptoms, hopefully without producing any increase in adaptive demands on an already extended system.

Which of these tactics are being employed in Goldstein's treatment approach in which drug-induced biochemical manipulation is being carried out, and does this address causes or symptoms?

The particular philosophical perspective adopted by the practitioner/therapist will determine his judgment on this question. Some may see the rapid symptom relief claimed for the majority of these patients as justifying the approach. Others might see this as offering short-term benefits, not addressing underlying causes, and leaving the likelihood of a return of the original symptoms, or of others evolving, a probability. These issues will be explored in relation to this and other approaches to treatment of FMS in later chapters.

ASSOCIATED CONDITIONS

A number of other conditions exist which have symptom patterns which mimic many of those observed in FMS, in particular:

- chronic myofascial pain syndrome (MPS) involving multiple active myofascial trigger points and their painful repercussions
- chronic fatigue syndrome (CFS) which has amongst its assortment of symptoms almost all those ascribed to FMS, with greater emphasis on the fatigue elements rather than the pain ones.

MPS, FMS and CFS – their similarities, and the sometimes great degree of overlap, as well as their differences – will be examined in detail in later chapters.

THEORIES OF CAUSATION

A variety of theories as to the causation of FMS have emerged, with many of these overlapping and some being essentially the same as others, with only slight differences in emphasis as to aetiology, cause and effect. FMS is variously thought to involve any of a combination of the following (as well as other) causative features, each of which raises questions as well as suggesting answers and therapeutic possibilities:

- FMS could be a neuroendocrine disturbance, particularly involving thyroid hormone imbalances (see Ch. 10) (Honeyman 1997, Lowe 1997) and/or hypophyseal growth hormone imbalances (possibly as a direct result of sleep disturbance – a key feature of FMS) (Moldofsky 1993). The question which then needs to be asked is, what produces the endocrine disturbance? Is it

genetically determined as some believe, or is it the result of deficiency, toxicity, allergy or infection?

- Duna proposes that disordered sleep leads to reduced serotonin production, and consequent reduction in the pain-modulating effects of endorphins and increased 'substance P' levels, combined with sympathetic nervous system changes resulting in muscle ischaemia and increased sensitivity to pain (Duna & Wilke 1993). This hypothesis starts with a symptom, sleep disturbance, and the logical question is what produces this?
- Muscle microtrauma may be the cause, possibly due to genetic predisposition (and/or growth hormone dysfunction), leading to calcium leakage, and so increasing muscle contraction and reducing oxygen supply. An associated decrease in mitochondrial energy production would lead to local fatigue and an inability for excess calcium to be pumped out of the cells, resulting in local hypertonia and pain (Wolfe et al 1992). The question as to why muscle microtrauma occurs more in some people than in others, or why repair is slower, requires investigation.
- FMS may be a pain modulation disorder resulting at least in part from brain (limbic system) dysfunction and involving mistranslation of sensory signals and consequent misreporting (Goldstein 1996). Why and how the limbic system and neural networks become dysfunctional is the key to this hypothesis (promoted by Goldstein, as discussed above).
- FMS may be a congenitally acquired disorder, possibly related to inadequate thyroid regulation of gene transcription, with an autosomal dominant feature (Pellegrino et al 1989, Lowe et al 1997). As will be outlined, some research studies have found evidence of predisposition towards FMS. The questions this raises include: which factors exacerbate these predispositions, and can anything be done about this?
- The underlying cause of FMS is seen by some to result from the (often combined) involvement of allergy, infection, toxicity and nutritional deficiency factors which themselves produce the major symptoms of FMS (and CFS) such as fatigue and pain, or which are associated with

endocrine imbalances and the various consequences outlined above such as thyroid hormone dysfunction and/or sleep disturbance (Abraham et al 1981, Cleveland et al 1992, Vorberg 1985, Fibromyalgia Network Newsletters 1990–94, Robinson 1981, Bland 1995). The list of possible interacting features such as these, which frequently seem to coexist in someone with FMS, offers the possibility of intervention strategies which seem to focus on causes rather than effects. These will be examined in later chapters.

• Many FMS patients demonstrate low carbon dioxide levels when resting – an indication of possible hyperventilation involvement. The symptoms of hyperventilation closely mirror those of FMS and CFS and the pattern of upper chest breathing which it involves severely stresses the muscles of the upper body which are most affected in FMS, as well as producing major oxygen deficits in the brain and so influencing its processing of information such as messages received from pain receptors (Janda 1988, King 1988, Lum 1981). When hyperventilation tendencies are present, they can be seen in some instances to be a response to elevated acid levels (because of organ dysfunction perhaps) or they can be the result of pure habit. Breathing retraining can, in some FMS patients, offer a means of modifying symptoms rapidly (Readhead 1984).

• Psychogenic (or psychosomatic) rheumatism is the name ascribed to FMS (and other non-specific chronic muscle pain problems) by those who refuse to see an organic origin for the syndrome. Until the 1960s it was suggested that such conditions be treated as 'psychoneurosis' (Warner 1964). There are, in FMS as in all chronic forms of ill health, undoubtedly elements of emotional involvement, whether as a cause or as an effect. These impact directly on pain perception and immune function, and, whether causative or not, benefit from appropriate attention, assisting both in recovery and rehabilitation (Melzack & Wall 1988, Solomon 1981).

• FMS is seen by some to be an extreme of the myofascial pain syndrome (MPS), where numerous active myofascial triggers produce pain both locally and at a distance (Thompson 1990). Others see FMS and MPS as distinctive, but

recognise that 'it is not uncommon for a patient with myofascial pain syndrome to progress with time to a clinical picture identical to that of FMS' (Bennett 1986a). Among the most important practical pain-relieving approaches to FMS will be the need to identify and deactivate myofascial trigger points which may be influencing the overall pain burden. A number of different approaches, ranging from electro-acupuncture to manual methods, will be detailed, (see Chapter 7).

• Trauma (e.g. whiplash) seems to be a key feature of the onset in many cases of FMS, and especially cervical injuries, particularly those involving the suboccipital musculature (Hallgren et al 1993, Bennett 1986b). Recognition of mechanical, structural factors allows for interventions which address their repercussions, as well as the psychological effects of trauma.

• There is an 'immune dysfunction' model for myalgic encephalomyelitis (ME) – that uniquely British name for what appears to be an amalgam of chronic fatigue syndrome and fibromyalgia. This proposes a viral or other (vaccination, trauma, etc.) initial trigger which may lead to persistent overactivity of the immune system (over-production of cytokines). Associated with this there may be chemical and/or food allergies, hypothalamic disturbance, hormonal imbalance and specific areas of the brain (e.g.limbic system) 'malfunctioning'. The primary feature of this model is the overactive immune function, with many of the other features, such as endocrine imbalance and brain dysfunction, secondary to this (Macintyre 1993).

THE MUSCULOSKELETAL TERRAIN OF FMS

Current research and clinical consensus seems to indicate that FMS is not primarily a musculo-skeletal problem, although it is in the tissues of this system that its major symptoms manifest: 'Fibromyalgia is a chronic, painful, musculo-skeletal condition characterised by widespread aching and points of tenderness associated with: 1) changed perception of pain, abnormal sleep patterns and reduced brain serotonin, and 2) abnormalities of microcirculation and energy metabolism in muscle' (Eisinger et al 1994). These characteristics, involving abnormal micro-circulation and energy deficits, are the prerequisites for the evolution of localised areas of myofascial distress and neural hyper-reactivity (i.e. trigger points), and, as indicated, one of the key questions to be answered in any given case is the degree to which the person's pain is deriving from myofascial trigger points – or other musculoskeletal sources–since these may well be more easily modified than the complex underlying imbalances which are producing, contributing to, or maintaining the primary FMS condition.

EARLY RESEARCH

A great deal of research into FMS (under different names – see Box 1.1), and of the physiological mechanisms which increase our understanding of the FMS phenomenon, has been conducted over the past century (and earlier) and is worthy of review. Additional research in parallel with that focused on chronic muscular pain may clarify processes at work in this complex condition.

Korr's work on facilitation

Amongst the most important researchers in the area of musculoskeletal dysfunction and pain over the past half century has been Professor Irwin Korr, whose work in explaining the facilitation phenomenon offers important insights into some of the events occurring in FMS and, more specifically, in myofascial pain settings – needless to say these often overlap. As suggested above, in a clinical context it is vital to know what degree of the pain being experienced in FMS is the result of myofascial pain, since this part of the pain package can relatively easily be modified or eliminated.

Neural structures can become hyper-reactive in either spinal and paraspinal tissues or in almost any other soft tissue. When they are found close to the spine they are known as areas of segmental facilitation. When they occur in ligaments, tendons or periosteal tissues, they are called trigger points; if situated in muscles or in fascia they are termed 'myofascial' trigger points.

Professor Michael Patterson (1976) explains the concept of segmental (spinal) facilitation as follows:

The concept of the facilitated segment states that because of abnormal afferent or sensory inputs to a particular area of the spinal cord, that area is kept in a state of constant increased excitation. This facilitation allows normally ineffectual or subliminal stimuli to become effective in producing efferent output from the facilitated segment, causing both skeletal and visceral organs innervated by the affected segment to be maintained in a state of overactivity. It is probable that the somatic dysfunction with which a facilitated segment is associated, is the direct result of the abnormal segmental activity as well as being partially responsible for the facilitation. (Patterson 1976)

Emotional arousal is also able to affect the susceptibility of neural pathways to sensitisation. The increase in descending influences from the emotionally aroused subject would result in an increase in toxic excitement in the pathways and allow additional inputs to produce sensitisation at lower intensities. This implies that highly emotional people, or those in a highly emotional situation, would be expected to show a higher incidence of facilitation of spinal pathways or local areas of myofascial distress (Baldry 1993).

This has a particular relevance to fibromyalgia, where heightened arousal (for a variety of possible reasons, as will become clear), in addition to possible limbic system dysfunction, leads to major influences from the higher centres (Goldstein 1996). Since the higher brain centres do influence the tonic levels of the spinal paths, it might be expected also that physical training and mental attitudes would tend to alter the tonic excitability also, reducing the person's susceptibility to sensitisation from everyday stress. Thus the athlete would be expected to withstand a comparatively high level of afferent input prior to experiencing the self-perpetuating results of sensitisation. This, too, has a relevance to fibromyalgia, where there exists ample evidence of beneficial influences of aerobic training programmes (McGain 1986).

In early studies by the most important researcher into facilitation, Irwin Korr (1970, 1976), he demonstrated that a feature of unilateral segmental facilitation was that one side would test as having normal skin resistance to electricity compared with the contralateral side, the facilitated area, where a marked reduction in resistance was present. When 'stress' – in the form of needling or heat – was applied elsewhere in the body, and the two areas of the spine were monitored, the area of facilitation showed a dramatic rise in electrical (i.e. neurological) activity. In one experiment volunteers had pins inserted into a calf muscle in order to gauge the effect on the paraspinal muscles, which were monitored for electrical activity. While almost no increase occurred in the normal region, the facilitated area showed greatly increased neurological activity after 60 seconds (Korr 1977) (see Fig. 1.4). This and numerous similar studies have confirmed that any form of stress impacting the individual – be it climatic, toxic, emotional, physical or anything else – will produce an increase in neurological output from facilitated areas.

Not only myelinated fibres

Research by Ronald Kramis has shown that, in chronic pain settings, non-nociceptive neurons can become sensitised to carry pain impulses (Kramis 1996).

Hypersenstisation of spinal neurons may actually involve non-nociceptive neurons altering their phenotype so that they commence releasing substance P. This, it is thought, may play a significant part in FMS pain perception, as increased levels of substance P in the cerebrospinal fluid maintain heightened amplification of what would normally be registered as benign impulses. The research suggests that impulses from associated conditions such as ongoing viral activity, 'muscular distress' or irritable bowel may be adequate to maintain the central pain perception.

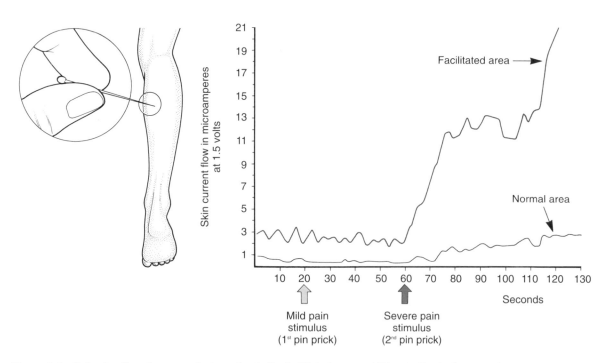

Figure 1.4   Pain stimuli produce a marked reaction in the facilitated area and little reaction in the normal area.

Local facilitation

Apart from paraspinal tissues, where segmental facilitation as described above manifests, localised areas of neural facilitation can occur in almost all soft tissues: these are called myofascial trigger points.

Much of the basic research and clinical work into this aspect of facilitation has been undertaken by doctors Janet Travell and David Simons (Travell 1957; Travell & Simons 1986, 1992; see also Ch. 6). Travell and Simons are on record as stating that if a pain is severe enough to cause a patient to seek professional advice (in the absence of organic disease), it usually involves referred pain, and therefore a trigger area is probably a factor. They remind us that patterns of referred pain are constant in distribution in all people, and that only the intensity of referred symptoms/pain will vary.

The implication for the fibromyalgia patient is the possibility (according to Travell and Simons this is a veritable certainty) that their pain has as part of its make-up the involvement of myofascial trigger points, which are themselves areas of facilitation. As such, these, and therefore the pain (and tingling, numbness, etc.) which they produce, will be exaggerated by *all* forms of stress influencing that individual patient. Travell has confirmed that her research indicates that the following factors can all help to maintain and enhance myofascial trigger point activity:

- Nutritional deficiencies (especially vitamins C and B-complex, and iron)
- Hormonal imbalances (low thyroid hormone production, menopausal or premenstrual dysfunction)
- Infections (bacteria, viruses or yeasts)
- Allergies (wheat and dairy in particular)
- Low oxygenation of tissues (aggravated by tension, stress, inactivity, poor respiration) (Travell & Simons 1986, 1992).

This list corresponds closely with factors which are key aggravating agents for many (most) people with fibromyalgia, suggesting that the connection between facilitation (trigger point activity) and FMS is close (Starlanyl & Copeland 1996).

Myofascial trigger points are, however, not the cause of fibromyalgia, and myofascial pain syndrome is not FMS, although they may coexist in the same person at the same time. Myofascial trigger points do undoubtedly frequently contribute to the painful aspect of FMS, and as such are deserving of special attention.

As will be explained in later chapters, there are a number of ways in which deactivation or modulation of myofascial trigger points can be achieved. Some practitioners opt for approaches which deal with them manually, while others prefer electro-acupuncture methods or a variation on that theme, with yet others suggesting that reduction in the number and intensity of stress factors – of whatever type – offers a safer approach to reducing the influence of facilitation on pain.

Following this introduction to the concept of hyper-reactive, sensitised (facilitated) neural structures, it would be justifiable to enquire as to whether or not what is happening in the brain and in the neural network, as described by Goldstein, is not simply facilitation on a grand scale? The outline of some of the leading current hypotheses as to the aetiology of FMA in Chapter 4 may shed light on this possibility.

OTHER EARLY RESEARCH INTO FMS

Early FMS research has been presented in summary form in Box 1.1. Aspects of that research, and how some of it correlates with more recent findings, are outlined below.

M. Gutstein, a Polish physician who emigrated to the UK prior to the Second World War, was a remarkable researcher who published papers under different names (M. G. Good for example) before, during and following the war. In them he clearly described the myofascial trigger point phenomenon, as well as what is now known as fibromyalgia, along with a great many of its predisposing and maintaining features.

Gutstein (1956) showed that conditions such as ametropia (an error in the eye's refractive power occurring in myopia, hypermetropia and astigmatism) may result from changes in the neuromuscular component of the craniocervical area as well as more distant conditions involving the pelvis or shoulder girdle. He stated: 'Myopia is the long-term effect of pressure of extra-ocular muscles in the convergence effort of accommodation involving spasm of the ciliary muscles, with resultant elongation of the eyeball. A sequential relationship has been shown between such a condition and muscular spasm of the neck.'

Gutstein termed reflex areas he identified 'myodysneuria' and suggested that the reference phenomena of such spots or 'triggers' would include pain, modifications of pain, itching, hypersensitivity to physiological stimuli, spasm, twitching, weakness and trembling of striated muscles, hyper- or hypotonus of smooth muscle of blood vessels and of internal organs, and/or hyper- or hyposecretion of visceral, sebaceous and sudatory glands. Somatic manifestations were also said to occur in response to visceral stimuli of corresponding spinal levels (Gutstein 1944). In all of these suggestions Gutstein seems to have been in parallel with the work of Korr.

Gutstein/Good's method of treatment involved the injection of an anaesthetic solution into the trigger area. He indicated, however, that where accessible (e.g. muscular insertions in the cervical area) the chilling of these areas combined with pressure would yield good results.

In this and much of what he reported in the 1940s and 1950s Gutstein was largely in agreement with the research findings of John Mennell (1952) as well as with Travell & Simons, as expressed in their major texts on the subject (Travell & Simons 1986, 1992). He reported that obliteration of overt and latent triggers in the occipital, cervical, interscapular, sternal and epigastric regions was accompanied by years of alleviation of premenopausal, menopausal and late menopausal symptoms (Good 1951). He quotes a number of practitioners who had achieved success in treating gastrointestinal dysfunctions by deactivating trigger areas. Some of these were treated by procainization, others by pressure techniques and massage (Cornelius 1903). He also reported the wide range of classical fibromyalgia symptoms and features, suggesting the name myodysneuria for this syndrome, which he also termed 'non-articular rheumatism' (Gutstein 1955).

In describing myodysneuria (FMS) Gutstein demonstrated localised functional sensory and/or motor abnormalities of musculoskeletal tissues and saw the causes of such changes as multiple (Gutstein 1955). Most of these findings have been validated subsequently, in particular by the work of Travell and Simons. They include:

- Acute and chronic infections, which he postulated stimulated sympathetic nerve activity via their toxins
- Excessive heat or cold, changes in atmospheric pressure and draughts
- Mechanical injuries, both major and repeated minor microtraumas – now validated by the recent research of Professor Philip Greenman of Michigan State University (Hallgren et al 1993).
- Postural strains, unaccustomed exercises, etc., which could predispose towards future changes by lowering the threshold for future stimuli (in this he was agreeing with facilitation mechanisms as described above)
- Allergic and endocrine factors which could cause imbalances in the autonomic nervous system
- Congenital factors which made adaptation to environmental stressors difficult
- Arthritic changes which could impose particular demands on the musculoskeletal system's adaptive capacity
- Visceral diseases which could intensify and precipitate somatic symptoms in the distribution of their spinal and adjacent segments.

We can see from these examples of Gutstein's thinking strong echoes of the facilitation hypothesis in osteopathic medicine.

Gutstein's diagnosis of myodysneuria was made according to some of the following criteria:

- A varying degree of muscular tension and contraction is usually present, although sometimes adjacent, apparently unaffected tissue is more painful
- Sensitivity to pressure or palpation of affected muscles and their adjuncts
- Marked hypertonicity may require the application of deep pressure to demonstrate pain.

Travell and Bigelow later produced evidence supporting much of what Gutstein had reported. They indicate that high intensity stimuli from active trigger areas produce, by reflex, prolonged vasoconstriction with partial ischaemia in localised areas of the brain, spinal cord, or peripheral nerve structures.

A widespread pattern of dysfunction might then result affecting almost any organ of the body. These early research findings correlate well with modern fibromyalgia and chronic fatigue research and the hypothesis of 'neural network disorders' as described by Goldstein (1996), and in British and American research utilising SPECT scans, which show clearly that severe circulatory deficits occur in the brain stem and in other areas of the brain of most people with CFS and FMS (Costa 1992).

Gutstein's suggested pathophysiology of fibromyalgia/fibrositis/myodysneuria

The changes which occur in tissue involved in the onset of myodysneuria/fibromyalgia, according to Gutstein, are thought to be initiated by localised sympathetic predominance, associated with changes in the hydrogen ion concentration and calcium and sodium balance in the tissue fluids (Petersen 1934). This is associated with vasoconstriction and hypoxia/ischaemia. Pain resulted, he thought, by these alterations affecting the pain sensors and proprioceptors.

Muscle spasm and hard, nodular, localised tetanic contractions of muscle bundles, together with vasomotor and musculomotor stimulation, intensified each other, creating a vicious cycle of self-perpetuating impulses (Bayer 1950). Varied and complex patterns of referred symptoms might then result from such 'trigger' areas, as well as local pain and minor disturbances. Sensations such as aching, soreness, tenderness, heaviness and tiredness may all be manifest, as may modification of muscular activity due to contraction, resulting in tightness, stiffness, swelling and so on.

It is clear from this summary of his work that Gutstein was describing fibromyalgia, and many of its possible causative features.

In Chapter 2 examination will be offered of what FMS is and what it is not, with suggestions for differential diagnosis.

REFERENCES

Abraham G et al 1981 Serum and red cell magnesium levels in patients with PMT. American Journal of Clinical Nutrition 34(11): 2364–2366

American College of Rheumatology 1990 Criteria for the classification of fibromyalgia. Arthritis and Rheumatism 33: 160–172

Baldry P 1993 Acupuncture trigger points and musculoskeletal pain. Churchill Livingstone, London

Bayer H 1950 Pathophysiology of muscular rheumatism. Zeitschrift fur Rheumaforschung 9: 210

Bennett R 1986a Fibrositis: evolution of an enigma. Journal of Rheumatology 13(4): 676–678

Bennett R 1986b Current issues concerning management of the fibrositis/fibromyalgia syndrome. American Journal of Medicine 81(S3A): 15–18

Bland J 1995 A medical food supplemented detoxification programme in the management of chronic health problems. Alternative Therapies 1: 62–71

Block S 1993 Fibromyalgia and the rheumatisms. Controversies in Rheumatology 19(1): 61–78

Cleveland C et al 1992 Chronic rhinitis and under recognised association with fibromyalgia. Allergy Proceedings 13(5): 263–267

Consensus document on FMS: the Copenhagen declaration. 1992 Lancet 340(September 12)

Cornelius A 1903 Die Neurenpunkt Lehre. George Thiem, Liepzig, vol. 2

Costa D 1992 Report. European Journal of Nuclear Medicine 19(8): 733

Crissinger K 1990 Pathophysiology of gastrointestinal mucosal permeability. Journal of Internal Medicine 228: 145–154

Croft P et al 1992 Is the hip involved in generalized osteoarthritis ? British Journal of Rheumatology 31: 325–328

Duna G, Wilke W 1993 Diagnosis, etiology and therapy of fibromyalgia. Comprehensive Therapy 19(2): 60–63

Eisinger J, Plantamura A, Ayavou T 1994 Glycolysis abnormalities in fibromyalgia. Journal of the American College of Nutrition 13(2): 144–148

Fibromyalgia Network Newsletters 1994–99 Reports on nutritional influences: October 1990–January 1992, Compendium No. 2, January 1993, May 1993 Compendium, January 1994, July 1994 (Back issues are available from the Network at PO Box 31750, Tucson, Arizona 85761-1750)

Goldstein J 1996 Betrayal by the brain: the neurological basis of CFS and FMS and related neural network disorders. Haworth Medical Press, New York

Good M G 1951 Objective diagnosis and curability of non-articular rheumatism. British Journal of Physical Medicine and Industrial Hygiene 14: 1–7

Gutstein R 1944 The role of abdominal fibrositis in functional indigestion. Mississippi Valley Medical Journal 66: 114–124

Gutstein R 1955 A review of myodysneuria (fibrositis). American Practitioner and Digest of Treatments 6(4)

Gutstein R 1956 The role of craniocervical myodysneuria in functional ocular disorders. American Practitioner's Digest of Treatments November

Hallgren R, Greenman P, Rechtien J 1993 MRI if normal and atrophic muscles of the upper cervical spine. Journal of Clinical Engineering 18(5): 433–439

Honeyman G 1997 Metabolic therapy for hypothyroid and euthyroid fibromyalgia: two case reports. Clinical Bulletin of Myofascial Therapy 2(4): 19–49

Janda V 1988 Muscles and cervicogenic pain and syndromes. In: Grant R (ed) Physical therapy of the cervical and thoracic spine. Churchill Livingstone, London, pp 153–166

King J 1988 Hyperventilation – a therapist's point of view. Journal of the Royal Society of Medicine 81(September): 532–536

Korr I 1970 Physiological basis of osteopathic medicine. Postgraduate Institute of Osteopathic Medicine and Surgery, New York

Korr I 1976 Spinal cord as organiser of disease process. Academy of Applied Osteopathy Yearbook 1976

Korr I (ed) 1977 Neurobiological mechanisms in manipulation. Plenum Press, New York

Kramis R 1996 Non-nociceptive aspects of musculoskeletal pain. Journal of Orthopaedic & Sports Physical Therapy 24(4): 255–267

Lowe J 1997 Results of open trial of T3 therapy with 77 euthyroid female FMS patients. Clinical Bulletin of Myofascial Therapy 2(1): 35–37

Lowe J, Cullum M, Graf L, Yellin J 1997 Mutations in the c-erb-Ab$_1$ gene: do they underlie euthyroid fibromyalgia? Medical Hypotheses 48(2): 125–135

Lum L 1981 Hyperventilation an anxiety state. Journal of the Royal Society of Medicine 74(January): 1–4

McCain G 1986 Role of physical fitness training in fibrositis/fibromyalgia syndrome. American Journal of Medicine (S3A): 73–77

McClean G, Wesseley S 1994 Professional and popular view of CFS. British Medical Journal 308: 776–777

Macintyre A 1993a What causes ME? Journal of Action for ME 14: 24–25

Macintyre A 1993b The immune dysfunction hypothesis. Journal of Action for ME 14: 24–25

Melzack R, Wall P 1988 The challenge of pain. Penguin, New York

Mennell J 1952 The science and art of manipulation. Churchill Livingstone, London

Moldofsky HL 1993 Fibromyalgia, sleep disorder and chronic fatigue syndrome. CIBA Symposium 173: 262–279

Patterson M 1976 Model mechanism for spinal segmental facilitation. Academy of Applied Osteopathy Yearbook 1976, Carmel

Pellegrino M, Waylonis G Sommer A 1989 Familial occurrence of primary fibromyalgia. Archives of Physical Medicine and Rehabilitation 70(1)

Petersen W 1934 The patient and the weather: autonomic disintegration. Edward Brothers, Ann Arbor

Readhead C 1984 Enhanced adaptive behavioural response in patients pretreated by breathing retraining. Lancet 22(September): 665–668

Robinson M 1981 Effect of daily supplements of selenium on patients with muscular complaints. New Zealand Medical Journal 93: 289–292

Selye H 1952 The story of the adaptation syndrome. ACTA, Montreal

Simons D 1988 Myofascial pain syndromes: where are we? Where are we going? Archives of Physical Medicine and Rehabilitation 69: 207–211

Solomon G 1981 Psychoneuroimmunology. Academic Press, New York

Starlanyl D, Copeland M E 1996 Fibromyalgia and chronic myofascial pain syndrome. New Harbinger Publications, Oakland, CA

Tagesson C 1983 Passage of molecules through the wall of the intestinal tract. Scandinavian Journal of Gastroenterology 18: 481–486

Thompson J 1990 Tension myalgia as a diagnosis at the Mayo Clinic and its relationship to fibrositis, fibromyalgia and myofascial pain syndrome. Mayo Clinic Proceedings 65: 1237–1248

Travell J 1957 Symposium on mechanism and management of pain syndromes. Proceedings of the Rudolph Virchow Medical Society

Travell J, Bigelow N Role of somatic trigger areas in the patterns of hysteria. Psychosomatic Medicine 9(6)

Travell J, Simons D 1986 Myofascial pain and dysfunction. Williams & Wilkins, Baltimore, vol. 1

Travell J, Simons D 1992 Myofascial pain and dysfunction. Williams & Wilkins, Baltimore, vol. 2

Tuncer T 1997 Primary FMS and allergy. Clinical Rheumatology 16(1): 9–12

van Why R 1994 FMS and massage therapy. Self published

Vorberg G 1985 Ginko extract – a longterm study of chronic cerebral insufficiency. Clinical Trials Journal 22: 149–157

Warner E (ed) 1964 Saville's system of clinical medicine, 14th edn. Edward Arnold, London, p 918

Wolfe F, Simons D et al 1992 The fibromyalgia and myofascial pain syndromes. Journal of Rheumatology 19(6): 944–951

Wolfe F, Anderson J, Ross K, Russel I 1993 Prevalence of characteristics of fibromyalgia in the general population. Arthritis and Rheumatism 36: S48(abstract)

2

Fibromyalgia's symptom patterns: causes or effects?

PREVALENCE OF ASSOCIATED CONDITIONS

The overlap between fibromyalgia syndrome (FMS) and other conditions, some of which closely mimic its defining features (chronic fatigue syndrome for example), and some which are more obviously distinctive, adds a confusing element to the understanding of this syndrome.

In later chapters particular attention is given to the similarities and differences which exist between FMS and CFS (see Ch. 5), and the similarities and differences which exist between FMS and myofascial pain syndrome (MPS) (see Ch. 6).

This chapter elaborates on some of the long list of other named conditions which have as a major part of their symptom picture comparable patterns to those associated with FMS. In Chapter 3 some of the major associated symptoms of FMS are evaluated in more detail in terms of their possible contribution to the overall aetiological progression of the syndrome.

Firstly, considering a number of frequently associated and overlapping conditions, a comparison can be made between their presence in the general population and their presence in patients with a diagnosis of either FMS or CFS. The list of associated conditions in Table 2.1, based on the research of Professor Daniel Clauw, shows those which are more prevalent in FMS (which is estimated to affect 2% of the population) than in the general population (or where appropriate – e.g. dysmenorrhoea – the general female population). The conditions are listed in alphabetical order, not in any order of importance in terms of symptom severity (Clauw 1995).

Table 2.1 Prevalence of associated conditions

Condition	% in CFS/FMS	% in general population
Chronic headache	50%	5%
Dysmenorrhoea	60%	15%
Endometriosis	15%	2%
Interstitial cystitis	25%	under 1%
Irritable bladder/urethral pain	15%	under 1%
Irritable bowel syndrome	60%	10%
Mitral valve prolapse	75%	15%
Multiple chemical sensitivities	40%	5%
Restless legs syndrome	30%	2%
Temporomandibular joint syndrome	25%	5%

Clauw states that it is his opinion that FMS/CFS represent a 'constellation' of many overlapping chronic pain disorders, many of which are difficult to treat satisfactorily:

• Many of these conditions have similar characteristics including, among others, pain and/or fatigue of a chronic nature.
• The patient population affected is predominantly female. This is one of the key defining differences between FMS and myofascial pain syndrome, which has no gender preference; another is the fact that people with MPS have no particular predilection towards the associated conditions which are characteristic of FMS.
• These associated symptoms are seen to occur to a significantly greater degree amongst fibromyalgia patients than in the general population, and many of them seem to be linked to neuroendocrine disturbance.

Dr Jay Goldstein (1996) enfolds all the symptoms of FMS – and a great many more – into a model which he has called 'neurosomatic disorders' (see Ch. 4, Aetiological models). He states that: 'Neurosomatic disorders are the the most common group of illnesses for which patients consult physicians (Yunus 1994). Fatigue, depression, anxiety, diffuse pain, cognitive dysfunction, and the other neurosomatic disorders present to different specialists in different ways and the

final diagnosis often depends on the orientation and speciality of the doctor.'

The associated symptoms listed in Table 2.1, which favour females and which are found in a large proportion of FMS/CFS patients, are not necessarily the major symptoms associated with FMS.

SYMPTOMS AS AETIOLOGICAL FACTORS

Many of the conditions associated with FMS/CFS are the end result of different causal factors, whether of a biochemical/toxic, neurological or infectious (or other) nature, for example chronic headaches, restless legs or interstitial cystitis. They are unpleasant, may irritate, depress and disturb the individual, but do not themselves act as causes of further pathology or significant metabolic disturbance.

On the other hand some symptoms do just that – they are not only major irritants but also act as the direct cause of further disturbance and imbalance. Sleep disturbance for example, an extremely common associated symptom of FMS, which can itself result from numerous stress-related causal factors, leads to a number of direct secondary changes, including reduced protein synthesis, decreased growth hormone secretion, reduced overnight oxygen haemoglobin saturation, reduced immune activity and perturbation of the hypothalamic–pituitary–adrenal axis. The obvious effects of these changes include, among other things, symptoms such as general malaise and increased pain perception (see Fig. 3.6B, Ch. 3, for a schematic representation of the changes relative to sleep disturbance, and full citations). The less obvious effects of such changes, if they become chronic – for example disruption of serotonin status – could well be implicated in the evolution of fibromyalgia symptoms.

Irritable bowel syndrome (IBS) is a common associated symptom of FMS and may itself derive from a wide range of causal factors (including stress, food intolerance, infection, disturbed gut flora resulting at times from the after-effects of antibiotics, enzyme deficiencies, serotonin deficiency and others). The obvious end result of IBS is a thoroughly disturbed digestive function which may involve irritated gut mucosa, malabsorption, dysbiosis and toxicity, as well as an increased likelihood of food intolerances – a suspected cause of both myalgia and fatigue (see Fig. 3A, Ch. 3, for a schematic representation of the possible interrelationship between IBS and FMS). The less obvious effects of the disruption of digestive function may involve nutritional deficiencies and stress on the organs of detoxification – liver and kidneys for example – with further ramifications in terms of declining health levels.

One of Selye's most important findings is commonly overlooked when the concurrent impact of multiple stressors on the system is being considered (1974). Shealy (1984) summarises as follows:

Relative values for various stressors can only be estimated since individual responses will depend upon the level of accommodation at a given time. Selye has emphasised the fact that any systemic stress elicits an essentially generalised reaction, with release of adrenaline and glucocorticoids, in addition to any specific damage such stressor may cause. During the stage of resistance (adaptation) a given stressor may trigger less of an alarm; however, Selye insists that adaptation to one agent is acquired at the expense of resistance to other agents. That is, as one accommodates to a given stressor, other stressors may require lower thresholds for eliciting the alarm reaction. Of considerable importance is Selye's observation that concomitant exposure to several stressors elicits an alarm reaction at stress levels which individually are sub-threshold. That is, one third the dose of histamine, one third the dose of cold, one third the dose of formaldehyde, elicit an alarm reaction equal to a full dose of any one agent.

Consider these findings of Selye when the multiple stressors involved in the aetiology and symptomatology of FMS are considered – as symptoms themselves become stressors to add to the load being adapted to (see Fig. 2.1).

As indicated, a number of the more important conditions associated with FMS, including IBS and sleep disturbance, will be considered in greater detail in Chapter 3, in so far as their existence seems to have a clear aetiological importance in the evolution of FMS/CFS. Some of the 'causal symptoms' which receive this more detailed attention are well researched, in that their links with FMS/CFS are reasonably clear. The links of others to FMS/CFS, however, despite a great deal of anecdotal evidence, remain somewhat speculative.

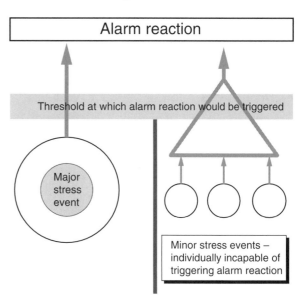

A combination of minor stresses, each incapable of triggering an alarm reaction in the general adaptation syndrome can, when combined or sustained, produce sufficient adaptive demand to initiate that alarm. In fibromyalgia a combination of major and minor biochemical, biomechanical and psychosocial stressors commonly seem to be simultaneously active.

Figure 2.1 Alarm reaction.

In this latter group can be included hyperventilation and hypoglycaemic tendencies, neither of which appear often in mainstream research or review literature, but which feature large in unconventional assessment of causal features of both FMS and CFS. These topics will be elaborated on in Chapter 4, which summarises the various hypotheses as to FMS causation.

FIBROMYALGIA NETWORK SURVEY

The evidence collected by one physician regarding the characteristic features of her FMS and CFS patients, both before and during their illness, is outlined below (One physician's findings). However, before seeing Dr Jessop's data, the evidence collected by the leading American patient advocacy organisation for FMS, the Fibromyalgia Network, offers useful information (Fibromyalgia Network Newsletter 1997).

In October 1997 the newsletter of the network published raw data compiled from the more than 6000 responses they had received to a survey questionnaire, as follows:

- 6240 patients responded
- 97% had a diagnosis of FMS and 28% had a diagnosis of CFS (with an overlap of a double diagnosis in fully a quarter of the respondents)
- Average age 52.6 years
- 95% female
- Duration of illness average 12.2 years
- 7.2 years on average was taken before a diagnosis was offered.

FMS diagnosis

Those patients with an FMS diagnosis reported the following percentage of additional diagnoses:

- IBS or irritable bladder 64%
- Headaches 59%
- Chemical sensitivities 26%
- Osteoarthritis 20%
- Thyroid disease 19%.

Known triggers

When asked for known triggering events, 59% indicated they could identify the trigger and the following were listed:

- Physical trauma 39% (of the 59%)
- Major emotional trauma such as bereavement 27%
- Infection 15%
- Surgery 9%
- Exposure to chemical agent or drug 5%.

Improvement (or lack of it) of those with FMS

Asked about improvement or lack of it since their diagnosis, those with FMS offered these responses:

- 0.2% had fully recovered
- 31% had improved
- 20% were unchanged
- 40% were worse
- 9% had become disabled.

Associated symptoms of those with FMS

The associated symptoms reported by the FMS responders (97% of the survey) were:

- Memory and concentration difficulties 86%
- Major discomfort following exertion 89%
- Waking tired in the morning 89%
- Unable to work because of FMS 40%
- Percentage of time spent in pain 76%
- Percentage of body in pain 71%.

Patient satisfaction

Which health care disciplines were the most helpful and knowledgeable regarding the condition? The percentage attending each health care discipline is given in parentheses; the disciplines are listed in descending order of patient satisfaction:

- Rheumatologists (51%)
- Physical medicine and rehabilitation specialists (13%)
- Neurologists (10%)
- Chiropractors (6%)

- Internists (27%)
- Family physicians (46%).

What helps most?

When asked what was the most helpful on a scale of 1 to 10 (with 10 being the most helpful) the responses were that:

- Drug and non-drug therapies rated 4.8
- Educational material rated 7.4.

ONE PHYSICIAN'S FINDINGS

San Francisco physician Carol Jessop has studied over 1000 people suffering from FMS or CFS who were referred to her following diagnosis by consulting rheumatologists or neurologists (Fibromyalgia Network Newsletters 1990–94). There is no distinction in the figures offered by Dr Jessop between patients with a diagnosis of FMS and those with CFS. Nevertheless, there is much to learn from the general information offered regarding this mixed population (CFS and FMS) as to their current symptoms, and from some of the clinical signs noted by her. Finally, and perhaps most significantly, the major symptoms existing in patients prior to the onset of their illness are listed.

Current symptoms

The commonest current symptoms reported by Jessop's patients were:

- Chronic fatigue   100%
- Cold extremities   100%
- Impaired memory   100%
- Frequent urination   95%
- Depression*   94%
- Sleep disorder   94%
- Balance problems   89%
- Muscle twitching   80%

---

* Jessop regarded the depression noted in her patients as almost always being reactive rather than a true clinical depression. She noted that no more than 8% of her patients had required prior medical attention for depression before the onset of CFS or FMS.

- Dry mouth   68%
- Muscle aches   68%
- Headache   68%
- Sore throat   20%

Common signs

Jessop reported the following findings amongst this group of patients (1324 patients, of whom 75% were female, average age 39):

- Elevated temperature   10%
- Normal temperature   25%
- Subnormal temperature   65%
- Low blood pressure   86%
- Yeast infections (tongue/mouth)   87%
- Tender thyroid   40%
- White spots on nails[†]   85%
- Tender neck muscles   91%
- FMS tender spots   86%
- Abdominal tenderness   80%
- Swollen lymph nodes   18%

Laboratory findings

Jessop reported the following summary of laboratory findings from 880 of this particular patient group:

- 82% had yeast cultured from purged stool samples
- 30% had parasites in their purged stool samples
- 38% were found to be deficient in magnesium using a 3 day loading test and two 24-hour urine samples
- 32% had low zinc levels using blood tests.

Symptoms before the onset of CFS or FMS

Jessop's patients' symptoms *before* the onset of their CFS or FMS were:

- 89% irritable bowel symptoms
- 80% 'constant gas' or bloating

[†]These white flecks are thought to relate to zinc deficiency (Davies & Stewart 1987).

- 58% constipation
- 40% heartburn
- 89% recurrent childhood ear, nose, throat infections
- 40% recurrent sinusitis
- 30% recurrent bronchitis
- 20% recurrent bladder infections
- 90% of the females had PMS prior to CFS/FMS
- 65% reported endometriosis
- 30% dysmenorrhoea
- 22% had generalised anxiety disorders prior to their illness
- Sleep problems were present in only 1% before CFS/FMS.

Analysis of this information and comparison with the list of commonly associated FMS symptoms helps to focus on underlying processes. For example:

- Only 1% reported prior sleep problems whereas by the time a diagnosis of FMS or CFS was made the sleep patterns of over 90% were severely disrupted.
- The high level of patients displaying subnormal temperatures, as well as the 'tender thyroid' observation, suggests thyroid dysfunction, something which has attracted a great deal of research (see Ch. 10).
- The high incidence of chronic genitourinary symptoms suggests additional (apart from thyroid) endocrine imbalances.
- The high levels of preexisting ENT, sinus, respiratory, bladder and other infections suggests either a degree of immune function inefficiency or allergy involvement and, almost certainly, high usage of antibiotics with consequent bowel flora damage. The link between these elements and the elevated levels of gastrointestinal symptomatology seems obvious. How these factors link with food intolerances, malabsorption possibilities (and consequent nutrient deficiencies) and general biochemical imbalances is a field of study in itself which is summarised in Chapter 3 (see also Fig. 2.2).

As will become evident in later chapters, these areas of possible involvement in the aetiology and/or maintenance of FMS (thyroid dysfunction, generalised endocrine imbalance, immune system deficiency, possible infection link, high use of antibiotics, bowel dysbiosis possibly involving ecological damage to the gut flora, allergy, etc.) are all possible factors in what a leading researcher into FMS, Mohammed Yunus MD, has called 'dysfunctional spectrum syndrome' (Yunus 1997).

WHY MUSCLE PAIN?

A great deal of research has been undertaken in order to better understand the morphological, biochemical and physiological changes found in the soft tissues of people with FMS as well as in the body as a whole. Such research has helped towards a greater understanding of *what* is happening, but has failed thus far to offer a clear picture of *why* it is happening, apart from gathering an ever lengthening list of possible factors as being involved, ranging from the psychological to the biochemical to the structural, or any combination of these.

Much attention is paid in research to the varying levels in different tissues of substance P, serotonin, cytokines, growth hormone and specific enzymes, and to the minutiae of the biochemistry of the tissues involved, in order to understand the mechanisms of pain in FMS. These represent the 'sharp end' of the pain picture as distinct from the broad hypothetical models which attempt to explain why these biochemical changes have occurred. Some of the most important hypothetical models are examined in Chapter 4. What they all have in common is an attempt to develop a model which draws together a collection of possible aetiological features which negatively influence neural, endocrine, immune, circulatory or other systems and functions, with an end-point of FMS (or CFS).

In a major review article on the pathogenesis of FMS, Swedish physician Karl Henriksson (1993) states that: 'There is no single cause for a pain condition such as FMS. The pathogenesis is a chain of events. Some links are still missing, and some links are weak.' Figure 2.2 shows some of these possible interacting pathogenic factors.

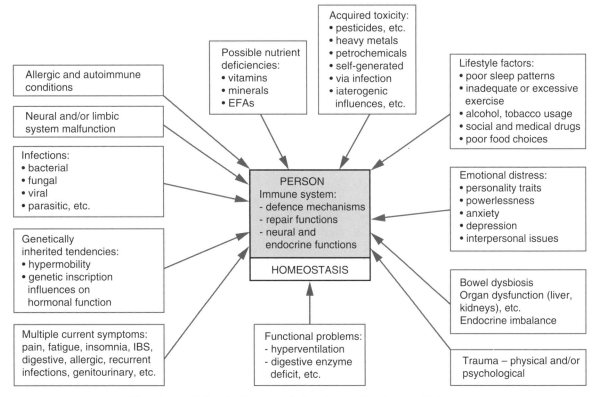

Figure 2.2 Multiple stressors in fibromyalgia.

What finally triggers FMS when these or other interacting stressors have loaded the 'variably genetically impaired' (Klimas 1994)) homeostatic mechanisms of the body with adaptive demands for an appropriate length of time?

It seems that a viral (Oldstone 1989, Joly 1991), or a traumatic (physical or emotional (Fry 1993, Bremner 1995, Waylonis 1994, Buskila 1997)) or some other incident can trigger the already compromised individual into a frank expression of dysfunction and pain.

As Goldstein (1996) explains: 'Those with a strong tendency to be afflicted with CFS/FMS may have had the disorder since childhood. Others may require one or more triggering stim-uli such as child abuse, viral infections, surgery, pronounced physical or mental overexertion [or trauma], childbirth or emotional stress.'

Selye, in his original research, showed that stressors, whether physical (trauma, inactivity, infection, weather, etc.), chemical (alcohol, caffeine, drugs, toxins, etc.) or psychological (fear, anger, grief, anxiety, etc.) could elicit a stress response which included serotonin, ACTH and beta endorphin and possibly prostaglandin E_1 release in the brain, followed by the adrenal response and glycogen release. Over time, the effects of stress would result in 'break down' in the 'weakest organ' or weakest organ system, whatever the total stress. The ultimate effects of the stress of life would negatively influence genetic or acquired susceptibilities (Selye 1950).

On which subject Randolph (1976), one of the primary workers in the evolution of clinical ecology, reminds us that the unique characteristics of the individual will determine the way in which symptoms evolve: 'It is well known that different persons may develop rhinitis, asthma, hives, eczema, colitis, urgency and tenesmus, fatigue, headache, fluid retention, myalgia, arthralgia, depression or other behavioural or psychotic manifestations from the impingement of a given environmental substance.'

This is not quoted to suggest that all the symptoms of FMS (or CFS) necessarily derive from allergy/sensitivity, although clearly in given circumstances they might be a key feature (see Ch. 3), but to emphasise that there is not a linear and predictable outcome in terms of what symptoms will emerge in response to different stressors or aetiological factors in different people.

A combination of the individual's unique characteristics together with the stressor elements (biochemical, biomechanical, psychosocial) determine illness expression. The examples which Randolph offers do, however, have very strong echoes of the main symptom picture of FMS and CFS, and the possibility of allergy/sensitivity involvement needs to be borne in mind when the aetiological elements of the condition are considered. In Chapter 3 a more detailed examination is offered of some of the associated conditions, such as sleep disorder, IBS and allergy. An attempt is made to link these dysfunctional features with what is known to be happening in the bodies of people with FMS – the biochemistry of pain, fatigue, 'brain fog', etc.

SELYE'S MESSAGE (Selye 1952, 1946)

As the often complicated biochemical pictures of what is happening in the tissues of people with FMS emerge, and as broad hypothetical models which try to explain them are considered, a therapeutic model may be usefully restated (see Fig. 2.4).

The catalogue of information derived from research into FMS and its associated conditions offers insights into what may be happening in the body and why. And while these insights allow the practitioner/therapist a huge range of treatment options, it is worth considering that these can only be focused in a limited number of ways; that is, towards:

- Enhancing immune, defence, repair, detoxification functions
- Reducing the biochemical, biomechanical and psychogenic stress load
- Symptomatic palliation.

In his early research, Selye demonstrated that homeostatic mechanisms, when operating optimally, dealt efficiently with many of the stressor elements. When overloaded – when adaptive demands are beyond the ability of the homeostatic repair and defence systems to maintain normal function – symptoms appear and ill health evolves (see Figs. 2.3A, 2.3B and 2.3C).

At this stage *heterostasis* is the label Selye offered for the situation. In a heterostatic setting 'something' needs to be brought into the equation from an external source, to assist restoration of homeostatic efficiency. This 'something' is treatment (externally applied or self-generated), which either reduces the stressor influences ('lightens the load') or enhances homeostatic defence and repair functions.

Apart from these choices, all that can usefully be done is to reduce the intensity of symptoms, hopefully without adding further toxic or other stresses to the adaptation demands oppressing the body/mind complex.

Selye reminds us of a further twist to this saga:

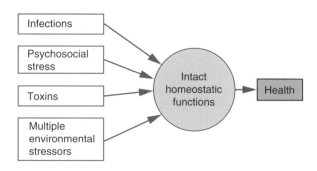

Figure 2.3A Homeostasis.

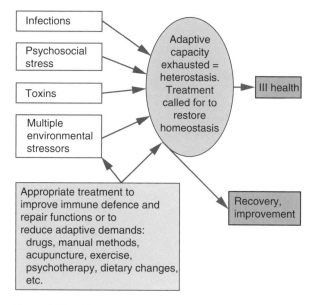

Figure 2.3B Heterostasis.

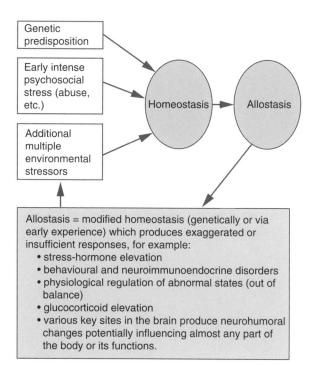

Figure 2.3C Allostasis (Sapolsky 1990, 1994, McEwan 1994).

the fact that since stress is defined as anything which demands an adaptive response, *all* forms of treatment should be seen as forms of stress. Only those treatment methods which are appropriate, which 'provoke' a beneficial adaptive (homeostatic) response, and which do not further compromise the already extended defence/repair potentials are useful in promotion of a healing response. All other treatments either make matters worse or offer no benefits.

Selye showed that while in many instances a mild degree of therapeutic stimulus achieved a positive response from the organism, the same stimulus amplified made matters worse (see Fig. 2.4). When confronted with an individual with FMS, whose adaptive coping agencies are working overtime, whose energy reserves are low, whose vulnerability and susceptibility to stress of any sort is great, the practitioner/therapist should tailor therapeutic interventions to meet the needs of what is clearly a limited adaptive capacity; to do as little as possible rather than as much as may seem necessary all at once. Clinically this may mean:

- Very precise interventions, slowly modulating stressors and augmenting function, while safely modifying symptoms.

Or it may call for:

- Very general, 'constitutional' approaches which do not have a specific aim but which allow homeostatic mechanisms to operate more efficiently. Examples of this include relaxation and meditation methods, although there are many others (outlined in Ch. 11 where treatment options are considered; see also Box 2.1).

The suggestion which Selye's observations on 'treatment as a potentially useful stressor' leads to is that the more compromised the defence/repair functions are, and the greater the levels of dysfunction and pain being experienced, the more limited (in dosage, degree, intensity, number, etc.) any therapeutic intervention should initially be – or the more general and nonspecific it should be (see Fig. 2.4).

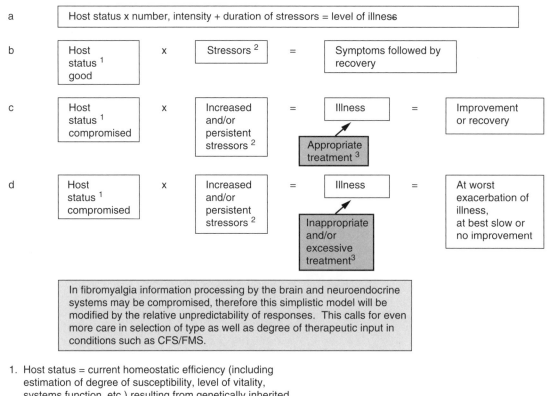

a   Host status x number, intensity + duration of stressors = level of illness

b | Host status [1] good | x | Stressors [2] | = | Symptoms followed by recovery |

c | Host status [1] compromised | x | Increased and/or persistent stressors [2] | = | Illness | = | Improvement or recovery |

Appropriate treatment [3]

d | Host status [1] compromised | x | Increased and/or persistent stressors [2] | = | Illness | = | At worst exacerbation of illness, at best slow or no improvement |

Inappropriate and/or excessive treatment[3]

In fibromyalgia information processing by the brain and neuroendocrine systems may be compromised, therefore this simplistic model will be modified by the relative unpredictability of responses. This calls for even more care in selection of type as well as degree of therapeutic input in conditions such as CFS/FMS.

1. Host status = current homeostatic efficiency (including estimation of degree of susceptibility, level of vitality, systems function, etc.) resulting from genetically inherited and acquired influences and characteristics
2. Stressors = infection, psychosocial stress, trauma, toxicity, etc.
3. Treatment (itself a form of stress) = improving host status or moderating stressors or palliation of symptoms

Figure 2.4   A therapeutic intervention model for FMS.

In caring for people with FMS, interventions (whether externally applied or self-generated) which ignore the underlying dysfunctional patterns existing in the digestive, immune, neuroendocrine and other systems, or which attempt to force an improvement in symptoms without taking into account the fact that treatment is itself a form of stress (due to the demands treatment of any sort makes on adaptive functions) may at worst produce harmful results, or at best offer only short-term benefits.

Box 2.1 Potentially useful complementary health care measures

Potentially useful complementary health care measures to be utilised in concert with standard medical methods which impose as little additional stress on the already distressed system as possible could include:

- Nutritional support and balanced eating patterns
- Attention to possible allergies and intolerances
- Stress reduction methods including counselling, psychotherapy
- Behaviour modification
- Relaxation methods including meditation, autogenic training, guided imagery, etc.
- Physical conditioning – aerobics, stretching methods (Pilates, yoga, etc.)
- Breathing retraining
- Structural normalisation (osteopathy, chiropractic, etc.) with emphasis on deactivation of myofascial trigger points and minimal microtrauma to soft tissues

- Non-toxic antifungal, antiviral, antibacterial, antiparasitic medications (herbal and standard pharmacological) as appropriate
- Probiotics to assist in bowel flora normalisation if needed
- Acupuncture and Traditional Chinese Medicine
- Immune support including herbs, nutrients, psychoneuroimmunology, fasting, etc.
- Detoxification methods
- Endocrine support
- Homoeopathic constitutional treatment
- Hydrotherapeutic – hyperthermic methods
- Non-specific 'constitutional' methods including bodywork (massage), Reiki, etc.
- Reflexology, aromatherapy
- Healing

REFERENCES

Bremner J 1995 MRI-based measurement of hippocampal volume in patients with combat-related post-traumatic stress disorder. American Journal of Psychiatry 152: 973–981

Buskila D 1997 Increased rate of FMS following cervical spine injury. Arthritis and Rheumatism 40(3): 446–452

Clauw D 1995 Fibromyalgia: more than just a musculoskeletal disease. American Family Physician (1 Sept 1995)

Davies S , Stewart A 1987 Nutritional medicine. Pan, London

Fibromyalgia Network Newsletter 1997 Survey Results (October): 11–13

Fibromyalgia Network Newsletters 1992–94: (October 1990–January 1992 Compendium No. 2), January 1993, (May 1993 Compendium), January 1994, July 1994 (Back issues are available from the Network at PO Box 31750, Tucson, Arizona 85761-1750)

Fry R 1993 Adult physical illness and childhood sexual abuse. Journal of Psychosomatic Research 37(2): 89–103

Goldstein J 1996 Betrayal by the brain: the neurological basis of CFS and FMS and related neural network disorders. Haworth Medical Press, New York

Henriksson K 1993 Pathogenesis of fibromyalgia. Journal of Musculoskeletal Pain 1(3/4): 3–16

Joly E 1991 Viral persistence in neurons explained by lack of major histocompatibility class 1 expressions. Science 253: 1283–1285

Klimas N 1994 Immune correlates in CFS and FMS. Presented at Fourth Annual Conference of Medical Neurobiology of CFS and FMS. CFIDS Chronicle (Summer): 1–11

McEwan B 1994 The plasticity of the hippocampus is the reason for its vulnerability. Seminars in Neuroscience 6: 197–204

Oldstone M 1989 Viral alterations of cell function. Scientific American 261(2): 42–49

Randolph T 1976 Adaptation to specific environmental exposures enhanced by individual susceptibility. In: Dickey L (ed) Clinical ecology. Charles C Thomas, Springfield, Illinois, Ch. 6

Sapolsky R 1990 Hippocampal damage associated with prolonged glucocorticoid exposure in primates. Journal of Neuroscience 10: 2897–2902

Sapolsky R 1994 Individual differences and the stress response. Seminars in Neuroscience 6: 261–269

Selye H 1946 The general adaptation syndrome and the diseases of adaptation. Journal of Allergy 17: 231–247, 289–323, 358–398

Selye H 1950 The physiology and pathology of exposure to stress. ACTA, Montreal

Selye H 1952 The story of the adaptation syndrome. ACTA, Montreal

Selye H 1974 Stress without distress. Lippincott, Philadelphia

Shealy C N 1984 Total life stress and symptomatology. Journal of Holistic Medicine 6(2): 112–129

Waylonis G 1994 Post-traumatic fibromyalgia. American Journal of Physical Medicine and Rehabilitation 73(6): 403–412

Yunus M 1994 Psychological aspects of FMS – a component of the dysfunctional spectrum syndrome. In: Masi A (ed) Fibromyalgia and myofascial pain syndromes. Baillière, London

Yunus M 1997 FMS – clinical features and spectrum. The fibromyalgia syndrome. Haworth Press, Binghamptom, NY

3

Conditions associated with fibromyalgia

The possible interconnections between the pathophysiology of FMS and a number of its associated conditions are evaluated in this chapter. The specific connections between FMS and myofascial pain syndrome are examined in depth in Chapter 6 and thyroid dysfunction as a possible associated and contributory condition is covered in detail in Chapter 10 (summarised below).

ALLERGY/CHEMICAL SENSITIVITY

What degree of chemical (ingested, inhaled, etc.) sensitivity exists in patients with FMS? How much does the immune system's reaction to foods or environmental chemicals influence the pain and other symptoms being experienced?

A study in Seattle evaluated the similarities and differences among three groups of patients referred to a university-based clinic with diagnosis of either chronic fatigue syndrome (CFS), fibromyalgia syndrome (FMS) or multiple chemical sensitivities (MCS). The variables assessed included demographic features, symptom characteristics, psychological complaints, measures of health locus of control and health care information. What emerged was a picture of three conditions which were frequently difficult to distinguish from one another, irrespective of the original diagnosis, particularly in terms of demographic characteristics and symptom patterns. Fully 70% of the patients with an FMS diagnosis and 30% of those with multiple chemical sensitivities met all the criteria for CFS.

The researchers state that: 'Patients with CFS and FMS frequently reported symptoms compatible with Multiple Chemical Sensitivities'. Their conclusion was: 'The demographic and clinical factors and health locus of control do not clearly distinguish patients with CFS, FMS and MCS. Symptoms typical of each disorder are prevalent in the other two conditions' (Buchwald 1994).

A recent Turkish study evaluated the frequency of major symptoms as well as allergy in a group of more than 30 patients with a diagnosis of 'primary fibromyalgia' compared with matched (age and sex) controls (Tuncer 1997). Symptom prevalence in the FMS group (apart from pain which was 100%) was migraine 41%, IBS 13%, sleep disturbance 72%, and morning stiffness 69%. There was a frequent finding of allergy history in the FMS group, with elevated (though not significantly) IgE levels. 66% of the FMS patients tested were positive for allergic skin tests.

A study at the school of medicine of East Carolina University in 1992, involving approximately 50 people with hay fever or perennial allergic rhinitis, found that approximately half those tested fitted the ACR criteria for FMS (Cleveland 1992).

One question which these three studies raise is whether the allergy factors are causal or, together with other FMS symptoms, represent common results of an underlying feature – possibly increased intestinal permeability or immune system over-reactivity – or some other common central causal phenomenon such as Goldstein's 'neurosomatic disorder' (Goldstein 1996).

Dr Anne Macintyre, medical adviser to ME Action, an active patient support group for patients with chronic fatigue conditions in the UK, supports an 'immune dysfunction' model as the underlying mechanism for CFS(ME)/FMS (see Chs 4 and 5 for more on this hypothesis). She states: 'The immune dysfunction in ME may be associated with increased sensitivities to chemicals and/or foods, which can cause further symptoms such as joint pain, asthma, headache and IBS' (Macintyre 1993).

Dr Theron Randolph has, over many years, recorded a sequence of changes which may occur clinically as an individual passes through stages of 'reaction' to chemicals (in food or as hydrocarbons in the environment, for example) (Randolph 1976). He divides these reactions into those which relate to the active stimulation of an immune reaction by the allergen and those which relate to withdrawal from it (see Fig. 3.1 for a schematic representation of the 'reaction cycle').

During some of the stages, most notably 'systemic allergic manifestations', most of the major symptoms associated with FMS may become apparent, including widespread pain, fatigue, mental confusion, insomnia and irritable bowel. Randolph used the knowledge of these 'stages', both in active test situations as well as in assessing a patient's reported symptom patterns in relation to possible allergy connections. Randolph notes that health care professionals seldom see patients at levels zero or +1, where adaptation to their allergens (from their perspective) is not causing problems, and may be felt to be mildly beneficial ('alert, responsive, witty', etc.). It is when maladaptation exists, where more pronounced symptoms emerge of a physical or psychological nature (stage '++' or '– –' or more) that help may be sought, and allergy might usefully be suspected (see Table 3.1).

Where particular food allergens are consumed daily, reactions are usually not acute, but may be seen to be chronically present. The clinical ecology model suggests that the individual may by then have become 'addicted' to the substance and that the allergy is then 'masked' by virtue of regular and frequent exposure to it – preventing the withdrawal symptoms which would appear if exposure was stopped, as detailed in Table 3.1.

Feingold states:

If a reacting individual associates the stimulatory effect [of an allergen] with a given exposure, he tends to resort to this agent as often as necessary 'to remain well'. The coffee addict for example who requires coffee to get started in the morning, tends to use it through the day as often as necessary and in the amount sufficient to keep going. Over a period of time, a person so adapting tends to increase the frequency of intake and the amount per dose to maintain the relatively desirable effect. The same holds true for other common foods. (Feingold 1973)

Why does the individual fail to maintain adaptation?

Over time adaptive responses may become less predictable, and the suggestion is that this may relate to additional 'load' (as outlined in Ch. 1, Fig. 1.2 and Ch. 2, Fig. 2.2). Randolph states that: 'This development may be induced and maintained by an increase in the total load of specific materials to which adaptation is being attempted. Nonspecific exposures, such as concurrence of an infectious process, especially a viral infection, may also induce specifically maladapted responses.'

Research over the past 20 years has confirmed much of Randolph's work and has elaborated on what might be happening in relation to allergy, in so far as myalgic pain is concerned (summarised in Fig. 3.2).

Allergy–hyperventilation synergy and confusion

A section later in this chapter (p. 37) looks at possible connections between dysfunctional breathing patterns such as hyperventilation and FMS; a further complicating element exists – the way in which some forms of allergic response, or intolerance/sensitivity, can produce symptoms which include breathing dysfunction, so that causes become blurred.

An element of this confusion arises because hyperventilation increases circulating histamines, making allergic reactions more violent and possibly more likely (Barelli 1994). Dr Jonathan Brostoff (1992) states that some experts are dismissive of the concept of food intolerance and believe that large numbers of people so diagnosed are actually hyperventilators. He considers that: 'hyperventilation is relatively uncommon and can masquerade as food sensitivity'.

We therefore have two phenomena - allergy and hyperventilation – both of which can produce symptoms reminiscent of the other (including many associated with FMS), each of which can exacerbate the effects of the other (hyperventilation by maintaining high levels of histamine and allergy by provoking breathing dysfunc-

tion), and both of which commonly coexist in individuals with CFS and FMS.

Allergy and muscle pain

In Randolph's model (see Fig. 3.1 and Table 3.1) the phase he calls 'systemic allergic reaction' is characterised by a great deal of pain, either muscular and/or joint-related, as well as numerous symptoms common in FMS.

In Chapter 1 (Box 1.1), note was made of the pioneering work in the 1920s and 1930s by Dr A. H. Rowe, who demonstrated that widespread chronic muscular pains – often associated with fatigue, nausea, gastrointestinal symptoms, weakness, headaches, drowsiness, mental confusion and slowness of thought as well as irritability, despondency and widespread bodily aching – commonly had an allergic aetiology. He called the condition 'allergic toxaemia' (A. H. Rowe 1930, A. Rowe 1972).

Randolph in particular has studied the muscular pain phenomenon in allergy and his plea for this possibility to be considered by clinicians is based on long experience of it being ignored:

The most important point in making a tentative working diagnosis of allergic myalgia is to think of it. The fact remains that this possibility is rarely ever considered and is even more rarely approached by means of diagnostico-therapeutic measures capable of identifying and avoiding the most common environmental incitants and perpetuants of this condition – namely, specific foods, addictants, environmental chemical exposures and house dust. (Deamer 1971)

Randolph points out that when a food allergen is withdrawn from the diet it may take days for the 'withdrawal' symptoms to manifest: 'During the course of comprehensive environmental control [fasting or multiple avoidance] as applied in clinical ecology, myalgia and arthralgia are especially common withdrawal effects, their incidence being exceeded only by fatigue, weakness, hunger and headache.'

The myalgic symptoms may not appear until the second or third day of avoidance and start to recede after the fourth day. He warns that in testing for (stimulatory) reactions to food allergens

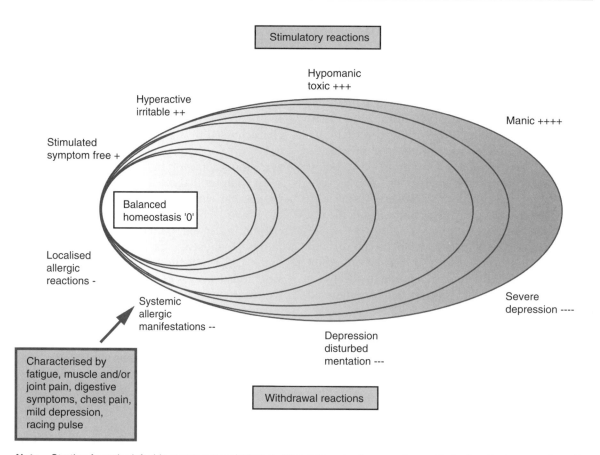

Stimulatory reactions

Hypomanic
toxic +++

Hyperactive
irritable ++

Manic ++++

Stimulated
symptom free +

Balanced
homeostasis '0'

Localised
allergic
reactions -

Severe
depression ----

Systemic
allergic
manifestations --

Depression
disturbed
mentation ---

Characterised by
fatigue, muscle and/or
joint pain, digestive
symptoms, chest pain,
mild depression,
racing pulse

Withdrawal reactions

Note – Starting from the left side centre move clockwise. Stimulatory reactions reach a particular level before merging with a corresponding withdrawal level, then receding. See Table 3.1 for more detail of individual stages

Figure 3.1   Schematic representation of the reaction cycle (adapted from Randolph 1976, p 157).

(as opposed to the effects of withdrawal), the precipitation of myalgia and related symptoms may not take place for between 6 and 12 hours after ingestion (of an allergen-containing food), which can confuse matters as other foods eaten closer to the time of the symptom exacerbation may then appear to be at fault.

Other signs which can suggest that myalgia is allied to food intolerance include the presence of a common FMS associated symptom, restless legs, a condition which also commonly coexists with and contributes to insomnia (see below) (Ekbom 1960).

When someone has an obvious allergic reaction to a food this may well be seen as a causal event in the emergence of other symptoms. If, however, the reactions occur many times every day, and responses become chronic, the cause and effect link may well be more difficult to make.

If symptoms such as muscular pain may at times be seen to be triggered by food intolerance or allergy, the major question remains – what is the cause of the allergy? One possibility is that the gut mucosa may have become excessively permeable, so allowing large molecules into the

Table 3.1   Clinical stages and features of allergic reactions (adapted from Randolph 1976, p 159)

Levels of ecological disturbance	Key signs and symptoms
+4 Manic	Distraught, excited, agitated, enraged, panicky; circuitous or one-track thoughts, <u>muscle twitching, jerking of extremities</u> (convulsive seizures, altered consciousness may develop)
+3 Hypomanic, toxic, anxious, egocentric	Aggressive, loquacious, clumsy (ataxic), feartul/apprehensive; alternating chills and flushing, ravenous hunger, excessive thirst; giggling or pathological laughter
+2 Hyperactive, irritable	Tense, jittery, talkative, argumentative, sensitive, over-responsive, self-centred, hungry and thirsty, possibly flushing, sweating and chilling, <u>insomnia</u>
+1 Stimulated – relatively symptom free	Active, alert, lively, responsive and enthusiastic with unimpaired ambition, energy, initiative, and wit; considerate of views and actions of others (this phase is often regarded as 'normal' behaviour)
0 Balanced, normal, homeostasis	Normal behaviour, asymptomatic
–1 **Localised allergic reactions**	<u>Running and stuffy nose</u>, clearing throat, coughing, wheezing, (asthma), itching, eczema and hives, <u>gas, diarrhoea, constipation</u> (colitis), <u>urgency and frequency of urination</u>, various eye and ear related symptoms
–2 **Systemic allergic reactions**	<u>Tired, dopey, somnolent, mildly depressed, oedematous with painful syndromes (headache, neckache, backache, neuralgia, myalgia, myositis, chest pain</u>, arthralgia, arteritis) and <u>cardiovascular effects (racing pulse,</u> etc.)
–3 **Depression, disturbed mentation**	<u>Confused</u>, indecisive, moody, sad, sullen, withdrawn or apathetic, emotional instability and <u>impaired attention, concentration, comprehension and thought processes (aphasia, mental lapses</u> and blackouts)
–4 Severe depression, possibly altered consciousness	Nonresponsive, lethargic, disorientated, melancholic, incontinent, regressive thinking, paranoid orientations, delusions, hallucinations, sometimes amnesia and finally comatose

NOTES:
The table should be read from the middle – from the notation marked '0' reading upwards for symptoms considered predominantly **stimulatory,** and downwards (from '0') for symptoms which are considered predominantly related to **withdrawal.**
All the terminology and the descriptors are those of Randolph (1976).
The symptoms which are commonly associated with FMS are underlined.
Marked changes in pulse rate or skipped beats may occur at any level of the sequence of reactions.

bloodstream where a defensive reaction is both predictable and appropriate. Is a 'leaky gut' then a cause of some people's allergy? And if so, what caused the leaky gut (Paganelli 1991, Troncone 1994)? These issues are addressed later in this chapter in relation to irritable bowel syndrome and bowel dysbiosis.

Allergy, hyper-reactive immune function and muscle pain

As part of the allergy link with myalgic pain, the immune system may be seen to be reacting to multiple or chronic infections as well as to a range of antigens, maintaining cytokine production at an excessively high level (Fig. 3.2).

A viral connection is often suggested in the aetiological progression to FMS and CFS. Anne Macintyre, previously quoted, offers research evidence for this, and states:

The onset of ME usually seems to be triggered by a virus, though the infection may pass unnoticed. Most common in the UK are enteroviruses including coxsackie B and Epstein–Barr virus (Gow 1991) ... Many people say they were fit and well before a viral infection which started their ME. But it is possible that in many such patients there have been other factors such as emotional stress, pesticide exposure, surgical or accidental trauma [see Whiplash below] some months before the triggering infection. (Macintyre 1993; see also notes on viral activity in FMS later in this chapter)

Because of the very close similarities between the complex aetiologies and symptoms of CFS (ME/post viral fatigue syndrome) and FMS,

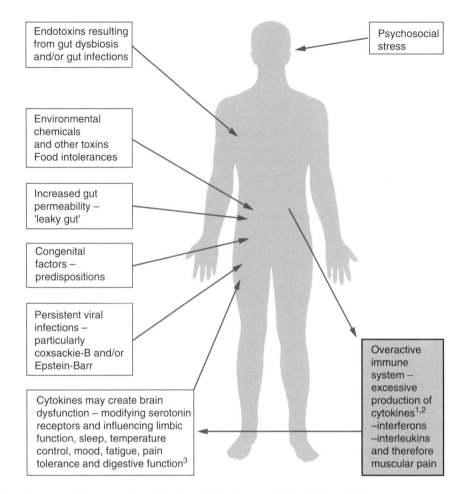

Figure 3.2 The allergy–myalgia connection ([1]Oldstone 1989, [2]Landay 1991, [3]Bakheit 1992).

the use of examples relating to one condition seem appropriate when considering the other (see Ch. 5).

Immune hyperactivity may therefore continue due to a persistent viral presence, or the existence of some other toxic immune stimulant (pesticides for example) or to repetitive allergic responses, as suggested by Randolph. If so, high levels of cytokines resulting from excessive immune activation will produce a variety of flu-like symptoms (Oldstone 1989).

Brain function may also be affected if, for example, interleukin-1 passes the blood–brain barrier, as has been shown to be possible. Interleukin-1 (a cytokine) seems to modify brain function by modulating serotonin receptor sites

(Bakheit 1992). If such changes occur in the hypothalamus, which seems plausible, a wide range of involuntary bodily functions could be affected, including endocrine production, sleep, temperature control, digestion, cardiovascular function, etc. (Goldstein 1993, Demitrack 1991). The interconnectedness of dysfunctional patterns involving the immune system and bodywide systems and functions can be seen to be possible in such a scenario (see Fig. 3.2).

TREATMENT FOR 'ALLERGIC MYALGIA'?

Randolph states his position: 'Avoidance of incriminated foods, chemical exposures and sometimes lesser environmental excitants.' How this is achieved in a setting other than a clinic or hospital poses a series of major hurdles for the practitioner and for the patient. It makes perfect sense – if foods or other irritants can be identified – for these to be avoided, whether or not underlying causes (such as possible gut permeability issues) can be, or are being, addressed.

According to the Fibromyalgia Network, the official publication of fibromyalgia/chronic fatigue syndrome support groups in the USA, the most commonly identified foods which cause problems for many people with FMS and CFS (ME) are wheat and dairy products, sugar, caffeine, Nutra-Sweet®, alcohol and chocolate (Fibromyalgia Network 1993).

Maintaining a wheat-free, dairy-free diet for any length of time is not an easy task, although many manage it. Issues involving patient compliance (or 'adherence' as it is now more politically correct to term it) deserve special attention as the way information is presented and explained can make a major difference in the determination displayed by already distressed patients as they embark on potentially stressful modifications to their lifestyles (see Ch. 8 and Ch. 11, p. 146).

Other therapeutic choices

Pizzorno (1996) has reviewed a range of detoxification and bowel enhancement methods which have been tested both clinically and in controlled studies, which demonstrate that if the bowel mucosa can be assisted to heal, gut flora replenished, liver function improved, allergens restricted, nutritional status evaluated and if necessary supplemented, marked improvements can be achieved in patients with chronic symptoms such as those evident in the discussion of allergy, including chronic myalgic pain conditions (Pizzorno 1996).

Information regarding elimination, rotation and exclusion patterns of eating are offered in Chapter 12, as are detoxification measures which have been shown effectively to reduce the degree of reactivity of sensitive individuals to their allergens (Randolph's 'excitants') (Bland 1995).

ANXIETY/HYPERVENTILATION

People suffering with FMS show a significantly higher degree of anxiety when compared with normal controls or with patients with other painful conditions such as rheumatoid arthritis. People who are anxious tend to breathe dysfunctionally, and the breathing patterns involved – largely upper chest with minimal diaphragmatic involvement – can exacerbate FMS and CFS symptoms, and may actually cause or aggravate many of them (Uveges 1990, Dailey 1990).

The repercussions of chronic dysfunctional breathing – with a hyperventilation tendency – can severely compromise the musculoskeletal structures involved, and can also produce widespread dysfunctional influences, as outlined below.

Notes on the physical manifestations of emotional turmoil

British physician Philip Barlow (Barlow 1959) who was a student of F. Methias Alexander, developer of Alexander technique, noted in 1959 that: 'There is an intimate relationship between states of anxiety and observable (and therefore palpable) states of muscular tension.' EMG readings have shown a statistical correlation between unconscious hostility and arm tension as well as leg muscle tension and sexual concerns (Malmo 1949, Sainsbury 1954). Wolff (1948) demonstrated that the majority of patients with headache showed, 'marked contraction in the muscles of the neck ... most commonly due to sustained contractions associated with emotional strain, dissatisfaction, apprehension and anxiety.'

Barlow explains:

Muscle is not only the vehicle of speech and expressive gesture, but has at least a finger in a number of other emotional pies for example, breathing regulation, control of excretion, sexual functioning and above all an influence on the body schema through proprioception. Not only are emotional attitudes, say, of fear and aggression, mirrored immediately in the muscle, but also such moods as depression, excitement and evasion have their characteristic muscular patterns and postures.

Assessment by means of palpation and observation, insofar as it relates to emotional states, requires that practitioners/therapists acquire the ability to observe patterns of use, posture, attitudes, tics and habits. They need also to be able to feel for changes in the soft tissues which relate to emotionally charged states, acute or chronic. And most importantly they need to be able to discern inappropriate muscular activity during upper chest breathing, epitomised by the extreme of hyperventilation.

Acute hyperventilation pattern

It is not hard to see the physical signs of acute hyperventilation as the rate of breathing and the excursion of the rib cage are characteristic, producing a heaving of the upper chest. When this is the result of emotion rather than activity there is a reduction in diaphragmatic activity with less expansion of the lower ribs. The upper ribs are pulled into inspiration, quickly followed by a fall on expiration.

Chronic hyperventilation pattern

This is easy to miss during observation, with the breathing rate often no more than the upper limit of normal, around 16 per minute. The more usual rate, however, is between 20 and 25 per minute in chronic hyperventilation in which a pattern of sighing and arrhythmic, shallow breathing is common. Upper rib movement is marked, with breath holding during activity (standing from sitting for example) and often during mental concentration.

Definition of hyperventilation (Timmons 1994)

Breathing in excess of metabolic requirements, i.e. ventilation is excessive relative to the rate of CO_2 production, leading to fall in pCO_2 below normal range (arterial hypocapnia), hypoxia.

Background to upper chest breathing

Breathing is the interface between mind and body, and any prolonged dysfunction such as 'upper chest breathing' (hyperventilation) in which 'psychology overwhelms physiology' represents a damaging pattern of behaviour with consequences which are biologically unsustainable, and which may influence a wide array of mind/body functions producing muscular imbalances, weaknesses, shortening and fibrosis, and impacting on spinal, neck, rib, shoulder function, leading to pain, headaches, etc. as well as to increased energy usage.

Biochemical effect of hyperventilation

As a tendency towards upper chest breathing becomes more pronounced, biochemical imbalances occur when excessive amounts of carbon dioxide are exhaled, leading to relative alkalosis, automatically producing a sense of apprehension and anxiety. This frequently leads on towards panic attacks and phobic behaviour, recovery from which is possible only when breathing is normalised (King 1988, Lum 1981).

Since carbon dioxide is one of the major regulators of cerebral vascular tone, any reduction due to hyperventilation patterns leads to vasoconstriction which could account in large part for the 'foggy brain' symptom so often complained of (see Fig. 3.3).

Along with heightened arousal/anxiety and cerebral oxygen lack there is also a tendency for what oxygen there is in the bloodstream to become more tightly bound to its haemoglobin carrier molecule, leading to decreased oxygenation of tissues. All this is accompanied by a decreased threshold of peripheral nerve firing.

Symptoms

In modern inner cities in particular, and late 20th century existence in general, there exists a vast expression of respiratory imbalance ('paradoxical breathing'), in which breathing function is seen to be at least an associated factor in most chronically fatigued and anxious people and almost all people subject to panic attacks and phobic behaviour; many of these also display symptoms of irritable bowel, multiple musculoskeletal symptoms and a tendency to be easily aroused emotionally, with mood swings, 'foggy brain' (concentration and memory impairment) and a sense of oppression/heaviness in the chest. 'I can't take a proper breath', 'I keep sighing', 'I feel as though there is a rock on my chest'... are all key expressions which are repeated over and over again at consultation.

Breathing exercises alone cannot work adequately to correct such dysfunctional patterns because the individual in the state described above will have developed structural modifications (short, tight muscles, restricted rib and spinal structures, etc.) which simply cannot allow a more desirable pattern to be imposed or relearned unless and until the restricted areas are stretched, relaxed and released, at least partially. Frank hyperventilation has been deeply studied with regard to its relationship to both physical and emotional symptoms, most notably in regard to anxiety and panic attacks (Bass & Gardner 1985, Perkin et al 1986).

Lum has discussed a vicious cycle of events:

Although Kerr et al (1937) pointed out that the clinical manifestations of anxiety were produced by hyperventilation, it was Rice (1950) who turned this concept upside down by stating that the anxiety was produced by the symptoms and, furthermore, that patients could be cured by eliminating faulty breathing habits. Lewis identified the role of anxiety as a trigger, rather than the prime cause. Given habitual hyperventilation, a variety of triggers, psychic or somatic, can initiate the vicious cycle of increased breathing, symptoms, anxiety arising from symptoms exacerbating hyperventilation and thus generating more symptoms and more anxiety.

Effects of hyperventilation

- Reduction in pCO_2 causes respiratory alkalosis via reduction in arterial carbonic acid, which leads to major systemic repercussions.
- The first and most direct response to hyperventilation is cerebral vascular constriction, reducing oxygen availability by about 50%.
- Of all body tissues, the cerebral cortex is the most vulnerable to hypoxia, which depresses cortical activity, causing dizziness, vasomotor instability, blurring of consciousness ('foggy brain') and vision. Many of these symptoms are noted in most cases of FMS.
- Loss of cortical inhibition results in emotional lability.

Neural repercussions

- Loss of CO_2 ions from neurons during moderate hyperventilation stimulates neuronal activity, producing muscular tension and spasm, speeding spinal reflexes, and producing heightened perception (pain, photophobia, hyperacusis) – of major importance in chronic pain conditions such as FMS.
- When hypocapnia is more severe or prolonged it depresses neural activity until the nerve cell becomes inert.
- What seems to occur in advanced or extreme hyperventilation is a change in neuronal metabolism; anaerobic glycolysis produces lactic acid in nerve cells, lowering pH, which then diminishes neuronal activity so that in extreme hypocarbia, neurons become inert. Thus, in the clinical condition, initial hyperactivity gives way to exhaustion, stupor and coma (Lum 1981).

Tetany

- Tetany is secondary to alkalosis; muscles which maintain 'attack-defence' mode – hunched shoulders, jutting head, clenched teeth, scowling – are those most likely to be affected, and these are common sites for pain in FMS.
- Painful nodules develop and are easily felt in nape of neck, anterior chest and shoulder girdle.
- Temporal headache centred on painful nodules in the parietal region are common.
- Also present in some, but not all, are painful legs.
- 'The whole body expresses tension and patients cannot relax in any position'.
- Sympathetic dominance is evident by virtue of dilated pupils, dry mouth, sweaty palms, gut and digestive dysfunction, abdominal bloating, tachycardia.
- Allergies and food intolerances are common due to increased circulating histamines.

Hyperventilation symptoms

Table 3.2 summarises the symptoms self-reported by 400 consecutive patients who were referred for a diagnosis of hyperventilation syndrome (Grossman & De Swart 1984).

Table 3.2   Self-reported symptoms in hyperventilation syndrome (Grossman & de Swart 1984)

	% HVS	% Non-HVS
Feeling of suffocation	54.5	41.0
Restless/panic	54.5	38.5
Pounding heart	50.0	27.0
Headaches	47.0	51.0
Tiredness	64.0	55.5
Tenseness	51.5	36.5
Hands tremble	38.5	25.0
Feeling of heat	42.0	34.0
Tingling in feet	20.0	17.0

The usefulness of a questionnaire to identify hyperventilation (the Nijmegen Questionnaire) was evaluated by Dutch physicians (van Dixhoorn et al 1985). They compared the results of use of the questionnaire when completed by 75 confirmed HVS patients and 80 non-HVS individuals. There were three dimensions measured in the questionnaire: breath shortness, peripheral tetany and central tetany: 'All three components had an unequivocally high ability to differentiate between HVS and non-HVS individuals. Together they provided a 93% correct classification. Statistical double cross validation resulted in 90–94% correct classifications. The sensitivity of the Nijmegen Questionnaire in relation to diagnosis was 91% and the specificity 95%.'

The signs and symptoms which the Nijmegen Questionnaire looks to might therefore usefully be used as a starting point (see also Fig. 3.3). Any patients, especially those whose symptom presentation includes FMS/CFS, who display or who report a number of the following signs or symptoms might be considered as suitable candidates for respiratory treatment:

- A feeling of constriction in the chest
- Shortness of breath
- Accelerated or deepened breathing
- Unable to breathe deeply
- Feeling tense (the questionnaire avoids the use of the word anxiety)

- Tightness around the mouth
- Stiffness in the fingers or arms
- Cold hands or feet
- Tingling fingers
- Bloated abdominal sensation
- Dizzy spells
- Blurred vision
- Feeling of confusion or losing touch with environment.

Structural considerations

Garland (1994) summarises the structural modifications which inhibit successful breathing retraining as well as psychological intervention, including:

- Visceral stasis/pelvic floor weakness
- Abdominal and erector spinae muscle imbalance
- Fascial restrictions from the central tendon via the pericardial fascia to the basiocciput
- Upper rib elevation with increased costal cartilage tension
- Thoracic spine dysfunction and possible sympathetic disturbance
- Accessory breathing muscle hypertonia and fibrosis involving shortening of muscles such as sternomastoid, scalenes and upper trapezius (see Whiplash below)
- Promotion of rigidity in the cervical spine with promotion of fixed lordosis

• Reduction in mobility of second cervical segment and disturbance of vagal outflow.

These changes, Garland states:

...run physically and physiologically against biologically sustainable patterns, and in a vicious circle promote abnormal function which alters structure which then disallows a return to normal function. In hyperventilation, where psychology overwhelms physiology, if assistance can be given to the individual by minimising the effect of somatic changes [as described above] and if these structural changes can be provided with an ability to modify, therapeutic interventions via breath retraining and counselling will be more effective.

Summary

There is a clear link between abnormal breathing patterns, excessive use of the accessory breathing muscles, upper chest breathing, etc. and increased muscle tone, which is itself a major cause of fatigue and pain, over and above the impact on the wider economy of the body of reduced oxygenation, particularly to the brain, and the unbalanced, malcoordinated patterns of use which stem from the structural and functional changes detailed by Garland.

Patients with this pattern of breathing will probably be fatigued, plagued by head, neck, shoulder and chest discomfort and a host of minor musculoskeletal problems as well as feeling apprehensive or frankly anxious. Many will have digestive symptoms such as bloating, belching and possibly hiatal hernia symptoms etc. associated with aerophagia which commonly accompanies this pattern of breathing, as well as a catalogue of other symptoms.

There is always a spectrum in such cases, with some being patent and obvious hyperventilators, others being borderline, and many being somewhere on their way towards a point where they will indeed show evidence of arterial hypocapnia and thus achieve the status of 'real' hyperventilators. The fact is that, just as in the case of FMS and the 'tender point count', before someone displays all the required (for a diagnosis) symptoms they will have been progressing towards that state for some time. It is important in conditions such as CFS and FMS to recognise

people who are borderline hyperventilators, and to address this.

Upper chest breathing: further implications and connections

Dr Janet Travell has confirmed that among the many factors which help to maintain and enhance trigger point activity is the low oxygenation of tissues which is aggravated by muscular tension, stress, inactivity and poor respiration. Travell and Simons also discuss 'Paradoxical breathing' in their *Trigger Point Manual* (Travell & Simons 1983):

In paradoxical respiration the chest and abdominal functions oppose each other; the patient exhales with the diaphragm while inhaling via the thoracic muscles, and vice versa. Consequently a normal effort produces inadequate tidal volume, and the accessory respiratory muscles of the upper chest, including the scalenes, overwork, to exchange sufficient air. The muscular overload results from the failure to coordinate the different parts of the respiratory apparatus.

As is made clear in Chapter 6, in which FMS and myofascial pain syndrome are compared, anything which exacerbates trigger point activity should be minimised ('lessen the load') as this will reduce overall pain input as well as improving coping mechanisms (reduced anxiety levels) and general function (more efficient oxygenation).

Why do people hyperventilate?

Lum (1984) discusses the reasons for people becoming hyperventilators: 'Neurological considerations can leave little doubt that the habitually unstable breathing is the prime cause of symptoms. Why they breathe in this way must be a matter for speculation, but manifestly the salient characteristics are pure habit.'

Breathing retraining has been used to correct hyperventilation. Lum reported that in one study more than 1000 patients were treated using breathing retraining, physical therapy and relaxation. Symptoms were usually abolished in 1–6 months with some younger patients requiring only a few weeks. At 12 months, 75% were free of all symptoms, 20% had only mild symptoms and about one patient in 20 had intractable symptoms.

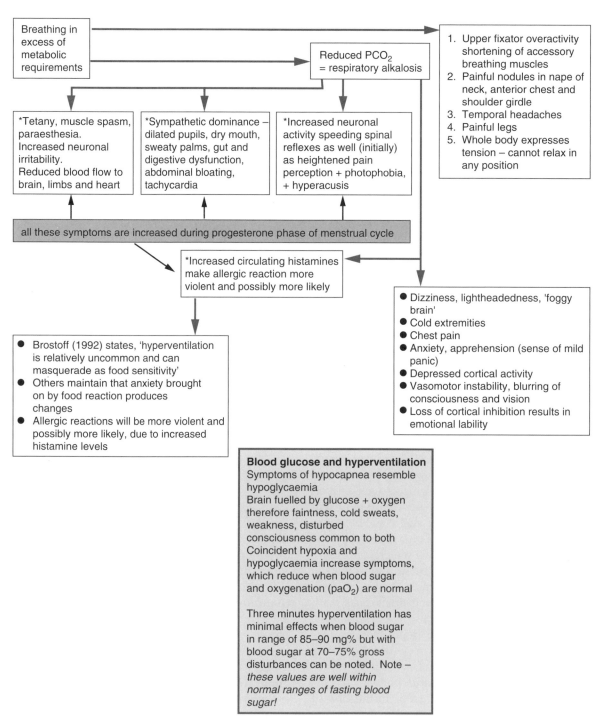

Figure 3.3   Breathing and the FMS connection (Lum 1994, Brostoff 1992).

Anti-arousal breathing technique

Ample research evidence exists to indicate that arousal levels can be markedly reduced via the habitual use of specific patterns which can be incorporated into breathing retraining. Cappo and Holmes (1984), Grossman et al (1985), among others, have shown that breathing retraining is a valid approach.

Cappo and Holmes have incorporated into their methodology a form of traditional yoga breathing which produces specific anti-arousal benefits. The pattern calls for a ratio of inhalation to exhalation of 1:4 if possible, but in any case for exhalation to take appreciably longer than inhalation (see Ch. 12 for details of this approach)

IRRITABLE BOWEL SYNDROME

The most frequent gastrointestinal problem for which specialist advice is sought is irritable bowel syndrome (IBS). The major symptoms include abdominal discomfort or pain, intermittent diarrhoea or constipation, bloating and distension. It is thought that an initial distinction can be made between IBS and organic bowel disease by virtue of the presence (in IBS) of the associated symptoms of urinary frequency, premature satiety, backache and fatigue (Maxton et al 1991). Just as in FMS (and CFS), the patient with IBS is far more likely to be a young adult female, displaying no clear laboratory evidence for the problem and with no obvious pathology (Yunus 1989).

There are various schools of thought as to the cause(s) of IBS:

• Stress-related influences including anxiety/hyperventilation (Nyhlin 1993).
• Allergy, sensitivity influences (particularly wheat, corn, dairy products, coffee, tea, citrus fruits) possibly effected by enzyme or HCl imbalances (Jones et al 1982).
• Infection and possible overgrowth, by fungi and/or bacteria; or parasitic infection (particularly *Giardia*, threadworms, *Ascaris* and *Amoeba*). Yeast overgrowth in particular has been blamed for damaging gut mucosa and precipitating malabsorption, and consequent allergic responses, including IBS symptoms (Holti 1966, Alexander 1967, Phaosawasdi 1986). British physicians Stephen Davies and Alan Stewart state: 'Apart from the simple matter of overgrowth with candida, some people are hypersensitive to it. . . . the main places candida takes hold are the GI tract, the mouth and the vagina. It has been reported that some people with the symptoms of IBS are allergic to the yeast' (Alexander 1975, Davies & Stewart 1988).

• Antibiotics usage can trigger a sequence which results in yeast overgrowth followed by bowel irritability. Dr John Henry (1995), chief medical editor for the British Medical Association's book, *A new Guide to Medicines and Drugs*, who is not antagonistic to the use of antibiotics, says: 'A risk of antibiotic treatment, especially if it is prolonged, is that the balance of micro-organisms normally inhabiting the body may be disturbed. In particular antibiotics may destroy bacteria that limit the growth of Candida, a yeast often present in the body in small amounts. This can lead to overgrowth of Candida in the mouth, vagina, or bowel.' Dr Joseph Pizzorno, of Bastyr University, Seattle, indicates the implications of this as follows:

In a study of 55 injured patients admitted to the trauma service of a hospital, all were given broad spectrum antibiotic therapy during some point of their stay. 67% developed elevated candida antigen levels in their blood during their hospital stay, indicating that candida were overgrowing in their intestines (and/or the vagina in women). The researchers also found that the white blood cells of patients with candida antigens were not able to inhibit candida albicans growth as effectively as white blood cells from patients who did not have candidal antigens in their blood. In other words, when patients receive antibiotics, the level of candida in their intestines increases so much, and the intestines become so damaged, that fragments of the candida leak into their bloodstream and inhibit the function of their immune system. (Pizzorno 1996)

• When such local gut irritation (caused by hypersensitivity of gastrointestinal mechano- and chemoreceptors caused by initial trauma) prevails, it is thought that visceral hyperalgesia may occur leading to central sensitisation (visceral afferents influence dorsal horn neurons which subsequently affect the hypothalamus) (Mayer 1993).

• This (visceral hyperalgesia) model is what Goldstein (1996) calls a 'bottom-up' version of what he sees as a 'top-down' process in his neurosomatic model of FMS aetiology (see Ch. 4): 'Thalamic and dorsal horn dysregulation in IBS would stem from prefrontal cortical dysfunction in this paradigm. There is no ... reason to complicate matters by invoking some peripheral lesion, although some may occur, just as primary immune dysfunction may occasionally cause CFS, and post-traumatic myofascial pain syndrome may produce fibromyalgia.'

In considering the merits of the sensitisation model, in which visceral irritants are seen to create central dysfunctional behaviour (termed in this hypothesis 'visceral hyperalgesia'), recall the research of Korr (described in Ch. 1) relating to facilitation. The process of localised or segmental facilitation as it occurs in the neural structures operating in the musculoskeletal system, in response to repetitive stress, seems to have strong echoes as to what is hypothesised to be happening in the brain in response to visceral dysfunction.

Is Goldstein's central dysfunction merely evidence of a facilitated brain?

Questions to ask in irritable bowel syndrome

In order to make sense of a patient's irritable bowel condition the following differentiations need to be made by means of questioning, examination, testing and, if necessary, hospital investigation:

• Is the problem related to gynaecological, urinary, liver or biliary, musculoskeletal or purely gastrointestinal factors?
• Is it modified by menstruation, defecation, urination, certain foods (fatty, etc.), work, rest?
• Do emotions relating to work, family, relationships, other factors influence the problem?
• Is there evidence of infection, inflammation, trauma, neoplasm, metabolic disturbance, degenerative disease?

Treatment should depend upon the answers to these questions.

How common is IBS in association with FMS?

A study in 1996 in Ankara, Turkey, noted the coexistence of these conditions in many patients, and surveyed the prevalence of IBS symptoms in 75 patients with FMS and 50 normal controls. 42% of the FMS patients displayed IBS symptoms as against 16% of the controls. The researchers question whether a common pathogenic mechanism exists for both conditions. Goldstein ('top-down') would certainly suggest this to be so, whereas others ('bottom-up') might see the IBS – whatever its aetiology – as part of the cause of FMS.

In Chapter 2 it was noted that Dr Clauw found 60% of his surveyed FMS patients to have IBS symptoms, while Dr Jessop observed that of her well over 1000 patients with CFS and FMS, fully 82% had yeast cultured, and 30% had parasites in their purged stool samples (Clauw 1995, Fibromyalgia Network Newsletter 1990–94).

Prior to the onset of their CFS/FMS, Jessop's patients were recorded as having had a high proportion of IBS (89%) with 80% reporting a history of 'constant gas' or bloating, and 58% chronic constipation.

Figure 3.4 outlines a schematic representation of possible connections between bowel dysfunction in general and IBS in particular. Goldstein's neurosomatic model is outlined in Chapter 4.

DEPRESSION

Many of the symptoms of FMS are similar to those experienced during depression, and there is ample evidence that mild antidepressant medication assists in symptom relief (sleep and pain) of many patients with FMS (but by no means all).

Is FMS a form of depression?

Several major reviews have concluded that there is indeed an association between depressive ill-

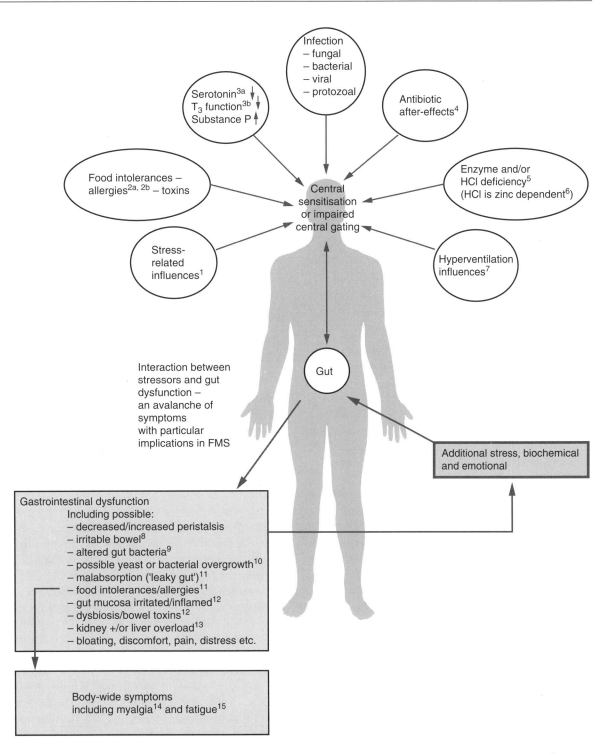

Figure 3.4   Stressors and gut dysfunction ([1]Langeluddecke 1990, [2a]Dickey 1976, [2b]Russell 1965, [3a]Haseqawa 1988, [3b]Lowe 1997, [4]Ball 1997, [5]Barrie 1995, [6]Cho 1991, [7]Timmons 1994, [8]Sivri 1996, [9]Ninkaya 1986, [10]Simon 1981, [11]Warshaw 1974, [12]Chadwick 1992, [13]Liehr 1979, [14]Tuncer 1997, [15]Rae 1992)

ness and conditions such as FMS. What this 'association' is is not clear, however. Some suggest, despite some equivocal evidence, that there exists a direct association (Hudson 1996), while others feel that both depressive illness and FMS (as well as CFS, IBS, premenstrual dysphoric disorder, migraine and atypical facial pain) may possibly share a common aetiological step (Gruber 1996).

The argument for a connection between FMS and depressive illness is based on:

- They have an overlapping symptomatology
- They both display similar patterns of comorbid disorders
- Patients with FMS report high rates of depressive disorders amongst relatives
- Depressives and FMS patients demonstrate similar responses to psychological tests and rating scales, as well as high lifetime rates for mood disorders.

Further support comes from the evidence that antidepressant medications, irrespective of their chemical class, are generally useful in treatment of FMS and associated conditions, although prescribed beneficially in very low doses as compared with amounts employed in treating major depressive illnesses.

A Turkish study attempted to evaluate the relationship between FMS and the intensity of anxiety and depression, as well as establishing whether there was a connection between psychological disturbances and duration and severity of pain. The psychological states of 30 FMS patients and 36 healthy controls were evaluated utilising the Beck Depression Inventory, the State and Trait Anxiety Inventory, and the Beck Hopelessness Scale. The findings showed a significant difference between the psychological status of FMS patients and the controls as measured by the Beck Depression Inventory and the Trait Anxiety Inventory – which correlated with pain severity. The conclusion was that somatic expression of depression was an important difference between the two groups. As to the link with anxiety trait, the researchers concluded that, 'the difference between state and trait anxiety inventory reflects that current anxiety is not secondary to

pain but trait anxiety is possibly causally related to pain.'

Several thoughts emerge from this study, including:

- The depression noted could well represent a response to the painful symptoms and disability.
- The anxiety trait as a possible aetiological factor. This links well with possible hyperventilation involvement, since the connection between overbreathing and anxiety is well established (see notes above on hyperventilation).

There also exists a strong degree of argument against a direct depression–FMS connection:

- As noted, dosage of antidepressants which assist in FMS (though not always) are lower than would be used in treatment of depression.
- There is little correlation between improved psychological status following antidepressant medication and the physical symptoms being experienced.

For example, a study conducted at a Toronto hospital examined and compared psychological adjustment and family functioning in patients with primary juvenile fibromyalgia and juvenile rheumatoid arthritis. There were almost no differences noted in the psychological adjustment of either the children or their parents, or in the ratings of family functioning or coping strategies. It was noted that a number of psychological adjustment, pain, fatigue and coping variables were significantly associated with functional disability, irrespective of the underlying condition. The conclusion of the researchers was that FMS is not a psychogenic condition (Reid 1997).

Mohammad Yunus (1994a) makes a number of important observations. He states that although up to 35% of FMS patients in some studies are reported to display significant psychological distress, most such reports are based on patients at speciality rheumatology clinics where psychological problems may well be over-represented due to referral bias. Referring to 'psychological stress' in general, Yunus reports that patients with FMS show a significantly greater degree of mental stress, as well as 'life event' scores, compared with patients with rheumatoid arthritis or normal controls as evaluated by Hassles Scale and the Life Event Inventory (Dailey 1990). Yunus is clear that his investigation shows that, 'presently available data indicates that FMS is not a psychiatric condition. Studies by Clark et al (1985) and Yunus et al (1991) specifically suggest that psychological abnormality is not essential for the development of FMS. However, it is important to realise that pain and perhaps fatigue may be more severe and difficult to manage in a minority subgroup of patients with psychological distress. These patients need special understanding and management by a caring physician.'

Goldenberg (1994a) has investigated the question as to depression and FMS. Comparing FMS patients with CFS and rheumatoid arthritis patients he found that there may be a greater lifetime and family history of depression in FMS, compared to RA and controls, as well as greater levels of daily stress. He found, however, that most patients with FMS do not have psychiatric illness and was able to demonstrate that no correlation existed between FMS symptoms or treatment response, and psychological factors.

Goldenberg emphasises the importance of the high levels of daily stress, reminding us that there is a growing body of evidence which shows that stress levels, including adaptation to chronic illness, has a profound effect on immune function, making viral infection more likely (Cohen 1991), and that neurohormonal dysregulation can be shown to correlate with stress levels (Giep et al 1993).

Research at the University of Alabama compared current FMS patients with non-patients who were either normal and healthy, or who met the ACR criteria for FMS but who had not sought treatment for the past 10 years (Bradley et al 1994). The findings were that:

• FMS patients show significantly lower pain thresholds at tested points (tender points and control points) as well as reporting greater symptom severity and disability, compared with normal controls and the non-patient FMS individuals.
• FMS patients as compared with non-patients met the criteria for a greater number of lifetime psychiatric diagnoses.

• The findings support the concept that the high level of psychological distress is not a primary feature of FMS but that, in combination with high pain levels and disability, psychological distress may cause the individual to seek medical care.
• As compared with normal controls, both FMS groups demonstrated lowered pain thresholds and significantly higher levels of fatigue, suggesting that central factors such as sleep disorder or neuropeptide levels are contributory features of their problems.
• The researchers confirm that they have found that FMS patients show reduced regional cerebral blood flow to the caudate nucleus and that the degree of this strongly correlates with pain thresholds.

The arguments for and against a causal depression link with FMS remain unresolved. While there appear to be benefits from the use of low dosage antidepressants, which, in some patients, offer symptomatic relief, possibly improving sleep patterns and reducing fatigue and pain levels, this approach does not seem to be dealing with underlying causes.

DYSREGULATION OF BRAIN FUNCTIONS

The main brain centres involved in dysfunctional behaviour with direct influence on FMS and CFS can, according to Goldstein (1996), be influenced by 'many triggering agents in the predisposed individual', including viral infections which influence neural function, 'immunizations which deplete biogenic amines' (Gardier et al 1992), toxic organophosphates or hydrocarbons, trauma to the head, difficulties in delivery, electromagnetic fields, sleep deprivation, general anaesthesia, and stress (whether mental, emotional or physical). To these potential influences on brain circulation and function might be added the effects of hyperventilation as discussed above, as well as specific allergic reactions.

Goldstein (1996) has also examined the effects of certain childhood influences on eventual central control changes which help to explain some influences on his concept of a neurosomatic cause of FMS and CFS (and many other apparently nonorganic conditions). Some of his key observations are summarised below:

* Conventional EEG and brain electrical activity mapping (BEAM) show the left frontotemporal region of the brain to display abnormalities in the majority of people who have a history of childhood abuse.
* Evaluation of patients with CFS shows approximately 40% to have similar abnormalities in this region.
* Early childhood experience of major stress increases cortisol levels which can affect hippocampal function and structure (Sapolsky 1990, 1994), suggesting a natural plasticity which allows environmental influences to 'programme' evolving biological responses to stimuli which are threatening.
* In this way variations in genetic influences, as well as upbringing and exposure to stress, together help to produce the patterns whereby the individual responds to subsequent stress, allowing exaggerated (or insufficient) responses to emerge to stressful influences as the norm for the individual.
* This would become even more likely, it is suggested, if essentially non-stressful events are misinterpreted, leading to both behavioural and neuroimmunoendocrine disorders.
* In contrast to normal homeostatic responses (where changes in hormonal and other variables result in stabilisation via adaptation), these potentially pathological responses have been dubbed allostasis – the physiological regulation of abnormal states which are not in balance.
* Allostasis is seen to involve a degree of arousal – and consequent stress-hormone elevation – resulting from anticipated adversity, as well as a sense of events being unpredictable, with a feeling that little personal control is possible.
* These altered homeostatic (allostatic) responses are accompanied by a complex array of well researched biochemical modifications to the norm, involving glucocorticoid elevation at various key sites in the brain which, when abnormally influenced, produce a chain reaction of neurohumoral changes potentially influencing

almost any part of the body or its functions (McEwan 1994).

* For example, animal studies show that lesions in the ventromedial medulla result in depressed immune function (natural killer cells in particular), a feature of CFS.
* Dysfunction of this part of the brain also produces a reduction in growth hormone production with major implications for tissue repair.
* A change in the thermoregulatory setpoint is another result of dysfunction in this region of the brain, possibly accounting for temperature intolerance common in FMS and CFS.
* Goldstein reports 'constantly' seeing just such abnormalities in CFS and FMS patients – and has gone into great detail to explain the link between the pathophysiological changes affecting different brain regions as a result of this sequence of events, and many of the multiple symptoms experienced by CFS/FMS patients including pain, sleep disorders, poor cold tolerance, etc.
* In the section on fatigue and pain (below) some of Goldstein's additional evaluation of central dysfunctional influences will also be summarised, as will the work of other FMS researchers (see Fig. 4.5).

FATIGUE AND PAIN

Chronic fatigue is reported by approximately 90% of people with a diagnosis of FMS (and pain by 100%), and is one of the main presenting symptoms. Yunus believes that, as with global pain, the widespread and pervading nature of the fatigue complained of probably has a neurohumoral basis (Yunus 1994b). The similarities and differences between FMS and CFS are examined in Chapter 5: what is absolutely clear is that the differences between CFS and FMS are far fewer than the similarities and that they probably share common underlying causes.

As part of his 'neurosomatic' hypothesis (see Ch. 4, and the notes on early influences above) Goldstein has given a detailed description of the biochemical patterns which may be operating as a major part of chronic fatigue as it occurs in FMS and CFS. Reference to his book *Betrayal by the Brain* (Haworth Medical Press, 1996) is suggested for more detailed appreciation of the complexity of this explanation.

Goldstein's work, and that of others, indicates that:

- The ventromedial hypothalamus (limbic system) controls energy metabolism as well as regulating glucocorticoids and other stress hormones.
- This part of the brain is also involved in regulating, via sympathetic routes, glucose uptake by skeletal muscles as well as by brown adipose tissue and the heart.
- Muscular contraction induced by active (not passive) stretching or pressure influences ergoreceptors – unmyelinated and myelinated non-nociceptor nerve fibres – causing release of substance P and other neuropeptides in various brain sites (such as the ventrolateral medulla) and the spinal cord.
- Substance P in particular has been shown to be present in elevated amounts in both CFS and FMS patients where inappropriate excessive production occurs, post-exercise.
- Substance P is normally released by spinal cord tissues (afferent neurons) as a response to painful stimuli, therefore excessive levels would increase pain perception (Malmberg 1992).
- The neuromodulator serotonin, and tryptophan from which it derives, are both noted as being significantly reduced in FMS patients, and this has been shown to correlate with pain symptoms (Russell et al 1993).

Russell suggests a model for FMS in which abnormal levels of serotonin (low) and substance P (high) in the brain and spinal cord lead to a number of neuroendocrine, nociceptive and general functional abnormalities including sleep disturbance, exaggerated pain perception and dysfunctional bowel symptoms. Relative tryptophan deficiency could be responsible for poor protein synthesis and its consequences (Russell 1994a).

Block (1993) summarises the possible factors associated with the abnormal response to stress noted in FMS, which some of the findings highlighted above may help to explain:

1. Oversensitive nociceptors
2. Dysfunctional [levels of] neurohumoral transmitter substances or their receptors
3. Over efficient or poorly modulated pain pathways
4. Heightened cerebral perception of pain and/or increased reaction to pain
5. Diminished tolerance to pain or over-reporting of perceived pain
6. All of these elements influenced by psychological, physical or environmental stressors.

Russell has described the biochemical association between serotonin, substance P and the phenomenon of pain (see Fig. 3.5).

Serotonin is an inhibitory neurotransmitter involved in the initiation and maintenance of restorative sleep (Moldofsky 1982). It is also suggested that serotonin acts in the thalamus as a regulator of pain perception as well as its additional role as a regulator of hormonal release, including growth hormone. What has been established is that serum levels of serotonin are indeed lower in FMS patients than in controls (Russell et al 1992). These low levels observed in FMS patients could result from inadequate serotonin manufacture (in the intestinal tract, from tryptophan, derived from protein digestion), or from lower uptake of serotonin by platelet cells, or from less efficient platelet activation during clotting.

Additional research confirms that serum tryptophan levels are also lower in FMS patients and that tryptophan in FMS patients has more difficulty in crossing the blood–brain barrier (Yunus et al 1992).

Serotonin has a dampening influence on pain perception – the opposite of the influence of substance P, which assists in transmission of peripheral pain messages to the brain. Thus:

- If serotonin and substance P levels are normal the amplitude of pain messages will be moderated
- If serotonin levels are lower than normal, or if levels of substance P are higher than normal, pain transmission will be amplified.

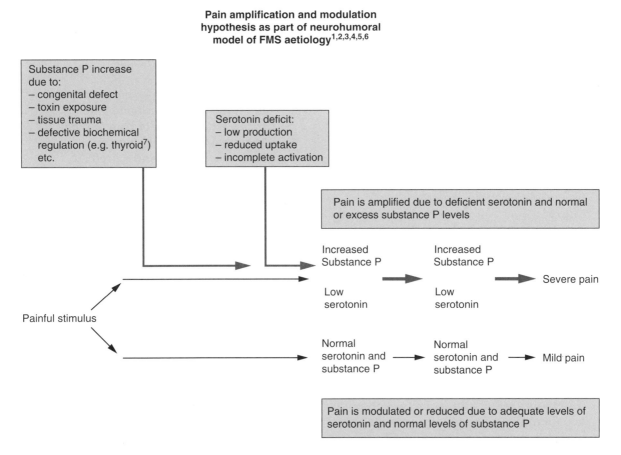

Figure 3.5 Biochemical association between serotonin, substance P and the phenomenon of pain. ([1]Russell et al 1992, [2]Russell et al 1993, [3]Yunus et al 1992, [4]Malmberg 1992, [5]Russell 1994b, [6]Moldofsky 1982, [7]Yellin 1997).

This would suggest that, even if only normal afferent pain messages ('discomfort') are being transmitted, these would be enhanced and might be perceived as intense discomfort or pain. Chemical communication processes would be presenting inaccurate information. It is suggested that antidepressant medication may help to retain greater levels of serotonin and so explain their apparent usefulness in FMS treatment.

These concepts, Russell suggests (Russell 1994), support a neurohumoral mechanism for the pathogenesis of FMS.

Summary

The circle of cause and effect seems to constantly be evaluated from different positions, with the same elements regularly appearing. Even Goldstein, who holds strongly to a primary central dysfunctional cause of all that follows in symptom terms in cases of FMS, acknowledges the numerous possible influences which can produce these dysfunctional neurohumoral patterns. His choice is to focus treatment using a variety of drugs (see Ch. 4) to help restore functional balance in the disturbed biochemistry he observes.

Others choose to see the neurohumoral and brain dysfunctions operating in FMS and CFS as being the result of other influences (including allergy, toxicity, infection, psychological stressors, etc.) acting on a possibly predisposed individual, which may be capable of being influenced by therapeutic intervention addressing the wider influences, the perpetuating factors (see Genetic hypothesis in Ch. 4 and Fig. 4.1).

SLEEP DISORDERS

Just how easily sleep disturbance can upset muscular status was demonstrated by Dr H. Moldofsky in a study in which six volunteers had their stage four sleep disrupted for three nights in a row. They all developed fatigue, widespread aching muscles and specific tenderness on palpation of the appropriate sites used to diagnose fibromyalgia (Moldofsky 1993).

Is sleep disturbance in FMS a result of influences which derive from higher centres, or is it a primary cause of the dysfunctional patterns which accompany it? Franklin Lue (Lue 1994) has reviewed some of the important issues around the FMS/sleep disturbance issue, summarised below:

• In pain clinics, those patients reporting sleep disturbance (70%) complain of more pain, disability and emotional distress than the 30% who do not complain of sleep problems.
• In FMS, patients' sleep disturbance is associated with greater pain and general symptom severity (e.g. fatigue) as well as greater morning stiffness.
• The intrusion of alpha-wave sleep during non-rapid eye movement (NREM) phases of sleep has been identified by a number of researchers as an index of non-restorative sleep in FMS; however, this feature is not universally accepted, partly because of a lack of standardisation in the measurement processes and their interpretation. Observation is also made of (some) people with alpha-wave disturbances in their sleep who are asymptomatic, and of people with severe FMS who have normal sleep patterns. The putative link between FMS and the alpha-wave intrusion phenomenon remains unproven at this stage, although there is little question that sleep disturbance is a major symptom of most people with FMS.
• Two key proposals for explaining the observed link between sleep disturbance and increased muscular pain are:
  — disruption of tissue repair and restoration (protein synthesis, energy ATP decrease)
  — disturbance of the immunomodulatory role of sleep (interleukin-1 levels decrease).
• Criticisms of these proposals have been noted, with the differences in sex hormones and the time of sleep both being seen to create sufficient variation to confuse any simplistic assessment of the influence of sleep on immune function in particular. 'Separating sleep and circadian changes is very difficult. Rhythmic variations – circannual, circadian and circahemidian – in immune functions have been reported in many studies' (Moldofsky 1993).
• The area of research into sleep patterns remains potentially useful but difficult.

A study which has looked at this phenomenon provides a further insight. Spanish researchers evaluated two features, possible sleep apnoea syndrome as well as oxygen saturation of haemoglobin in arterial blood ($SaO_2\%$) during sleep in normal controls and patients with FMS. They found that 'patients with FMS showed small overnight falls in $SaO_2\%$ and spent more time during the night in $SaO_2\%$ below 92% than did the control group. These alterations are not as a whole due to sleep apnoea and could be important in FMS musculoskeletal pathophysiology' (Alvarez et al 1996).

The significance of the $SaO_2\%$ finding, in terms of generation of pain, may well be significant; Travell and Simons have noted the relative importance in generation and maintenance of myofascial pain problems of tissue hypoxia (see Box 6.1)

A possibility exists that upper-chest breathing patterns persist throughout sleep, and are directly responsible for the observed reduction in $SaO_2\%$, discussed above. Goldstein (1996) reviews some of the influences of sleep on the biochemistry of the body in general, and in relation to FMS/CFS in particular:

• Slow-wave sleep induces the replenishment of astrocytic glycogen which is depleted during wakefulness.
• Reduction in cerebral glucose causes increased synthesis of adenosine, stimulating adenosine receptors, producing increased sleep need (EEG evidence exists for this).
• The levels of adenosine (an inhibitory neurotransmitter) are inversely related to ATP.

Therefore, lower levels of ATP (energy) increases adenosine, so promoting sleep onset as well as NREM sleep.

• Benington and colleagues (Benington & Heller 1995) call sleep disturbance a 'defect of adenosine metabolism'.

• Adenosine is formed from S-adenosylmethionine, which, when supplemented in several double-blind studies, has been shown to offer effective treatment of FMS (improved activity, reduced pain, fatigue and morning stiffness, as well as elevated mood) (Jacobsen 1991).

• Excessive levels of neuromodulators such as substance P can overcome the adenosine influence, and since substance P is known to be present in higher than normal levels in patients with CFS/FMS this might account for disturbed sleep patterns as well as associated symptoms such as bruxism, nightmares, restlessness, and sweating.

• The underlying cause of this disturbance could relate to one of number of causes of a complex nature which Goldstein details (Goldstein 1996, pp 113–118).

Figures 3.6A and 3.6B provide a framework of information regarding restorative and non-restorative sleep influences. Whether sleep disturbance is part of the aetiology of FMS or is an associated symptom resulting from a common central cause is not clear. Sleep enhancement strategies can be seen to be helpful in either case and these are outlined in Chapter 12.

THYROID DYSFUNCTION

A hypothesis exists, supported by placebo controlled, double-blind trials, which asserts that gene transcription inadequacy can result in an individual who is euthyroid, having symptoms of hypothyroidism and as a result, FMS. This hypothesis claims that all the symptoms of FMS can be accounted for via this explanation (see Ch. 4 for a summary and Ch. 10 for a detailed presentation of this hypothesis utilising triiodothyronine (T_3) in its treatment.

Pizzorno (1996) has outlined the importance of nutritional balance in reestablishing normal thyroid function. He states that apart from the more obvious insistence on adequate iodine intake, the amino acid tyrosine as well as zinc, copper and selenium are essential in order to ensure that adequate thyroid hormone secretion is achieved and that T_4 is capable of being converted to T_3.

See Pizzorno (1996, pp. 231–232) for more information.

TRAUMA (PARTICULARLY WHIPLASH)

Trauma is seen to be one of the major triggers for the onset of FMS. A diagnosis of 'secondary FMS' or 'post-traumatic FMS' distinguishes such patients from those who develop FMS spontaneously, without an obvious triggering event.

An Ohio study evaluated the progress of 176 individuals who had been seen between 1980 and 1990 with a diagnosis of post-traumatic FMS. They were examined and completed a lengthy questionnaire about symptoms and treatment experiences. Over 60% of these patients had been involved in a vehicle accident shortly before onset of their condition; 12.5% had had a work-related accident, 7% started symptoms following surgery, and just over 5% had suffered sports injuries, with the remainder having experienced a variety of traumas not fitting these categories.

Whiplash as a trigger

A study involving over 100 patients with traumatic neck injury as well as approximately 60 patients with leg trauma evaluated the presence of severe pain (fibromyalgia syndrome) an average of 12 months post-trauma (Buskila et al 1997). The findings were that 'almost all symptoms were significantly more prevalent or severe in the patients with neck injury ... The fibromyalgia prevalence rate in the neck injury group was 13 times greater than the leg fracture group.'

Pain threshold levels were significantly lower, tender point counts were higher and quality of life was worse in the neck injury patients as compared with leg injury subjects. Over 21% of the patients with neck injury (none of whom had chronic pain problems prior to the injury) developed fibromyalgia within 3.2 months of trauma as against only 1.7% of the leg fracture patients

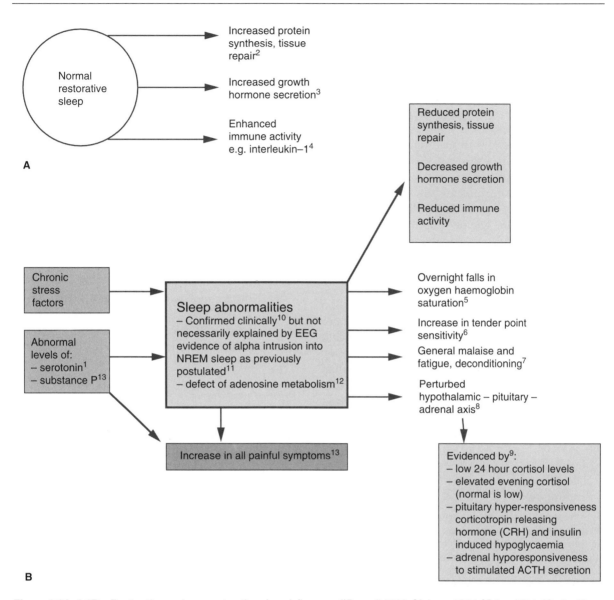

Figure 3.6A, 3.6B   Restorative and non-restorative sleep influences ([1]Russell 1993, [2]Adams 1997, [3]Griep 1994, [4]Gudewill 1992, [5]Alvarez 1996, [6]Jacobsen 1989, [7]Hawley 1988, [8]Bennett 1997, [9]Crofford 1994, [10]Affleck 1996, [11]Shaver 1997, Hrycaj 1993, [13]Benington & Heller 1995).

(not significantly different from the general population). The researchers make a particular point of noting that, 'in spite of the injury or the presence of FMS, all patients were employed at the time of examination and that insurance claims were not associated with increased FMS symptoms or impaired functioning.'

Why should whiplash-type injury provoke FMS more effectively than other forms of trauma? One answer may lie in a particular muscle, part of the sub-occipital group.

Rectus capitis posterior minor (RCPM)

A recent discovery revealed new anatomical knowledge. A human dissection performed using a saggital rather than a coronal incision, revealed that rectus capitis posterior minor (RCPM) has a unique connection to the dura at the atlanto-occipital junction. Subsequent research has shown it to have a major potential for symptom production – especially chronic pain – when damaged in whiplash-type injuries, or when it is severely stressed (Hack et al 1995).

The superior insertion of the muscle, which arises from a tendon on the atlas, is into the medial part of the inferior nuchal line on the occipital bone, between the nuchal line and the foramen magnum. The orientation of the muscle is described as being perpendicular to the dura, an arrangement which 'appears to resist movement of the dura towards the spinal cord'.

The dissection referred to above, in 1994, demonstrated that a connective tissue extension ('bridge') links this muscle to the dura mater which provides it with potentials for influencing the cranial reciprocal tension membranes directly. Because of its siting, close to the posterior cranial fossa and the cisterna magna, the relative 'health' of this muscle has particular implications relating to cerebrospinal fluid fluctuation. It might also have the potential to influence the functioning of the vertebral artery and the suboccipital nerve which could affect hypertonus of the region.

The researchers at the University of Maryland, Baltimore, state:

In reviewing the literature, the subject of functional relations between voluntary muscles and dural membranes has been addressed by Becker (1983) who suggests that the voluntary muscles might act upon the dural membranes via fascial continuity, changing the tension placed upon them, thus possibly influencing cerebro spinal fluid pressure. Our observation, that simulated contraction of the RCPM muscle flexed the posterior atlanto-occipital membrane–spinal dura complex and produced CSF movement, supports Becker's hypothesis.

They note that:

• During head extension and anterior translation the spinal dura is subject to folding, with the greatest amount occurring in the area of the atlanto-occipital joint (Cailliet 1991).
• A possible function of RCPM may be to resist dural folding, thus assisting in the maintenance of the normal circulation of the CSF.

• Trauma resulting in atrophic changes to the RCPM muscle could possibly interfere with this suggested mechanism (Hallgren et al 1993).
• The observed transmission of tension created in the spinal dura to the cranial dura of the posterior cranial fossa is consistent with the described discontinuity between the spinal and intracranial parts of the dura mater (Penfield & McNaughton 1940).
• Not only has the dura which lines the posterior cranial fossa been shown to be innervated by nerves that subserve pain (Kimmel 1961), but also it has been confirmed that pressure applied to the dura of the posterior cranial fossa in neurosurgical patients induces pain in the region of the posterior base of the skull (Northfield 1938).

The researchers postulated that the dura of the posterior cranial fossa can be irritated and become symptomatic if stressed to an unaccustomed extent by the RCPM muscle acting on the dura mater.

Further research

Additional research at the department of osteopathic medicine at Michigan State University, College of Osteopathic Medicine, utilising magnetic resonance imaging of both RCP major and minor, which was performed on six patients with chronic head and neck pain as well as on five control subjects, produced remarkable findings (Hallgren et al 1994).

• In the subjects with chronic pain the muscles were shown to have developed fatty degeneration in which muscle tissue had been replaced by fatty deposits.
• This was not seen in the control (normal) subjects.

The researchers suggest that the reduction in proprioceptive afferent activity in these damaged muscles may cause increased facilitation of neural activity which is perceived as pain.

Professor Philip Greenman, a major researcher in both the studies reported above, has found, utilising EMG testing, that rectus capitis posterior minor is not an extensor of the head, as is suggested by most physiology texts. When tested, the muscle does *not* fire during extension, but rather does so when the head is translated forwards, in a 'chin poking' manner, as would be the case, for example, if bilateral sternocleido-mastoid shortening existed, something which would commonly result from chronic upper-chest breathing which automatically involves the accessory breathing muscles such as sternoclei-domastoid (personal communication to the author, October 1997).

Greenman further suggests (personal communication to the author, October 1997) that denervation of the muscle may lead to the reported fatty degeneration, following severe trauma such as whiplash. He also states that in some instances he has observed that the muscle hypertrophies and is then involved in severe headache problems. It is also hypothesised that joint dysfunction in this region may contribute towards fatty degeneration of rectus capitis posterior minor, much as has been noted in the multifidus muscles of the low back when spinal joint damage or major restriction has occurred in that region.

C. Chan Gunn (Gunn 1983) observes that pain management is simplified when it is realised that, following trauma, three sequential stages may be noted:

1. Immediate: a perception of noxious input which is transient unless tissue damage is sufficient to cause the next stage
2. Inflammation: during which time algesic substances are released which sensitise higher threshold receptors
3. Chronic phase: where there may be persistent nociception (or prolonged inflammation). Hyperalgesia may exist where normally non-noxious stimuli are rendered excessive due to hypersensitive receptors.

This sequence seems to prevail in relation to rectus capitis posterior minor following whiplash, and treatment objectives should include attempts at desensitisation of the hyperalgesic structures.

A close similarity can be observed between facilitation concepts (as outlined in Ch. 1) and the sequence described by Gunn.

A number of possible links can be suggested between these musculoskeletal observations and some of the major symptoms of FMS:
• The link between cranial venous circulation as well as CSF circulation and a traumatically induced dysfunctional pattern in the upper cervical region has been suggested. This could relate to a number of the symptoms observed in FMS – most notably pain perception – as well as those hypotheses which are based upon brain/neurological dysfunction as a central aetiological feature.
• It seems probable that excessive demands on the stabilising function of the suboccipital extensor muscles and RCPM in particular (posturally induced 'chin poking' for example, aggravated by upper-chest breathing) could induce hypertrophy of RCPM and consequent headache symptoms – as noted by Greenman – without trauma.
• The findings in the whiplash study described above, and the MRI observations of Greenman and his colleagues regarding fatty degeneration of rectus capitis posterior minor following whiplash trauma, suggest that specific injury to this vulnerable cervical region offers a possible explanation for the onset of FMS in some patients.

VIRAL INFECTION

The possibility of viral infection being associated with the onset of FMS has been noted in several of the major associated conditions discussed in this and previous chapters: as a trigger impacting someone genetically predisposed to FMS, as a factor in promoting neurohumoral dysfunction, as a feature creating excessive immune response demands, as a precursor to widespread allergy and central neurological dysfunction, etc.

Goldenberg describes two possible pathways via which infection could be associated with FMS:

1. An infectious agent directly invades tissues or activates immune mediators (cytokines) and produces the symptoms of pain and neural dysfunction.

2. An infection triggers an adaptive response which leads to the symptom picture. In this model infection is just one possible trigger resulting in avoidance ('sickness') behaviour involving altered sleep patterns, emotional changes, increased muscle tension and reduced activity.

Goldenberg says that the first model is unsupported by any evidence of the presence of infectious agents in either peripheral tissues of the nervous system. The provocation of cytokine production (such as Interleukin-2) does, however, result in symptoms similar to FMS and CFS (Goldenberg 1994b).

Both models are worthy of further research, although Goldenberg is clear that, 'It is unlikely that a single infection is the cause of most cases of fibromyalgia. Studies of the complicated integration of mind, body and patient's psychological milieu are more likely to provide meaningful answers to all potential factors, including infections, that may be associated with fibromyalgia.'

British physician Anne Macintyre (Macintyre 1993), herself afflicted with myalgic encephalomyelitis, writes:

The incidence of new cases [of ME] peaks in late summer and autumn, coincident with the peak time of year for enteroviral infections. It is likely that enteroviral infection accounts for the majority of ME illness in this country [UK], even if other factors (stress, trauma) are present. There may also be a genetic predisposition, evidenced by the higher than expected number of parents with ME whose children also develop it some years after the parents. (Dowsett 1990)

Some of the major influences of viral infection suggested by various researchers to be linked to CFS/FMS are summarised below:

• HHV6, a lymphotrophic herpesvirus has been found to be more prevalent in FMS/CFS patients than in controls, with elevated antibody titers being observed (Buchwald et al 1992).

• British research implicates enteroviruses which have been found to be more prevalent in stools as well as muscle biopsies, with blood antigens also higher (Gow et al 1991, Behan 1993).
• Buskila (1990) and Simms (1992) have both reported on the presence of FMS symptoms in patients infected by HIV.
• Chronic coxsackie B virus infection has been shown to mimic FMS symptoms (Nash 1989).
• Parvovirus has likewise been associated with FMS (Leventhal 1991).

CONCLUSION

This chapter's review of some of the main symptoms of FMS and where they are thought to fit (by various experts, without any great consensus as yet) into the spectrum of cause and effect, should assist the review of hypotheses for the development of FMS (outlined in Ch. 4). A common feature of several hypotheses seems to involve abnormal response to stimuli:

• Of pain receptors following sensitisation or facilitation
• Of neurohumoral responses due to congenital or acquired abnormalities
• Of homeostasis which in some instances evolves to allostasis due to congenital or early stress influences
• Of central (limbic) processing of information.

To help FMS patients might involve: reducing allergic activity, improving breathing function, enhancing and normalising bowel function, promoting better sleep patterns, modifying the abnormal biochemistry, assisting circulation to and drainage from the brain, reducing dysfunctional muscular influences, especially in the upper cervical region. All or any of these measures should reduce the stressor load as well as improving aspects of homeostatic and immune function.

REFERENCES

Adams K 1977 Sleep is for tissue restoration. Journal of the Royal College of Physicians 11: 376–388

Affleck G 1996 Sequential daily relations of sleep, pain intensity and attention to pain among women with FMS. Pain 68(2–3): 363–368

Alexander J 1967 Thrush bowel infection. Current Med. Drugs 8: 3–11

Alexander J 1975 Allergy in the GI tract. Lancet ii: 1264

Alvarez L et al 1996 FMS overnight falls in arterial oxygen saturation. American Journal of Medicine 101(1): 54–60

Bakheit A 1992 Possible upregulation of 5HT receptors in patients with post viral fatigue syndrome. British Medical Journal 304: 1010–1012

Ball A 1997 Antibiotic toxicity. In: O'Grady F, Lambert H, Finch R, Greenwood D (eds) Antibiotic and chemotherapy, 7th edn. Churchill Livingstone, New York, Ch. 7

Barelli P 1994 Nasopulmonary physiology. In: Timmons B (ed) Behavioural and psychological approaches to breathing disorders. Plenum Press, New York

Barlow W 1959 Anxiety and muscle tension pain. British Journal of Clinical Practice 13(5)

Barrie S 1995 Heidelberg pH capsule gastric analysis. In: Pizzorno J, Murray M (eds) Textbook of natural medicine. Bastyr University Publications, Seattle

Bass C, Gardner W 1985 Respiratory and psychiatric abnormalities in chronic symptomatic hyperventilation. British Medical Journal (11 May): 1387–1390

Becker R 1983 In: Upledger J, Vredevoogd J (eds) CranioSacral therapy. Eastman Press, Seattle

Behan P 1993 Enteroviruses and post viral fatigue syndrome CFS. In: Bock G, Whelan J (eds) CIBA Foundation Symposium 173. Wiley, Chichester

Benington J, Heller H 1995 Restoration of brain energy metabolism as the function of sleep. Progress in Neurobiology 45(4): 347–360

Bennett R 1997 Hypothalamic-pituitary-insulin-like growth factor-1 axis dysfunction in patients with FMS. Journal of Rheumatology 24(7): 1384–1389

Bland J 1995 Medical food-supplemented detoxification program in management of chronic health problems. Alternative Therapies 1: 62–71

Block S 1993 Fibromyalgia and the rheumatisms. Controversies in Clinical Rheumatology 19(1): 61–78

Bradley L, Alarcon G, Triana M et al 1994 Health care seeking behaviour in FMS. Journal of Musculoskeletal Pain 2(3): 79–87

Brostoff J 1992 Complete guide to food allergy. Bloomsbury, London

Buchwald D 1994 Comparison of patients with CFS, FMS and MCS. Archives of Internal Medicine 154(18): 2049–2053

Buchwald D et al 1992 A chronic illness characterized by fatigue, neurologic and immunologic disorders and active human herpesvirus type 6 infection. Annals of Internal Medicine 116: 103–113

Buskila D 1990 FMS in HIV infection. Journal of Rheumatology 17: 1202–1206

Buskila D, Neumann L et al 1997 Increased rates of fibromyalgia following cervical spine injury. Arthritis and Rheumatism 40(3): 446–452

Cailliet R 1991 Neck and arm pain, 3rd edn. F. A. Davis, Philadelphia

Cappo B, Holmes D 1984 Utility of prolonged respiratory exhalation for reducing physiological and psychological arousal in non-threatening and threatening situations. Journal of Psychosomatic Research 28(4): 265–273

Chadwick R 1992 Role of gastrointestinal mucosa and microflora in bioactivation of dietary and environmental mutagens or carcinogens. Drug Metabolism Reviews 24: 425–492

Cho C 1991 Zinc: absorption and the role in gastrointestinal metabolism and disorders. Digestive Diseases 9: 49–60

Clark S, Campbell S, Forehand M et al 1985 Clinical characteristics of fibrositis. A blinded controlled study using standard psychological tests. Arthritis and Rheumatism 28: 132–137

Clauw D 1995 Fibromyalgia: more than just a musculoskeletal disease. American Family Physician (September 1)

Cleveland C 1992 Chronic rhinitis and under recognised association with fibromyalgia. Allergy Proceedings 13(5): 263–267

Cohen S 1991 Psychological stress and susceptibility to the common cold. New England Journal of Medicine 325: 606–612

Crofford L 1994 Neuroendocrine aspects of FMS. Journal of Musculoskeletal Pain 2(3): 125–133

Dailey P 1990 Psychological stress and FMS. Journal of Rheumatology 17: 1380–1385

Davies S, Stewart A 1988 Nutritional medicine. Pan, London

Deamer W 1971 Pediatric allergy: impressions gained over a 37 year period. Pediatrics 48: 930–938

Demitrack M 1991 Impaired activation of hypothalamic–pituitary–adrenal axis in patients with CFS. Journal of Clinical Endocrinology and Metabolism 73: 1224–1234

Dickey L 1976 Clinical ecology. Charles C Thomas, Springfield, Illinois

Dowsett E 1990 M.E. – a persistent viral infection? Postgraduate Medical Journal 66: 526–530

Ekbom K 1960 Restless legs syndrome. Neurology 10: 868

Feingold B 1973 Hyperactivity in children. Presentation at the Kaiser Foundation Hospital, Sacramento, California, 3 Dec 1973

Fibromyalgia Network Newsletters 1990–94. October 1990–January 1992, (Compendium No. 2), January 1993, May 1993 (Compendium), January 1994, July 1994

Fibromyalgia Network 1993 Newsletter (October): 12

Gardier A et al 1992 Effects of a primary immune response to T-cell dependent antigen on serotonin metabolism in the frontal cortex. Brain Research 645: 150–156

Garland W 1994 Somatic changes in hyperventilating subject – an osteopathic perspective. Presentation to Paris Symposium, 1994

Goldenberg D 1994a Psychiatric illness and FMS. Journal of Musculoskeletal Pain 2(3): 41–49

Goldenberg D 1994b Fibromyalgia and chronic fatigue syndrome. Journal of Musculoskeletal Pain 2(3): 51–55

Goldstein J 1993 Limbic aetiology of some CFS symptoms. Chronic fatigue syndromes. Haworth Medical Press, New York

Goldstein J 1996 Betrayal by the brain. Haworth Medical Press, Binghamptom, New York

Gow J 1991 Enteroviral sequences detected in muscles of patients with postviral fatigue syndrome. British Medical Journal 302: 692–696

Griep E 1994 Pituitary release of growth hormone and prolactin in primary FMS. Journal of Rheumatology 21(11): 2125–2130

Griep E, Boersma J, de Kloet E et al 1993 Altered reactivity of hypothalamic-pituitary adrenal axis in primary FMS. Journal of Rheumatology 20: 469–474

Grossman P, De Swart J 1984 Diagnosis of hyperventilation syndrome on the basis of reported complaints. Journal of Psychosomatic Research 28(2): 97–104

Grossman P et al 1985 Controlled study of breathing therapy for treatment of hyperventilation syndrome. Journal of Psychosomatic Research 29(1): 49–58

Gruber A 1996 Management of treatment-resistant depression in disorders on the interface of psychiatry and medicine. Psychiatry Clinics of North America 19(2): 351–369

Gudewill S 1992 Nocturnal plasma levels of cytokines in healthy males. Archives of Psychiatry and Clinical Neuroscience 242: 53–56

Gunn C C 1983 Three phases of pain. Acupuncture and Electro Therapeutics 8(3/4): 334

Hack G, Koritzer R, Robinson W, Hallgren R, Greenman P 1995 Anatomic relationship between rectus capitis posterior minor muscle and the dura mater. Spine 20 (23): 2484-2486 December

Hallgren R, Greenman P, Rechtien J 1993 MRI of normal and atrophic muscles of the upper cervical spine. Journal of Clinical Engineering 18(5): 433–439

Hallgren R, Greenman P, Rechtien J 1994 Atrophy of suboccital muscles in patients with chronic pain. Journal of the American Osteopathic Association 94(12): 1032–1038

Haseqawa H 1988 2,4-diamino-6-hydroxy-pyrimidine (DAHP) induces intestinal disorder in mice. Biological Chemistry 369: 532

Hawley D 1988 Pain, functional disability and psychological states – a 12 month study of severity in fibromyalgia. Journal of Rheumatology 1: 1551–1556

Henry J 1995 BMA's new guide to medicines and drugs. Dorling Kindersley, London

Holti G 1966 Candida allergy. In: Winner H, Hurley R (eds) Symposium on Candida infections. Churchill Livingstone, Edinburgh

Hrycaj P 1993 Platelet 3H-imipramine uptake receptor density and serum serotonin in patients with FM syndrome. Journal of Rheumatology 20: 1986–1987

Hudson J 1996 The relationship between FMS and major depressive disorder. Rheumatic Diseases Clinics of North America 22(2): 285–303

Jacobsen S 1989 Inter-relations between clinical parameters and muscle function in patients with primary FMS. Clinical and Experimental Rheumatology 7: 493–498

Jacobsen S 1991 Oral S-adenosylmethionine in primary FMS. Scandinavian Journal of Rheumatology 20(4): 294–302

Jones A et al 1982 Food intolerance – a major factor in pathogenesis of IBS. Lancet ii: 1115–1117

Kerr W et al 1937 Annals of Internal Medicine 11: 962

Kimmel D 1961 Innervation of the spinal dura mater and the dura mater of the posterior cranial fossa. Neurology 10: 800–809

King J 1988 Hyperventilation – a therapist's point of view. Journal of the Royal Society of Medicine 81(September): 532–536

Landay A 1991 Chronic fatigue syndrome – clinical condition associated with immune activation. Lancet 338: 707–711

Langeluddecke P 1990 Psychological factors in dyspepsia of unknown cause: a comparison with peptic ulcer. Journal of Psychosomatic Research 34(2): 215–222

Leventhal L 1991 FMS and parvovirus infection. Arthritis and Rheumatism 34: 1319–1324

Liehr H 1979 Progress in liver disease – endotoxins in liver disease. Grune and Straten, New York

Lowe J 1997 Effectiveness and safety of T3 therapy in FMS. Clinical Bulletin of Myofascial Therapy 2(2/3): 31–57

Lue F 1994 Sleep and fibromyalgia. Journal of Musculoskeletal Pain 2(3): 89–100

Lum L 1981 Hyperventilation an anxiety state. Journal of the Royal Society of Medicine 74(January): 1–4

Lum L 1984 Editorial. Hyperventilation and anxiety state. Journal of the Royal Society of Medicine 77 (January): 1–4

Lum L 1994 Hyperventilation syndromes. In: Timmons B Behavioural and psychological approaches to breathing disorders. Plenum Press, New York

McEwan B 1994 The plasticity of the hippocampus is the reason for its vulnerability. Seminars in Neuroscience 6: 197–204

Macintyre A 1993 What causes ME? The immune dysfunction hypothesis. Journal of Action for ME 14(Autumn): 24–25

Malmberg A 1992 Hyperalgesia mediated by spinal glutamate or substance P receptor blocked by spinal cyclooxygenase inhibition. Science 257: 1276–1279

Malmo R 1949 Journal of Psychosomatic Medicine 2 (9)

Maxton D et al 1991 More accurate diagnosis of IBS by use of non-colonic symptomatology. Gut 32: 784–786

Mayer E 1993 Basic and clinical aspects of chronic abdominal pain. Elsevier, New York

Moldofsky H 1982 Rheumatic pain modulation syndrome. Advances in Neurology 33: 51–57

Moldofsky H 1993 Fibromyalgia, sleep disorder and chronic fatigue syndrome. CIBA Symposium 173, 1993, pp 262–279

Nash P 1989 Chronic coxsackie B infection mimicking primary FMS. Journal of Rheumatology 116: 1506–1508

Ninkaya R 1986 Role of bifidobacteria in enteric infection. Bifidobacteria Microflora 5: 51–55

Northfield D 1938 Some observations of headache. Brain 61: 133–162

Nyhlin H 1993 Non-alimentary aspects of IBS. Journal of Psychosomatic Research 37(2): 155–162

Oldstone M 1989 Viral alteration of cell function. Scientific American 261: 34–40

Paganelli R 1991 Intestinal permeability in patients with chronic urticaria–angiodema with and without arthralgia. Annals of Allergy 66: 181–184

Penfield W, McNaughton F 1940 Dural headache and the innervation of the dura mater. Archives of Neurology and Psychiatry 44: 43–75

Perkin G et al 1986 Neurological manifestations of hyperventilation syndrome. Journal of the Royal Society of Medicine 79(August): 448–450

Phaosawasdi K 1986 Primary and secondary Candida oesophagitis. Illinois Medical Journal 169: 361–365

Pizzorno J 1996 Total wellness. Prima Publishing, Rocklin, California

Rae W 1992 Chemical sensitivity, vol. 1. CRC Press, Boca Raton, FL

Randolph T 1976 Stimulatory and withdrawal and the alternations of allergic manifestations. In: Dickey L (ed) Clinical ecology. Charles C Thomas, Springfield, Illinois, Ch. 12

Reid G et al 1997 Primary juvenile FMS: psychological adjustment, family functioning, coping and functional disability. Arthritis and Rheumatism 40(4): 752–760

Rice R 1950 American Journal of Medicine 8: 691

Rowe A H 1930 Allergic toxemia and migraine due to food allergy. California West Medical Journal 33: 785

Rowe A 1972 Food allergy – its manifestation and control. C. W. Thomas, Springfield, Illinois

Russell I 1994a Biochemical abnormalities in FMS. Journal of Musculoskeletal Pain 2(3): 101–105

Russell I 1994b Pathogenesis of FMS – neurohumoral hypothesis. Journal of Musculoskeletal Pain 2(1): 73–86

Russell I, Michalek J, Vipraio G et al 1992 Platelet 3H-imipramine uptake receptor density and serum serotonin levels in patients with FMS. Journal of Rheumatology 19: 104–109

Russell I, Vipraio G, Lopez Y et al 1993 Serum serotonin in FMS and rheumatoid arthritis and healthy normal controls. Arthritis and Rheumatism 36(9): S223

Russell J 1965 Eosinophilic infiltration of stomach and duodenum complicated by perforation. Postgraduate Medical Journal 41: 30

Sainsbury J 1954 Journal of Neurology, Neurosurgery and Psychiatry 17 (3)

Sapolsky R 1990 Hippocampal damage associated with prolonged glucocorticoid exposure in primates. Journal of Neuroscience 10: 2897–2902

Sapolsky R 1994 Individual differences and the stress response. Seminars in Neuroscience 6: 261–269

Shaver J 1997 Sleep, psychological distress and stress arousal in women with FMS. Res Nursing Health 20(3): 247–257

Simon G 1981 Intestinal flora in health and disease. In: Johnson L (ed.) Physiology of the gastrointestinal tract. Raven Press, New York, pp 1361–1380

Simms R 1992 FMS in patients infected with HIV. American Journal of Medicine 92: 368–374

Sivri A 1996 IBS and FMS. Clinical Rheumatology 15(3): 283–286

Timmons B (ed) 1994 Behavioural and psychological approaches to breathing disorders. Plenum Press, New York

Travell J, Simons D 1983 Myofascial pain and dysfunction, vol. 1. Williams and Wilkins, Baltimore, pp 364–365

Troncone R 1994 Increased intestinal sugar permeability after challenge in children with cow's milk allergy or intolerance. Allergy 49: 142–146

Tuncer T 1997 Primary fibromyalgia and allergy. Clinical Rheumatology 16(1): 9–12

Uveges J 1990 Psychological symptoms in primary FMS. Arthritis and Rheumatism 33: 1279–1283

van Dixhoorn J, Duivenvoorden H 1985 Efficacy of Nijmegen questionnaire in recognition of hyperventilation syndrome. Journal of Psychosomatic Research 29(2): 199–206

Warshaw A 1974 Protein uptake in the intestines – evidence of intact macromolecules. Gastroenterology 66: 987–992

Wolff J 1948 Headache and other head pain. Oxford University Press, Oxford

Yellin J 1997 Why is substance P high in fibromyalgia? Clinical Bulletin of Myofascial Therapy 2(2/3): 23–30

Yunus M 1989 Fibromyalgia and other functional syndromes. Journal of Rheumatology 16(S19): 69

Yunus M 1994a Psychological factors in FMS. Journal of Musculoskeletal Pain 2(1): 87–91

Yunus M 1994b FMS – clinical features and spectrum. Journal of Musculoskeletal Pain 2(3): 5–21

Yunus M, Ahles T, Aldag J, Masi A 1991 Relationship of clinical features with psychological status in primary FMS. Arthritis and Rheumatism 34: 15–21

Yunus W, Dailey J, Aldag J et al 1992 Plasma tryptophan and other amino acids in primary FMS. Journal of Rheumatology 19: 90–94

4

The causes of fibromyalgia: various hypotheses explored

Having examined some of the proposed and known influences of associated conditions and dysfunctional patterns – sleep, irritable bowel, allergy, hyperventilation tendency, etc. – on fibromyalgia, an awareness will have emerged of differing emphases ascribed to the roles of one or other of these associated conditions by leading researchers, depending to some extent upon their particular beliefs and interests.

Some conditions are seen to have the potential to have a (partially?) causal link, while others are merely expressions of dysfunction deriving from a common (or a different) set of aetiological factors impacting the individual, possibly associated with congenital predispositions.

There are a number of hypotheses which try to explain the evolution of FMS, and some of the leading ones are summarised in this chapter. Space does not permit a full elaboration on the minutiae of these concepts; however, it is hoped that the condensed form in which they are presented will allow the reader to form a view of FMS which makes sense, has scientific and clinical validity, and which above all helps in formulating strategies for therapeutic action.

The evidence seems to suggest that there may well be more than one form of FMS, with a genetic predisposition possibly being a basic requirement, followed by either a single major traumatic experience (physical or psychological), or an infection (viral as a rule), or the compound effect of multiple minor stresses.

We already see that FMS is sometimes described as primary (where no obvious predisposing trigger can be identified), while at others it is described as secondary FMS (where a trigger is a well established feature). The pathway which follows one or other of these possible aetiological patterns might then be the same, involving eventually a large degree of central dysfunction as proposed by Goldstein (see Neurosomatic hypothesis and Fig. 4.5, below), along with all that flows from this.

The following summaries are listed in alphabetical order rather than any hierarchy of importance or validity. In a sense they all (or almost all) have credibility and represent examples of the same phenomena being scrutinised and interpreted from differing perspectives.

CHRONOBIOLOGICAL HYPOTHESIS
(Moldofsky 1993)

Harvey Moldofsky MD, professor of psychiatry and medicine at the University of Toronto, has proposed a pathway to FMS which is the result of altered biological rhythms, including diurnal physiological functions, seasonal environmental influences and psychosocial and behavioural influences.

• He describes a 'non-restorative sleep syndrome' which is characterised by pain, fatigue and cognitive difficulties (often following a febrile illness) as well as irritable bowel problems.
• This non-restorative sleep syndrome is seen to emerge from central nervous system disturbances, associated with altered metabolic functions including those of serotonin, substance P, interleukin-1, growth hormone and cortisol.
• Moldofsky reports that environmental disturbances affect brain functions as well as somatic symptoms.
• Further, he states that altered sleep physiology along with the somatic and psychological symptoms may result from acute traumatic incidents, such as those involved in an accident.
• Moldofsky has traced the patterns of wellbeing (mood, capacity for intellectual function, performance skills, wakefulness and optimal behavioural functioning) experienced over a 24-hour period by normal healthy individuals and compared this with the common experience of patients with FMS and CFS.

• This research indicates that the norm is to wake refreshed and for a slow decline to occur throughout the day, with a minor improvement early evening. FMS patients, on the other hand, wake feeling 'awful' and slowly improve to midday (optimal function is between 10.00 a.m. and 2.00 p.m.) and then decline steeply until early evening when they plateau with feelings of greater exhaustion and pain.
• Increased sensitivity to dolorimeter pressure was observed in normal individuals when slow wave sleep was disturbed (by noise). Normal pain thresholds were restored by a night of undisturbed sleep.
• Moldofsky relates the altered pain sensitivity directly to intrusive alpha waves into the early hours of sleep. He reports that slow wave sleep has been shown to depend upon the presence of appropriate neurotransmitters and immunologically active peptides (including serotonin, interleukin-1 and factor S).
• He highlights the fact that with sleep disturbance growth hormone production decreases and indicates that while average 24-hour cortisol levels are unaffected by sleep deprivation, a change in pattern occurs so that instead of a late nocturnal increase (in cortisol) being noted, this occurs earlier when sleep is disturbed.
• Further research has indicated that seasonal variations, involving both climate and light availability, affect symptom severity more dramatically in patients with FMS than normal controls or individuals with rheumatoid arthritis. FMS symptoms were reported as being more intense between November and March (fall/winter); they improved between May and August (spring/summer).
• Moldofsky has evaluated the effects on sleep patterns of industrial or vehicle injuries, and subsequent development of FMS symptoms. In a longitudinal prospective study involving 150 individuals who had experienced industrial injury involving a similar degree of soft tissue strain or damage, he has shown that, over a period of 21 months, the symptoms of pain and fatigue in those who remain off work correlated directly with the degree of disturbance in their sleep patterns. He states: 'Study of the evolution

of pain symptoms and the ability to return to work are related to psychological distress, sleep disturbance and fatigue. The temporal patterns are consistent with the chronobiological theoretical model for understanding the evolution of persistent pain, fatigue and non-restorative sleep.'

• He suggests that a chronobiological model allows consideration of the dynamics of CNS mechanisms as they are involved in FMS. The model takes into account variations associated with biological rhythmic activity so that the involvement of behaviour, brain function and somatic factors can be evaluated over time.

GENETIC HYPOTHESIS

Goldstein's hypothesis, and those of many others, depends for cogency upon a genetic predisposition. Is there any evidence for this in FMS?

• There are, in some studies, clear indications of familial tendencies to the development of FMS (Pellegrino 1989).
• Israeli research by Dr Dan Buskila has concluded that FMS has a major genetic component (Fibromyalgia Network 1996a).
• FMS has been associated in some studies with joint laxity, and a Danish study noted that 43% of 42 FMS patients had generalised joint hypermobility, an apparently genetically acquired trait which is more common in females (Fibromyalgia Network 1996b).
• Mitral valve prolapse has been reported in 75% of patients with FMS, a far higher rate than that noted in the general population (Fibromyalgia Network 1995).
• Particular patterns of human leukocyte class II antigens were identified when the blood of over 100 patients with chronic fatigue syndrome was analysed and compared with healthy controls (Keller & Klimas 1994).
• When HLA typing was carried out by Mohammad Yunus, involving 4 multi-case families (in which at least two members of the same family have FMS), statistically significant genetic linkage was established. Such findings are thought to offer strong support for a genetic hypothesis in the aetiology of FMS (Fibromyalgia Network 1996b).

• Researchers at the University of Miami, led by immunologist Dr Nancy Klimas, have evolved a model for the evolution and perpetuation of CFS and FMS. This involves an initial predisposition followed by an 'etiological event'; this might involve a single trauma, or a reactivation of dormant viral activity, or a one-off infection. One or other such event seems to lead to a major ongoing immunological response which is perpetuated either by further activation of infectious agents (viral as a rule) or by a dysfunctional hypothalamic–pituitary–adrenal axis related to stress influence (Klimas 1995).

Comment

A genetic predisposition to FMS seems likely, and since at this time little can be done about this, therapeutic focus on the events which surround the triggering and perpetuation of the condition seems a reasonable clinical approach (see Fig. 4.1).

Klimas suggests that:

Treatment is basically symptomatic. Our concept is to treat anything we can. If someone has allergy we treat allergy. If someone has sleep disturbance we treat it. If we can take 20% of the miseries away by giving someone restorative sleep and we can eliminate 20% of the symptoms by treating their allergy overlay, then they are 40% better and that's significant.

These thoughts support the suggestions outlined in Figs.1.2 and 2.2 – i.e. 'lessen the load'.

INTEGRATED HYPOTHESIS

Robert Bennett, professor of medicine at Oregon Health Sciences University, Portland, Oregon, is one of the leading researchers into fibromyalgia. He observes that there are currently two broad ideas regarding the pathogenesis of FMS – those which hold to a central and those which support a peripheral aetiology (Bennett 1993).

His hypothesis attempts to blend these. He points out that, 'No global muscle defect has ever been demonstrated [in FMS]. On the other hand several studies suggest focal muscle changes in terms of: reduced high energy phosphates, scattered red-ragged fibres, focal changes in oxygen tension and repetitive '"contraction bands".'

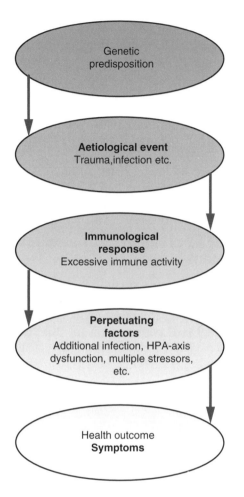

Figure 4.1 Genetic predisposition hypothesis.

These altered states of muscle may derive, he believes, from muscle microtrauma (MMT) following unaccustomed exercise. MMT results in changes which are well understood, particularly in relation to the changes seen in myofascial pain syndrome where, as myofascial trigger points evolve, taut bands appear due to a combination of Ca++ ion influx following tissue damage, contraction of the involved sarcolemmal units (so forming the bands) and an inability due to energy (ATP) deficit of the tissues to pump excess Ca++ out of the cells. Muscle spindle resetting is then thought to lead to stiffness sensations. Many of the features described in this model are noted to be prevalent in FMS patients (Jacobsen 1991).

Bennett suggests that this form of muscle response is genetically predetermined. 'It is envisaged that there is a genetic polymorphism in susceptibility to MMT and that fibromyalgia patients are at one extreme end of the curve. Most susceptible people will not develop FMS unless they also develop alpha–delta sleep anomaly ... an acquired central defect which may provide a "double-hit" in the form of impaired growth hormone secretion.' (See Fig. 4.2.)

Since growth hormone (released largely during stage 4 sleep) is essential for normal muscle repair and homeostasis, a combination of a deficit in this regard plus repetitive tendency to tissue damage may be the scenario for the onset of chronic muscular pain.

Aspects of these changes are discussed in greater detail in Chapter 6 which evaluates the relationship between myofascial pain and FMS.

IMMUNE DYSFUNCTION HYPOTHESIS (Oldstone 1989, Landay 1991, Bakheit 1992, Macintyre 1993)

As outlined in Chapter 3 (see Fig. 3.2), a general hypothesis exists in which 'something' or a variety of 'somethings' provoke the immune system into excessive responses, resulting in increased cytokine production. The nature of the potential triggers, and the variety of the possible subsequent negative results of overstimulated immune function are summarised in Figure 4.3 (see also Fig. 3.2).

NOCICEPTIVE HYPOTHESIS

If pain is the final major symptom of FMS, it may also be the cause. Wolfe (1994) in the USA and Croft (1992) in the UK, among many researchers, have contributed a wealth of information regarding FMS and its characteristics.

Croft observes a sequence of:

- No pain
- Increased tenderness
- Transient pain
- Chronic regional pain
- Chronic widespread pain
- Psychological distress
- FMS symptoms.

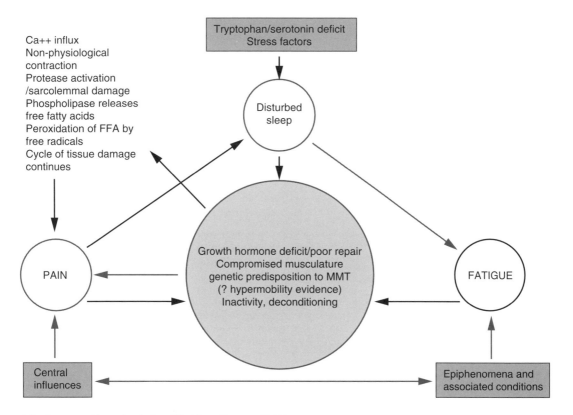

Ca++ influx
Non-physiological
contraction
Protease activation
/sarcolemmal damage
Phospholipase releases
free fatty acids
Peroxidation of FFA by
free radicals
Cycle of tissue damage
continues

Figure 4.2   Integrated hypothesis (modified from Bennett 1993).

Wolfe proposes that:

- Chronic pain stimuli lead to lowered pain threshold
- Pain amplification (lowered threshold) then progresses, influenced by genetic (especially childhood onset FMS), disease (mainly viral), sleep disturbance and psychological factors (psychosocial stress and the way with which it is coped)
- FMS evolves (see Fig. 4.4).

Wolfe suggests that there may be many fibromyalgias: 'Does the distressed older patient with chronic back and neck pain and FMS have the same disease process as the middle aged person developing the syndrome after an apparent viral illness? Are they the same as those with pain from childhood or with major psychological abnormalities? Do these subsets have the same

neurohumoral and biochemical changes that are said to be characteristic of FMS generally?'

NEUROSOMATIC HYPOTHESIS
(Goldstein 1996)

Goldstein has proposed a neurosomatic hypothesis to explain a wide range of disorders, including FMS (Fig. 4.5).

He explains a possible sequence:

- A variable genetic susceptibility. If this is strong, neurosomatic symptoms will develop early in life. If it is a weak 'predisposition', other factors are required to cause expression of the traits.
- If hypervigilance develops during the period between birth and puberty, this could lead to a tendency for misinterpretation of sensory input, associated with increased substance P levels

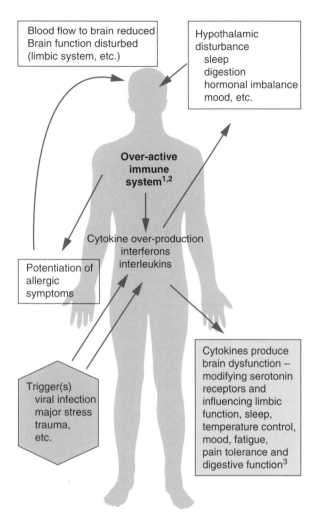

Blood flow to brain reduced
Brain function disturbed
(limbic system, etc.)

Hypothalamic
disturbance
  sleep
  digestion
  hormonal imbalance
  mood, etc.

**Over-active
immune
system[1,2]**

Cytokine over-production
interferons
interleukins

Potentiation of
allergic
symptoms

Trigger(s)
viral infection
major stress
trauma,
etc.

Cytokines produce
brain dysfunction –
modifying serotonin
receptors and
influencing limbic
function, sleep,
temperature control,
mood, fatigue,
pain tolerance and
digestive function[3]

Figure 4.3 Overactive immune system ([1]Oldstone 1989, [2]Landay 1991, [3]Bakheit 1992)

as well as transiently elevated cortisol, together with a 'downregulation' of the hypothalamic–pituitary–adrenal axis. Central norepinephrine levels could also be lowered adding to dysautonomia.

• Persistent infections in neurons and glia may occur (viral encephalopathy), possibly without an immune response. This would be 'largely genetically predetermined' or could be influenced by 'situational perturbations of an immune response'. Persistent CNS viral infections are seen to be capable of altering neurotransmitter production as well as modifying cellular behaviour.

• Due to reduction in 'neural plasticity' increased susceptibility to environmental stressors could develop. If these combined genetic and developmental influences (outlined above) interact, the flexibility of the brain to modify neural networks to cope with internal and external demands could be impaired.

Goldstein offers an example relating to the memory problems so common in patients with FMS (or as Goldstein calls them 'neurosomatic patients').

In order to encode a memory, a fragile neural network must be strengthened. This process may occur by augmenting secretion of glutamate from firing presynaptic neurons by secretion of a retrograde messenger such as nitric oxide (NO) by the post-synaptic neuron. NO diffuses in a paracrine manner into firing neurons in the locality, enhancing glutamate secretion. If insufficient glutamate or NO is secreted, neural networks will not be appropriately reorganised (strengthened) and encoding will be fragile. Neurosomatic patients have an impaired neural plasticity. Deficiency in the neurobiological encoding is one example of this pervasive disorder. Thus the individual who is predisposed to develop a neurosomatic disorder may have neural network function dysregulated by overtaxing his capacity for neural plasticity.

In this model allostasis is seen to be operating instead of homeostasis (see Fig. 2.3C). It is in this way that the multiple stressors influencing such patients are seen to produce their negative effects following anything which triggers and maintains increased hypothalamic activity – whether infection or exposure to chemical, physical or emotional stress.

Goldstein suggests utilising any of a very long list of medications, applied sequentially, until the neural behaviour is normalised and the patient is asymptomatic. This was discussed further in Chapter 3 (see Box 7.3 for a summary of Goldstein's hypothesis).

RETENTION HYPOTHESIS

R. Paul St Amand MD, assistant clinical professor of medicine at Harbor UCLA, suggests that FMS is a 'retention' disease similar to gout, but with a wider range of tissue involvement (St Amand

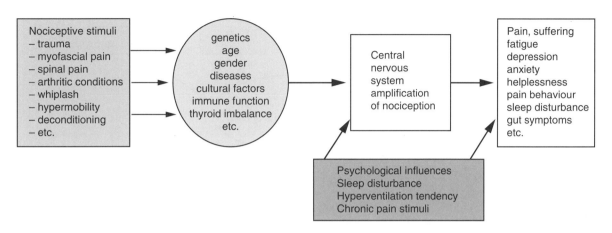

Figure 4.4   Nociceptive hypothesis (adapted from Wolfe 1994)

1997). He notes that although patients respond to uricosuric medications, urates are not involved: 'The ubiquitous symptoms and number of organs and systems affected [in FMS] point to a metabolic misadventure induced by an accumulation of an anion different from urates. This putative ion wreaks havoc throughout many systems and yet evokes no inflammatory response. It is obviously perceived as a normal tissue constituent.' The agent considered most likely to fit this description is inorganic phosphate.

The metabolic processes most affected include ATP generation, 'The most plausible theory of fibromyalgia is that of defective ATP generation from a fully operational citric acid (Krebs) cycle that produces heat instead of energy.' An as yet unidentified enzyme, receptor or pump defect is suggested as a reason for systemic accumulation of phosphate.

Treatment recommendation is for use of the expectorant guaifenesin, a weak uricosuric, along with calcium which lowers the required dosage. Results are claimed to be good, and without side-effects, despite the possibility of a period of aggravation of symptoms at the outset until dosage requirements are fine-tuned to meet individual needs.

It is suggested that inadequate production of energy, combined with 'overstimulated areas' which utilise excess energy, creates a relative hypoglycaemic effect as noted in many FMS patients ('40% of fibromyalgic females and 20% of males'). A rise in epinephrine has been noted prior to the greatest trough in blood sugar levels which requires separate (from medication) dietary control measures. This phenomenon, which is often accompanied by diverse symptoms including apparent panic attack (noted to be a 'carbohydrate intolerance'), is seemingly unresponsive to carbohydrate ingestion, due to ATP production inadequacy.

A double-blind, placebo controlled trial of use of guaifenesin was conducted at the University of Oregon in 1995, with no difference being noted between placebo and the medication group. The study has been criticised by St Amand for failing to fully implement precautions during the trial relating to the use by patients of salicylate containing substances (including cosmetics) which are said to block the effects of the medication, as well as the failure to exclude hypoglycaemics from the study (Bennett 1996).

STRESS HORMONE HYPOTHESIS

Don Goldenberg MD, professor of medicine at Tufts University School of Medicine, and endocrinologist Gail Adler MD are researching the hypothesis that FMS involves a deficiency in cortisol, whether triggered by an infection, trauma or psychosocial events. They observe that

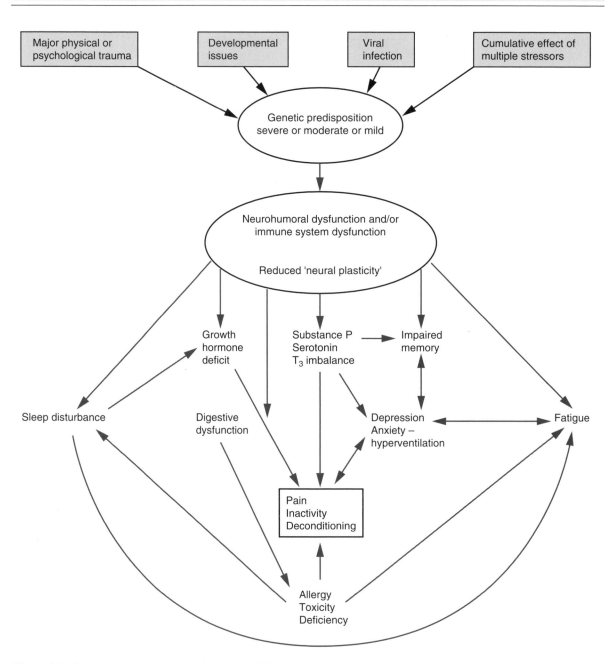

Figure 4.5 Neurosomatic hypothesis – hypothetical FMS evolution.

the symptoms of cortisol deficiency are very similar to those of FMS (see Fig. 4.6).

Since cortisol is produced in response to most stress events, including hypoglycaemic episodes, infection, inflammation, low blood pressure, exercise, and emotional stress, the need for its abundant presence is clear. Deficiency in cortisol is characterised by fatigue, weakness, muscle and joint pain, bowel symptoms, nausea, increased allergic reactions, mood disturbance.

The research into this hypothesis, which is ongoing, is evaluating:

- Whether FMS patients have inappropriately low cortisol levels in either stressed or unstressed situations over a 24-hour period and at known peak times in normal individuals
- Which sites within the hypothalamic–pituitary–adrenal axis might be associated with cortisol deficit
- The effects of induced hypoglycaemia as a stressor to provoke ACTH and cortisol release
- Pituitary production of ACTH in response to corticotropin-releasing hormone in people with and without FMS
- Adrenal response to ACTH in individuals with and without FMS.

THYROID HORMONE DYSFUNCTION HYPOTHESIS

- The symptoms of FMS closely resemble those of hypothyroidism (Wilke 1981, Sonkin 1985), including depression, mental fatigue, anxiety, poor memory, sleep disturbance, headaches, gastrointestinal dysfunction, menstrual irregularities, fatigue, hypoglycaemia, sensitivity to cold, increased susceptibility to infection, musculoskeletal symptoms and skin problems.
- A diagnosis of FMS is not an uncommon associated condition in many people with a diagnosis of hypothyroidism (Ferraccioli 1990).
- John Lowe DC, and colleagues, propose that when thyroid function is apparently normal (euthyroid) in patients with FMS, this (FMS) may be the result of a failure of normal thyroid hormone concentrations to regulate gene transcription (Lowe 1997).
- Inadequate gene transcription in a euthyroid individual might be the result of cellular resistance to thyroid hormone (Refetoff 1993).
- The clinical features of FMS might be seen to result from by-products of inadequate regulation of gene transcription, phosphodiesterase, Gi proteins and adrenoceptors (which are stated to occur in both hypothyroidism and cellular resistance to thyroid hormone).

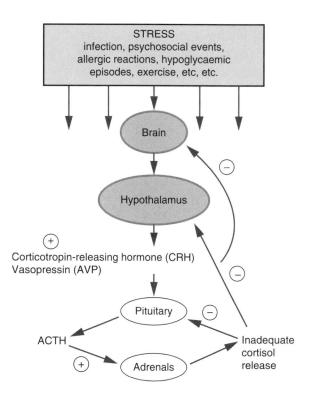

Figure 4.6   The stress hormone hypothesis (adapted from Adler (1995)).

- Various trials have been conducted which support this hypothesis involving medication with T_3 in excess of normal physiological dosages (Lowe et al 1997).
- No adverse effects were noted alongside the observed benefits of T_3 medication in five measures of FMS status in double-blind, placebo controlled studies.
- Yellin notes that, 'thyroid hormone regulates substance P in discrete nuclei of the brain, in the anterior pituitary, in the lumbar cord and the dorsal root ganglia ... inadequate regulation of gene transcription by thyroid hormone could not only account for high substance P levels but for all other objective findings and associated symptoms of FMS' (Yellin 1997).

See Chapter 10 for a full description of this hypothesis and treatment protocols.

SUMMARY

It is clear from examination of the various hypotheses outlined above that the same set of variables are being assembled in slightly different ways, with priorities varying, so that while the ingredients making up the mixture remain much the same, the flavour changes. Out of this cocktail of ingredients it is necessary to discern which elements are operating in any given case, and to work with what is possible, in terms of moderating the dysfunctional patterns at work.

In the next chapter focus is given to a comparison of CFS and FMS – similarities and differences.

REFERENCES

Adler G 1995 Fibromyalgia: is there a stress hormone imbalance? Fibromyalgia Association UK Newsletter, December 1995

Bakheit A 1992 Possible upregulation of 5HT receptors in patients with post viral fatigue syndrome. British Medical Journal 304: 1010–1012

Bennett R 1993 The origin of myopain: an integrated hypothesis of focal muscle changes and sleep disturbance in patients with FMS. Journal of Musculoskeletal Pain 1(3/4): 95–112

Bennett R 1996 Poster presentation of Oregon guaifenesin study. Academy of Rheumatology meeting, Orlando, Florida. In: Fibromyalgia Network Newsletter January 1997, p 12

Croft P, Cooper C, Wickham C, coggon D 1992 Is the hip involved in generalized osteoarthritis. British Journal of Rheumatology 31: 325–328

Ferraccioli G 1990 Neuroendocrineologic findings in primary FMS. Journal of Rheumatology 17: 869–873

Fibromyalgia Network 1995 Newsletter. October 1995, p 11

Fibromyalgia Network 1996a Report. January 1996, p 9

Fibromyalgia Network 1996b Report. January 1996, p 10

Goldstein J 1996 Betrayal by the brain. Haworth Medical Press, Binghampton, NY

Jacobsen S 1991 Single cell morphology of muscles in patients with muscle pain. Scandinavian Journal of Rheumatology 20: 336–343

Keller R, Klimas N 1994 Association between HLA class II antigens and CFS. Clinical Infectious Diseases 18(supp): S154–156

Klimas N 1995 Report to CFS patient conference. Charlotte, North Carolina, September 23 1995. In: Fibromyalgia Network Newsletter January 1996, p 12

Landay A 1991 Chronic fatigue syndrome – clinical condition associated with immune activation. The Lancet 338: 707–711

Lowe J 1997 The metabolic treatment of fibromyalgia. Hawthorne BioMedical Press, Houston

Lowe J, Garrison R, Reidman A, Yellin J, Thompson M, Kaufman D 1997 Effectiveness and safety of T_3 therapy for euthyroid fibromyalgia. Clinical Bulletin of Myofascial Therapy 2(2/3): 31–58

Macintyre A 1993 What Causes ME? Journal of Action for ME 14(Autumn): 24–25

Moldofsky H 1993 A chronobiological theory of fibromyalgia. Journal of Musculoskeletal Pain 1(3/4): 49–59

Oldstone M 1989 Viral alteration of cell function. Scientific American 261: 34–40

Pellegrino M 1989 Familial occurrence of primary fibromyalgia. Archives of Physical Medicine and Rehabilitation 70(1)

Refetoff S 1993 The syndromes of resistance to thyroid hormone. Endocrine Review 14: 348–399

St Amand R P 1997 The use of uricosuric agents in fibromyalgia: theory, practice and rebuttle of Oregon study. Clinical Bulletin of Myofascial Therapy 2(4): 5–17

Sonkin L 1985 Endocrine disorders and muscle dysfunction. In: Gelb B (ed) Clinical management of head, neck and TMJ pain and dysfunction. W. B. Saunders, Philadelphia

Wilke S 1981 Hypothyroidism with presenting symptoms of fibrositis. Journal of Rheumatology 8: 627–630

Wolfe F 1994 Fibromyalgia: on criteria and classification. Journal of Musculoskeletal Pain 2(3): 23–39

Yellin J 1997 Why is substance P high in fibromyalgia? Clinical Bulletin of Myofascial Therapy 2(2/3): 23–30

5

Chronic fatigue syndrome and fibromyalgia compared

DEFINITIONS

The history of FMS, of its associated conditions, and of the many hypotheses which try to explain it (and such associated conditions as CFS), represents a mosaic of interlocking elements and contributing features which seem to have a constantly shifting focus:

- Is this a biochemical (viral infection, toxic exposure, allergy, etc.) phenomenon with psychological as well as physical manifestations?
- Is this a psychosocial condition (anxiety, depression, etc.) which produces biochemical and musculoskeletal changes?
- Is this a biomechanical condition (acute whiplash, postural and respiratory dysfunction, etc.) with repercussions affecting the individual biochemically and emotionally?
- Or is this really a condition emerging out of a warped homeostatic function (allostasis, which is thought to result from excessive adaptation demands made on immature defence and immune capabilities early in life as a result of violent physical or emotional events (Goldstein 1996)) which subsequently affects all aspects of the mind/body complex?

In individual cases, one or other (or more than one) of these possibilities may operate. Certainly, if we look at the common associated conditions and contributing features, we can see that some degree of fatigue is bound to emerge from any of them, whether it be sleep disturbance, allergy, viral infection, depression, hyperventilation, irritable bowel, chronic pain or any combination of these.

It is also reasonable to ask whether the conditions defined as fibromyalgia (FMS) and chronic fatigue syndrome (CFS) are not in fact simply variations on the same theme, with similar aetiologies and symptoms. Does the diagnosis of one or the other depend more on which physician is making the assessment than on real differences which define each condition?

Experts differ in their answers to these questions. Wolfe suggests that, 'Chronic nociceptive stimuli can lead to lowered pain threshold and . . . [this] . . . might be influenced by genetic, disease and psychological factors.' The various hypotheses which explain these events and how they lead to FMS (see Ch. 4), Wolfe states, 'suggest that there may be many fibromyalgias' (Wolfe 1994).

Is the fatigued older patient with chronic neck and back pain and a diagnosis of FMS likely to be manifesting the same systemic dysfunctional neurohumoral processes as a younger patient whose symptoms are apparently associated with a viral infection, or a whiplash injury, or a major psychological illness – all of which may have chronic fatigue as one of the key presenting features?

It may be useful to refer back to the definition of fibromyalgia as officially specified by the American College of Rheumatologists (Ch. 1, and Box 1.2) and compare this with the summarised definition of CFS given below (as defined by the US Centers of Disease Control in 1988, revised 1994).

1. A new, unexplained, persistent or relapsing chronic fatigue which is not a consequence of exertion, is not resolved by bed rest, and which is severe enough to significantly reduce daily activity.

2. The presence of four or more of the following symptoms for at least 6 months:

- headaches
- concentration and short-term memory impairment
- muscular pain
- multiple joint pain NOT accompanied by swelling or redness
- poor and unrefreshing sleep
- post-exertion malaise lasting more than 24 hours
- tender lymph nodes in the neck or armpits.

Someone with the muscle and joint features of this selection of symptoms, together with (say) the sleep disturbance and fatigue traits, would easily fit an FMS diagnosis (if 11 of the tested sites were sufficiently painful). Similarly, someone with the full FMS set of attributes would almost certainly have enough of the CFS characteristics to qualify for such a diagnosis.

The similarities between fibromyalgia syndrome and chronic fatigue syndrome are listed in Table 5.1.

Goldenberg characterises these similarities as follows: 'Both are chronic disorders with no known cause, no highly effective therapy and similar clinical and demographic characteristics. Studies of potential pathophysiologic abnormalities have been strikingly similar, including studies of muscle and immune function, sleep, as well as neurohormone alteration (Goldenberg 1994a).

In his research Goldenberg has found that approximately 70% of patients with chronic fatigue (who meet CDC criteria for CFS diagnosis) also meet the ACR diagnostic criteria for FMS. All those patients with CFS who also reported chronic musculoskeletal pain met the FMS diagnostic criteria. He acknowledges, however, that other researchers have not found this same degree of overlap and believes that, 'studies of the complicated integration of mind, body and the patient's psychosocial milieu are most likely to provide meaningful answers to all potential factors, including infections, that may be associated with FMS'.

Table 5.1 Similarities between fibromyalgia syndrome and chronic fatigue syndrome (Block 1993, Yunus 1989, Goldenberg 1989)

	FMS	CFS
Age	Young adult	Young adult
Primary sex	Female	Female
Prevalence	Common	Common
Cause	Not known	Not known
Chronic	Yes	Yes
Laboratory studies	Normal	Normal
Pathological findings	None	None
Disabling	Yes	Yes

The extreme tiredness experienced in CFS and FMS is not a normal response to activity which soon passes: indeed the fatigue and muscular pain felt by people with CFS and FMS after even mild activity often increases for several days following activity, despite rest. Chronic fatigue is a major symptom of most people with fibromyalgia and it is certainly not easy to distinguish between people with CFS and FMS except that in the former the fatigue element is probably more dominant than the pain symptoms, while people labelled as having FMS have muscular pain as their main symptom.

Both groups of patients frequently suffer sleep disturbances, both suffer fatigue and are affected by weather changes, and muscular pain is a common feature of both.

ARE CFS PATIENTS MORE LIKELY TO HAVE AN INFECTION AETIOLOGY?

Despite the fact that the swollen glands, sore throats and low grade fever experienced by many people with CFS are also reported by many FMS sufferers, some experts hold that a viral or bacterial origin is more likely in CFS than FMS (although not all agree, see Russell's opinion below). What is the evidence?

Dr Harvey Moldofsky (1993) tested patients with a diagnosis of chronic fatigue syndrome and also FMS patients whose symptoms had commonly started after a flu-like infection, as well as those whose symptoms started in other ways. He found that the brain wave patterns, tender points, pain and fatigue were *virtually identical* in all these groups (Moldofsky 1989). Moldofsky's research further suggests that neuroendocrine imbalances affecting sleep/wake functions were a key feature of both conditions (Moldofsky 1993).

Don Goldenberg MD has compared 50 patients diagnosed as having FMS with 50 patients diagnosed with CFS and found that symptoms of sore throat (54%), rash (47%), chronic cough (40%), swollen lymph glands (33%), and recurrent low-grade fever (28%) were virtually the same in both groups. Since these symptoms are common amongst CFS patients it seemed to him likely that the diagnosis can often be interchangeable (Goldenberg 1993a).

To some specialists the possibility of viral infection being a key feature in the aetiology of CFS helps to define the difference between it and FMS, although numerous tests and trials have not as yet led to anything definitive being established in the way of a common infecting agent (Straus 1994).

Nevertheless, Dr I. Jon Russell asserts that FMS patients display little or no evidence of infection: 'I have over 400 fibromyalgia patients and I don't find patients with tender nodes or recurrent fevers. And I have chronic fatigue patients with both spouses involved and have never seen this in fibromyalgia' (Russell 1994).

The implication of Russell's statement is that infection seems to be a major aspect of CFS and not of FMS. Goldenberg, however, says that in FMS there is often strong evidence for an infectious link and reports on viral links with FMS including HIV, coxsackie and parvovirus (Goldenberg 1993). He also reports on the well-known association between Lyme disease and FMS: 'the development of fibromyalgia as a consequence of infection with *B. burgdorferi* is now considered the worst complication of the disorder' (Steere et al 1993).

Goldenberg is clear that, 'It is unlikely that a single infection is the cause of most cases of fibromyalgia. Studies of the complicated integration of mind, body and patient's psychological milieu are more likely to provide meaningful answers to all potential factors, including infections, that may be associated with fibromyalgia' (Goldenberg 1994b).

Dr Anne Macintyre states:

The onset of ME [the British name for severe chronic fatigue is myalgic encephalomyelitis – ME] usually seems to be triggered by a virus, though the infection may pass unnoticed (Gow 1991). . . . many people say they were fit and well before a viral infection which started their ME [CFS/FMS] but it is possible that in many such patients there have been other factors such as emotional stress, pesticide exposure, surgical or accidental trauma some months before the triggering infection. (Macintyre 1993)

Dr Macintyre, herself afflicted with ME, also writes that:

The incidence of new cases peaks in late summer and autumn, coincident with the peak time of year for enteroviral infections. It is likely that enteroviral infection accounts for the majority of ME illness in this country [UK], even if other factors (stress, trauma) are present. There may also be a genetic predisposition, evidenced by the higher than expected number of parents with ME whose children also develop it some years after the parents. (Dowsett 1990)

Some of the major (possible) influences of viral infection on FMS are summarised below:

- HHV6, one of the herpes viruses, is more commonly found in FMS/CFS patients than other people (Buchwald et al 1992).
- British research which examined stool samples and blood evidence implicates enteroviruses (Behan 1993, Gow et al 1991).
- Buskila (1990) and Simms (1992) have both reported on the presence of FMS symptoms in patients infected by HIV.
- Chronic coxsackie B virus infection has been shown to mimic FMS symptoms (Nash 1989).
- Parvovirus has likewise been associated with FMS (Leventhal 1991).

If a major part of the background to CFS and FMS is a dysfunctional pattern which involves immune function, then infection would be a logical association, and to an extent Goldstein, in his all-embracing concept of neurosomatic disorders (see Ch. 4 and Fig. 4.5), expresses such a viewpoint. He sees little if any difference between chronic fatigue syndrome and FMS aetiology and offers a detailed explanation of the complex biochemical changes involved in the origins and maintenance of these and other conditions as outlined in previous chapters (Goldstein 1996).

Other fibromyalgia experts do not believe that FMS and CFS are the same, although they may coexist in many patients. Drs Starlanyl and Copeland (1996) state: 'FMS has many subsets, depending on which neurotransmitters are affected. Some of these subsets are similar to CFS. People with well-managed FMS may have little or no fatigue at all.'

So the question remains, are these virtually the same condition, with a slight difference in the degree and emphasis on one symptom or another (particularly muscular pain and fatigue) or are there clinically relevant differences which impact on how the condition is treated? For example, it seems clear from evidence that aerobic exercise benefits FMS patients (Goldenberg 1993b, McCain et al 1988). The performance of aerobic exercise, however, remains impossible for many CFS patients, for whom the pathological degree of fatiguability and the repercussions of excessive effort are defining characteristics.

Straus for one also suggests that cognitive dysfunction (memory lapses, problems with calculating) as well as physical effort are far worse in CFS compared with FMS (Straus 1994).

Probably the most important warning that can be given to anyone who is chronically fatigued with ME or post-viral fatigue conditions, whatever the degree of muscular involvement, is that a return to normal activity should be cautious and slow. If symptoms eventually improve, the single most damaging mistake is to try to do too much too soon. The natural desire to return to full activity needs to be well curbed so that gains can be built on and not destroyed by excessive activity before stamina and strength are restored.

From the clinical perspective, this highlights a vital warning – that we should offer only a modulated and limited degree of treatment at any given time, and should avoid overloading adaptation mechanisms. This means making simple changes (whether lifestyle, dietary, medication, exercise or anything else) one at a time, with ample time allowed for accommodation to new patterns, encouraging a degree of very gradually incremental conditioning – exercise or activity – well within tolerance levels but with a view towards a gradually expanding degree of effort rather than a contracting one.

IS CFS THE SAME AS FMS?

While for many people the two labels attached to their distressing and disabling conditions are interchangeable, the answer would seem to be 'not always, and not quite'.

REFERENCES

Behan P 1993 Enteroviruses and post viral fatigue syndrome/CFS. In: Bock G, Whelan J (eds) CIBA Foundation Symposium 173. Wiley, Chichester

Block S 1993 Fibromyalgia and the rheumatisms. Controversies in Clinical Rheumatology 19(1): 68

Buchwald D et al 1992 A chronic illness characterized by fatigue, neurologic and immunologic disorders and active human herpesvirus type 6 infection. Annals of Internal Medicine 116: 103–113

Buskila D 1990 FMS in HIV infection. Journal of Rheumatology 17: 1202–1206

Dowsett E 1990 M.E. – a persistent viral infection? Postgraduate Medical Journal 66: 526–530

Goldenberg D 1989 Fibromyalgia and its relationship to chronic fatigue syndrome, viral illness and immune abnormalities. Journal of Rheumatology 16(S19): 92

Goldenberg D 1993a Fibromyalgia, chronic fatigue syndrome and myofascial pain syndrome. Current Opinion in Rheumatology 5: 199–208

Goldenberg D 1993b Fibromyalgia: treatment programs. Journal of Musculoskeletal Pain 1(3/4): 71–81

Goldenberg D 1994a FMS and CFS. In: Pillimer S (ed) The fibromyalgia syndrome. Haworth Medical Press, Binghampton, NY

Goldenberg D 1994b Fibromyalgia and chronic fatigue syndrome. Journal of Musculoskeletal Pain 2(3): 51–55

Goldstein J 1996 Betrayal by the brain. Haworth Medical Press, Binghampton, NY

Gow J 1991 Enteroviral sequences detected in muscles of patients with postviral fatigue syndrome. British Medical Journal 302: 692–696

Leventhal L 1991 FMS and parvovirus infection. Arthritis and Rheumatism 34: 1319–1324

McCain G et al 1988 Controlled study of supervised cardiovascular fitness training program. Arthritis and Rheumatism 31: 1135–1141

Macintyre A 1993 What causes ME? The immune dysfunction hypothesis. Journal of Action for ME 14: 24–25

Moldofsky H 1989 Non-restorative sleep and symptoms of febrile illness in patients with fibrositis and chronic fatigue syndrome. Journal of Rheumatolgy 16(S19): 150–153

Moldofsky H 1993 Fibromyalgia, sleep disorder and chronic fatigue syndrome. In: Bock G, Whelan J (eds) CIBA Foundation Symposium 173. Wiley, Chichester, pp 262–279

Nash P 1989 Chronic coxsackie B infection mimicking primary FMS. Journal of Rheumatology 116: 1506–1508

Russell I 1994 Biochemical Abnormalities in FMS. In: Pillimer S (ed) The fibromyalgia syndrome. Haworth Medical Press, Binghampton, NY

Simms R 1992 FMS in patients infected with HIV. American Journal of Medicine 92: 368–374

Starlanyl D, Copeland M E 1996 Fibromyalgia and chronic myofascial pain syndrome: a survivors manual. New Harbinger, Oakland, CA

Steere A et al 1993 The overdiagnosis of Lyme disease. Journal of the American Medical Association 269: 1812–1816

Straus S 1994 Chronic fatigue syndrome. In: Pillimer S (ed) The fibromyalgia syndrome. Haworth Medical Press, Binghampton, NY

Wolfe F 1994 Fibromyalgia: on criteria and classification. In: Pillimer S (ed) The fibromyalgia syndrome. Haworth Medical Press, Binghampton, NY

Yunus M 1989 Fibromyalgia and other functional syndromes. Journal of Rheumatology 16(S19): 69

6

Acupuncture treatment of fibromyalgia and myofascial pain

Peter Baldry

This chapter discusses the circumstances which led me to employ superficial dry needling (SDN) in the treatment of the myofascial pain syndrome (MPS) and subsequently in the treatment of the fibromyalgia syndrome (FMS). However, in order to explain the rationale for using this particular form of treatment in these two disorders it is first necessary to discuss their respective aetiologies and clinical characteristics.

MYOFASCIAL PAIN SYNDROME

MPS is a disorder in which pain of muscular origin is confined to one region of the body. This notwithstanding, it may in some cases affect several regions concomitantly. Factors responsible for the development of pain in this disorder include muscle trauma and muscle ischaemia. This is because either of these cause activity to develop in plexi of C (Group IV) nociceptor nerve endings at discrete sites known as trigger points.

Trigger points

The term trigger point (TrP) was first introduced by Steindler (1940), an American orthopaedic surgeon, because nociceptor activity at such a point triggers off the referral of pain to a site some distance from it (zone of pain referral). However, it was Janet Travell, an American physician, who brought the term into general use when, in the early 1950s, she showed that each muscle in the body has its own specific pattern of TrP pain referral (Travell & Rinzler 1952).

Diagnosis

The diagnosis of MPS depends on being able to demonstrate the presence of active pain-producing TrPs in muscles in any particular region of the body. The first physician to draw attention to this was John Kellgren when working under the direction of Sir Thomas Lewis at University College Hospital, London, in the 1930s (Kellgren 1938). Because of Kellgren's pioneer observations and Janet Travell's subsequent ones it is now recognised that a muscle containing an active pain-producing TrP and muscles in the zone to which this pain is referred are slightly tender, but the TrP itself, because of trauma or ischaemia-induced activity in its nociceptor nerve endings, is so exquisitely tender as to make it a point of maximum tenderness. It is because of a TrP's excessive tenderness that pressure applied to it causes the patient to flinch involuntarily and to cry out. The eliciting of these two reactions at a TrP site are essential requirements for the diagnosis of this disorder. The application of sustained pressure to a TrP also causes pain to be referred to a site some distance from it (zone of pain referral).

There are, in addition, two other signs which it may or may not be possible to elicit. One is the presence of a firm elongated band of muscle at the TrP site (palpable band). The other is being able to evoke a twitch at a TrP site when a finger is moved sharply across the palpable band containing it in a manner similar to that used for plucking a violin string (local twitch response). These signs, however, are of limited diagnostic value as it is only possible to elicit them when the muscle containing the TrP is situated near to the surface of the body. Furthermore, palpable bands are liable to be found in normal subjects (Wolfe et al 1992, Njoo & Van der Does 1994). It is now believed that a taut band does not, as previously assumed, develop in response to TrP activity but conversely is present prior to the development of it (Simons 1996).

FIBROMYALGIA SYNDROME
Diagnosis

Fibromyalgia syndrome (FMS) is by contrast a generalised pain disorder with a number of points of maximum tenderness scattered all over the body. These points in FMS have traditionally been called tender points (TPs) and the American College of Rheumatology's criteria for its diagnosis is that pain on palpation must be present at at least 11 of 18 specified TP sites (Wolfe et al 1990).

Points of maximum tenderness, tender points and trigger points

A TP's nociceptors in this disorder become activated and sensitised as a result of some as yet unknown systemic biochemical disorder. The difference between a TP and a TrP is that pressure applied to a TP causes pain to be felt locally around it, but pressure applied to a TrP causes pain to be referred to a site some distance from it (zone of pain referral). This has led to the clinical axiom that TPs are to FMS what TrPs are to MPS (McCain 1994). However, this unfortunately is an over-simplification because, as Margoles (1989) has shown from a study of a large number of patients with FMS, it is the rule rather than the exception for both TPs and TrPs to be present in this disorder. Also, Bengtsson et al (1986) have reported both TPs and TrPs to be present in it. And Bennett (1990), from studying the disorder for a considerable number of years, has been led to conclude that: 'Many patients with FMS have myofascial trigger points and many of the so-called tender points are in fact latent trigger points that have become symptomatic as a result of enhanced pain perception.'

Support for this belief has come from a survey carried out by Wolfe et al (1992) as this showed that taut bands, which are now generally agreed to be TrP precursors (Simons 1996), were present with nearly equal frequency in control subjects, MPS patients and FMS patients.

Concomitant MPS and FMS

It is not uncommon for a patient with MPS to develop, over the course of time, the characteristic symptoms of FMS (Bennett 1986a, 1986b).

Characteristic symptoms of FMS

Apart from pain, the two commonest symptoms are early morning stiffness of the muscles and non-restorative sleep. It is because of the latter that the patient wakes feeling as tired as before going to bed, despite having had a seemingly undisturbed night. These symptoms are not restricted to FMS. They may also be present in other rheumatological disorders, particularly rheumatoid arthritis, but their frequency in FMS is significantly higher.

Other symptoms include paraesthesiae, subjective swelling of joints, tension headaches, irritable bowel syndrome and dysmenorrhoea. In addition, there may be sympathetic over-activity giving rise to coldness of the extremities with 12% of FMS sufferers having a fully-developed Raynaud's syndrome (Wolfe et al 1990).

SUPERFICIAL DRY NEEDLING IN THE TREATMENT OF MYOFASCIAL PAIN SYNDROME

When Kellgren (1938) demonstrated that pain in what has since become called myofascial pain syndrome (MPS) emanates from TrPs, he found that he could alleviate the pain by injecting a local anaesthetic (procaine) into them. Many physicians continue to use this method.

However, because the injection of a local anaesthetic into a TrP may occasionally give rise to serious and, at times, life-threatening hypersensitivity reactions, Sola and Kuitert (1955) decided to see whether an injection of saline might be equally effective. Their experience of doing this in 100 consecutive cases of MPS at the United States Air Force hospital in Texas led them to state that, 'the use of normal saline has none of the disadvantages often associated with the use of a local anaesthetic but appears to have the same therapeutic value'. A year later, Sola and Williams (1956) were able to confirm this in 1000 patients with MPS treated at the same hospital. And subsequently Frost et al (1980), in a double-blind trial comparing the effectiveness of injecting either the local anaesthetic mepivacaine

or saline into TrPs, found, to their surprise, that the group in which saline was used did better, with 80% of them reporting relief from pain as compared to 52% of those given mepivacaine injections.

Over the years many other substances, including corticosteroids (Bourne 1984) and non-steroidal anti-inflammatory drugs (Frost 1986, Drewes 1993) have been injected into TrPs but there is no evidence to suggest that any of them give better results than those obtained with either a local anaesthetic or saline. The pain-relieving effect of such disparate substances therefore cannot be due to any specific properties each may possess but rather to the one factor common to them all, namely the nerve-stimulating effect of the needle through which they are injected.

ACUPUNCTURE

The insertion of needles into muscles for the relief of pain is not some new concept: as long ago as the 6th-century *AD* the Chinese physician Sun Ssu-Mo, in his books on acupuncture (*acus* (L) = needle), described how he treated pain of muscular origin by inserting needles into points of maximum tenderness, or what the Chinese call *ah shi* points (Lu & Needham 1980).

News about the Chinese practice of acupuncture first reached Europe in the 16th century but the seemingly esoteric concepts upon which most of it is based for long proved to be unacceptable to physicians trained in Western medicine. However, at the beginning of the 19th century, an English physician named Churchill decided to employ Sun Ssu-Mo's technique for the treatment of what he called rheumatalgia, and in 1828 published books describing this and the results obtained with it (Churchill 1821, 1828). These books only attracted a limited amount of interest, with no more than a few physicians following his example. The most famous of these was Sir William Osler, professor of medicine at Oxford University who, in his student textbook *The Principles and Practice of Medicine*, published in 1912, described how in the treatment of lumbago he inserted, 'needles of from three to four inches in length (ordinary bonnet needles sterilised will do) . . . into the lumbar muscles at the seat of the pain'.

Despite this, the medical profession in general continued to view such treatment with incredulity and nothing further was heard of it until much later, in the 20th century, when Travell and Rinzler (1952), during the course of describing specific patterns of pain referral from TrPs and how such pain may be alleviated by injecting a local anaesthetic into them, mentioned in passing that it is possible to achieve the same effect with dry needling. However, it has only been in the last 20 years, during which time time there have been considerable advances in knowledge concerning the neurophysiology of pain, that the scientific basis for this type of treatment has become increasingly widely accepted.

Dry needling

The first physician to use dry needling extensively for the deactivation of TrPs was Karel Lewit in Czechoslovakia. Lewit (1979) reported favourably on the use of the technique in a series of 241 patients with TrP pain treated in 1975 and 1976. Both he, and since then others (Jaeger & Skootsky 1987, Gunn 1989), have stressed that in their opinion deep dry needling is required, and that its effectiveness is related to the precision with which a needle is inserted into the intramuscularly-situated TrP.

Superficial dry needling

Although it is certainly essential to locate each TrP accurately, experience has led me to believe that it is not necessary to employ deep needling but easier, safer and just as effective to insert the needle into the superficial tissues overlying a TrP (Baldry 1993). My reason for adopting this superficial dry needling (SDN) technique is that when attempting to deactivate a TrP in the scalenus anterior muscle at the base of the neck some years ago, it seemed prudent to me, in view of the proximity of the apex of the lung, only to insert the needle for a short distance under the skin, and found that this was sufficient to relieve the pain referred down the arm from this TrP. Superficial needling at TrP sites elsewhere in the body was then tried and found to be equally effective. Not long after this Macdonald et al (1983) confirmed my findings by showing that it is possible to alleviate low-back pain by inserting needles to an approximate depth of only 4 mm at TrP sites.

Bowsher (1990) has now explained why SDN is all that is required by pointing out that the A-δ sensory afferents – which are the ones that need to be stimulated when deactivating a TrP – are present mainly, but not exclusively, in the skin and just beneath it.

In order to understand the neurophysiological basis for the use of SDN it has to be remembered that when a TrP is in an active phase, noxious information generated in it is conducted along thin unmyelinated C (Group IV) sensory afferents to a spinal cord's dorsal horn. From there this information is transmitted, via the contralaterally-situated ascending spinoreticular pathway, to the brain with, as a consequence, the development of pain. Alleviation of this pain may be brought about by inserting a needle into the tissues overlying the TrP and by this means stimulating medium-sized myelinated A-δ nerve fibres in the skin and subcutaneous tissues. This is because one of the effects of doing so is to cause activity to develop in inhibitory interneurons (IIs) situated in the dorsal horn. These IIs then release enkephalin and this opioid peptide blocks the TrP's C (Group IV) sensory afferents' input to the spinal cord.

Dry needle stimulation of A-δ nerve fibres causes activity to develop in these IIs because:

- These nerve fibres, on entering the spinal cord, give off branches which connect directly with the IIs
- The neospinothalamic tract up which pinprick information is conveyed to the brain gives off collaterals that project to the midbrain's periaqueductal grey area at the upper end of a descending pain-inhibitory system. Axons in this system at the dorsal horn level also connect with these IIs. (See Fig. 6.1 and Fig. 6.2.)

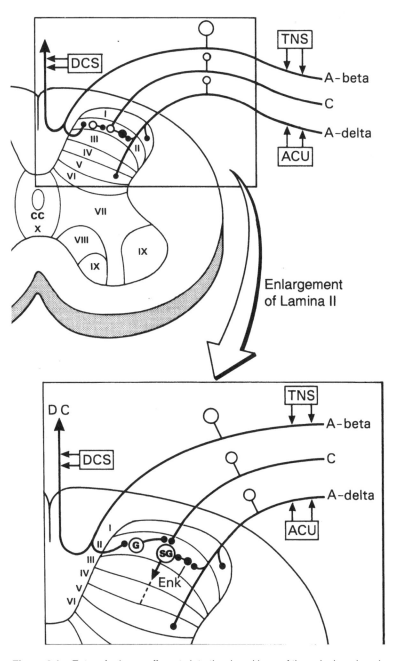

Figure 6.1 Entry of primary afferents into the dorsal horn of the spinal cord, and circuits involved in TENS and acupuncture. Roman numerals refer to laminae numbers. SG = Substantia gelatinosa cell. G = GABAergic interneuron, presynaptically inhibiting primary afferent C fibre terminal. Enk = Enkephalinergic interneuron, postsynaptically inhibiting substantia gelatinosa neuron. The enkephalinergic interneuron is not only activated, as shown, by A-delta primary afferent terminals, but also by serotoninergic fibres descending from the brainstem (see Fig. 6.2). CC = Central canal. DC = Dorsal column. DCS = Dorsal column stimulation. TNS = Low-threshold, high frequency stimulation. ACU = High-threshold, low frequency stimulation. Dr David Bowsher's diagram in Journal of British Medical Acupuncture Society 1990. Reproduced with permission.

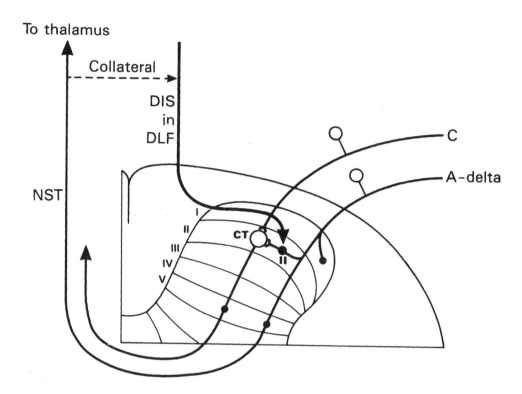

Figure 6.2 Diagram of dorsal horn to show the local intraspinal connection between A-delta nerve fibres and enkephalinergic inhibitory interneuron (II), whose function it is to inhibit activity in C afferent terminal cell (CT). Also, to show the indirect A-delta link with inhibitory interneuron via the collateral connecting the A-delta afferent's ascending pathway — the neospinothalamic tract (NST) with the descending inhibitory system in the dorsolateral funiculus (DIS in DLF).

Responsiveness to needle stimulation

The amount of needle stimulation required depends on an individual's responsiveness to it. It has been estimated that about 10% of adults and almost all children with TrP pain are strong responders so that with them it may be necessary to do no more than insert a needle into the tissues overlying a TrP and then to withdraw it immediately. With these strong reactors, if the stimulation given is greater than this, the pain, rather than being alleviated, may be exacerbated. The majority of people are average responders but even with them it may only prove necessary to leave a needle in situ for 30–60 seconds. There is also a small group of adults who are weak responders and therefore require exceptionally strong needle stimulation. With them the needle has to be left in situ for several minutes and the

strength of the stimulus may have to be increased by means of the needle being vigorously rotated.

When carrying out SDN for the first time there is no way of knowing whether the response to it will be strong, average or weak; it is therefore necessary to start with a light stimulus and for this to be increased only if it proves to be necessary. Initially, a needle should be inserted into the tissues overlying a TrP and left in situ for 30 seconds. Then, because the amount of stimulation required is the minimum necessary to abolish the TrP's exquisite tenderness, on withdrawing the needle, pressure as firm as before needling should be applied to the TrP to see whether or not this has been achieved. One 30-second period of needling is often all that is required but when appreciable tenderness is still found to be present the needle should be reinserted and left in situ for about 2–3 minutes. Very occasionally with a weak responder this is still insufficient and the needle then has to be once again reinserted and vigorously rotated in order to increase the strength of the stimulus.

SUPERFICIAL DRY NEEDLING IN THE TREATMENT OF FIBROMYALGIA

As previously stated, pain in MPS emanates from TrPs, and the most widely employed method of deactivating a TrP's nociceptors in this disorder is to inject a local anaesthetic into the TrP. This, however, has a number of potential complications. Not only may the local anaesthetic occasionally give rise to hypersensitivity reactions, but also the hollow needle used for injecting it has a cutting edge that is liable to damage blood vessels; because of this, there is a significant incidence of post-injection soreness. In addition, inserting a needle into a TrP gives rise to appreciable, albeit transient, pain, and the deep needling required for this is liable to damage important structures in the vicinity. These potential hazards preclude the technique from being employed in FMS, where the TPs and TrPs that have to be deactivated are usually not only extremely numerous but also widely scattered.

The discovery that TrPs in MPS may be simply, safely and successfully deactivated with SDN prompted me to see whether it would be equally effective in deactivating the TrPs and TPs present in FMS.

Because of the large number of scattered points that have to be deactivated, it might be thought that each treatment session would take a considerable amount of time. However, this is not usually so as FMS sufferers tend to be strong responders and often only require each point to be needled for a very brief period. Admittedly, the treatment involves both patient and doctor in a long-term commitment because, due to FMS invariably taking a chronic course, SDN has to be carried out once a week for 3–4 weeks and then at 4–6 week intervals on a long-term basis. Nevertheless, most patients find that this is worthwhile as the pain relief obtained appreciably improves the quality of their lives.

ELECTRO-ACUPUNCTURE

Electro-acupuncture (EA) with needles inserted into fibromyalgia tender points has been found to exacerbate the pain (Deluze et al 1992). This is presumably because, due to nociceptors at these tender points being in an activated and sensitised state, the stimulus provided by this means is too strong.

In contrast to this, EA with needles inserted into traditional Chinese acupuncture points has been shown to provide fibromyalgia sufferers with some reasonably long-lasting pain relief (Waylonis 1977, Deluze et al 1992). A trial is therefore needed to compare the effectiveness of this with that of manually inserting dry needles into the tissues overlying tender points. In the meantime the great advantage of using the latter technique is that it is far simpler to carry out and does not require the person employing it to have had training in traditional Chinese acupuncture.

SUMMARY

[See also additional information in Boxes 6.1 and 6.2] Two disorders, the regional myofascial pain syndrome (MPS) and the generalised fibromyalgia syndrome (FMS), have certain features in common. The pain in MPS develops as a result of muscle trauma or ischaemia-induced activation of nociceptors at points of maximum tenderness in muscles situated in one or other region of the body. Such points are called trigger points (TrPs) because the development of nociceptor activity at these points triggers off pain that is referred to sites some distance away (zones of pain referral).

The pain in FMS develops because of the activation of nociceptors at points of maximum tenderness in a large number of muscles throughout the body. It is believed that widespread nociceptor activity is due to some as yet unidentified systemic biochemical disorder. Points of maximum tenderness in FMS are of two types. Tender points (TPs), i.e. points where pain is felt locally at these sites alone; and trigger points (TrPs), i.e. points from which pain is referred to distant sites (zones of pain referral).

TREATMENT OF MPS

As pain in MPS emanates from nociceptors in TrPs it has for long been recognised that, in order to alleviate the pain, it is necessary to deactivate the TrP nociceptors. The original method, and one still widely used, is to inject a local anaesthetic into the TrP. This method, however, has certain disadvantages:

1. The irritant effect of the needle on nerves at the TrP site gives rise to appreciable, albeit short-lasting, pain.
2. The hollow needle through which the substance is injected has a cutting edge which is liable to damage blood vessels and, because of this, there is a significant incidence of bleeding into the tissues with consequent post-injection soreness.
3. Because the needle has to be inserted deeply into the substance of a muscle it is also liable to damage other structures in the vicinity.
4. In addition, there is a small but significant incidence of hypersensitivity reactions to the local anaesthetic.

It was next discovered that a TrP may be deactivated by inserting an acupuncture needle into it. The main advantage of this is that an acupuncture needle, whilst having a sharp point, has no cutting edge and therefore the incidence of bleeding into the tissues and post-treatment soreness is less.

It has subsequently been shown that a TrP may be deactivated by means of inserting an acupuncture needle into the skin or subcutaneous tissues overlying it. This superficial dry needling (SDN) technique has none of the disadvantages of the other two methods. It is therefore safer, simpler and seemingly equally effective.

SDN achieves its pain-relieving effect because it causes electrical activity to develop in A-∂ nerve fibres and one of the effects of this is to stimulate activity in opioid peptide mediated inhibitory interneurons in the spinal cord's dorsal horn. This in turn blocks the sensory afferent input to the spinal cord from C (Group IV) nociceptors at the TrP site in a muscle.

Treatment of FMS

A wide variety of therapies are employed in the treatment of FMS but as its pain, like the pain of MPS, emanates from nociceptors at points of maximum tenderness (TPs and TrPs), once the value of SDN in MPS had been demonstrated, it was decided to observe its effect on the pain of FMS. It has been found that SDN does not influence the protracted course taken by FMS but the pain relief achieved by carrying it out at intervals of 4–6 weeks on a long-term basis significantly improves the quality of life.

Box 6.1 Myofascial ('trigger point') pain and fibromyalgia syndrome
Leon Chaitow

In this chapter, Peter Baldry explains an effective means of pain control utilising acupuncture ('dry needling') methods. He also outlines a brief overview of myofascial trigger point characteristics. This boxed information offers a summary relating to the relationship between fibromyalgia syndrome (FMS) and myofascial pain syndrome (MPS). The historical linking of myofascial (trigger point) pain and fibromyalgia can be seen to date from the early years of research into these topics, and is summarised in Box 1.1. There we see researchers from the 1930s onwards (Kellgren, Gutstein, Travell and others) wrestling with the phenomenon of pain being referred from localised areas to distant target tissues, as a part of what was variously being termed fibrositis, or myalgia, or myodysneuria (Fig. 6.3).

If, as seems likely, a significant degree of the pain suffered by anyone with fibromyalgia results from myofascial trigger point activity, then, one way or another, this should be able to be eased, modified, abated, removed (see Box 6.2) (Fig. 6.4).

Trigger points are characterised by:
1. Localised, painful, discrete, palpable areas of altered soft tissue structure.
2. These lie in fine, taut bands which Simons hypothesises evolve in stressed tissues of some individuals who may be genetically predisposed to these changes.
3. These bands may be maintained by virtue of excessive calcium in the muscle cells, which cannot be 'pumped out' due to poor ATP (energy) levels. In time neural structures become sensitised (facilitated) and pain develops which is referred to distant sites where the cycle repeats itself. Travell & Simons (1986, 1993) have described the process of trigger point evolution as follows:
In the core of the trigger lies a muscle spindle which is in trouble for some reason. Visualise a spindle like a strand of yarn in a knitted sweater ... a metabolic crisis takes place which increases the temperature locally in the trigger point, shortens a minute part of the muscle (sarcomere) – like a snag in a sweater, and reduces the supply of oxygen and nutrients into the trigger point. During this disturbed episode an influx of calcium occurs and the muscle spindle does not have enough energy to pump the calcium outside the cell where it belongs. Thus a vicious cycle is maintained and the muscle spindle can't seem to loosen up and the affected muscle can't relax. (Travell & Simons 1986, 1993)
4. On pressure a trigger point is painful locally as well as referring pain to a distance ('target area') or radiating pain from itself. This is commonly referred to as 'regional' pain. The referred or radiating pain will often reproduce symptoms of which the patient is already aware.
5. Among the referred effects of an active trigger point, apart from pain, there may be numbness, tingling, weakness, lack of normal range of movement and altered sympathetic activity (Webber 1973).

6. A brisk stroke across the band evokes a response which is regarded as significant in identifying myofascial trigger point activity. To elicit the sign most effectively, one must place the relaxed muscle under moderate passive tension, and snap the band briskly with the palpating finger.
7. Activity involving the tissues housing the trigger usually increases the symptoms (pain, etc.), while rest usually eases them.
8. The premier researcher into pathophysiological processes involved in osteopathic manipulation, Irwin Korr PhD, has described a process he calls facilitation in which neural structures become sensitised and hyper-reactive in response to overuse, misuse or abuse. Myofascial trigger points would seem to fall into this definition (Korr 1970, 1976, 1977; see also Ch. 1).
9. The implications of hundreds of studies into the phenomenon of facilitation are that any form of stress impacting the individual, be it climatic, chemical, emotional, physical or anything else, will produce a rise in neurological output from facilitated areas (Beal 1983).
10. Wall & Melzack (1989), in their exhaustive investigation of pain, are clear that all chronic pain has myofascial trigger point activity as at least a part of its aetiology and that in many instances trigger points are major contributors to pain. These researchers have also shown that roughly 80% of major trigger point sites are on established acupuncture points.
11. Janet Travell MD (Travell 1957, Travell & Simons 1986, 1993) is on record as stating that if a pain is severe enough to cause a patient to seek professional advice (in the absence of organic disease), referred pain is likely to be a factor, and therefore a trigger area is probably involved.
12. A single trigger may refer pain to several reference sites and can give rise to embryonic or satellite triggers; for example Travell describes how a trigger in the distal areas of the sternomastoid muscle can give rise to new triggers in the sternalis muscle, the pectoral muscle and/or serratus anterior (Travell & Simons 1986).

Among the research into the connection between myofascial trigger point activity and fibromyalgia, are the following:
• Yunus (1993) suggests that: 'Fibromyalgia and Myofascial Pain Syndrome (MPS) [trigger point-derived pain] share several common features [and] it is possible that MPS represents an incomplete, regional or early form of fibromyalgia syndrome since many fibromyalgia patients give a clear history of localized pain before developing generalised pain.'
• Granges & Littlejohn (1993) in Australia have researched the overlap between trigger points and the tender points in fibromyalgia and come to several conclusions, including:
 a. Tender points in FMS represent a diffusely diminished pain threshold to pressure while trigger points are the expression of a local musculoskeletal abnormality

---

Box 6.1 (Contd.)   Myofascial ('trigger point') pain and fibromyalgia syndrome

b. It is likely that trigger points in diffuse chronic pain states such as FMS contribute only in a limited and localised way to decreasing the pain threshold to pressure in these patients
c. Taken individually, the trigger points are an important clinical finding in some patients with FMS, with nearly 70% of the FMS patients tested having at least one active trigger point
d. Of these FMS patients with active trigger points, about 60% reported that pressure on this trigger 'reproduced a localized and familiar [FMS] pain'.

• Researchers at Oregon Health Sciences University studied the history of patients with FMS and found that over 80% reported that prior to the onset of their generalised symptoms they suffered from regional pain problems (which almost always involve trigger points). Physical trauma was cited as the major cause of their pre-FMS regional pain. Only 18% had FMS which had started without prior regional pain (Fibromyalgia Network 1995).

• Research at UCLA has shown that injecting active trigger points with the pain-killing agent Xylocaine produced marked benefits in FMS patients in terms of pain relief and reduction of stiffness but that this is not really significantly apparent for at least a week after the injections. FMS patients reported more local soreness following the injections than patients with only myofascial pain but improved after this settled down. This reinforces the opinion of many practitioners that myofascial trigger points contribute a large degree of the pain being experienced in FMS (Hong 1996).

• Travell & Simons (1993) are clearly of this opinion, stating that: 'Most of these [fibromyalgia] patients would be likely to have specific myofascial pain syndromes that would respond to myofascial therapy.'

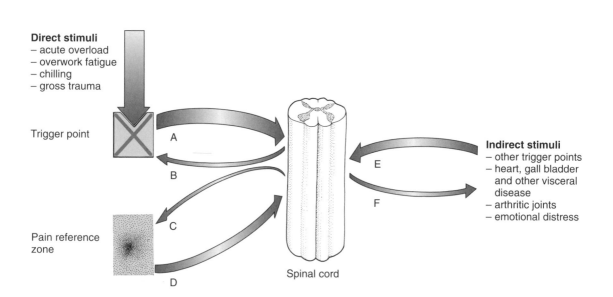

Figure 6.3   Direct stress influence can affect the hyper-reactive neural structure of a myofascial trigger point, leading to increased activity (A–B) as well as referring sensations (pain, paraesthesia, increased sympathetic activity) to a target area (C–D) which feed back into the cord to increase the background stress load. Other stimuli reach the cord from distant trigger points and additional dysfunctional areas (E–F).

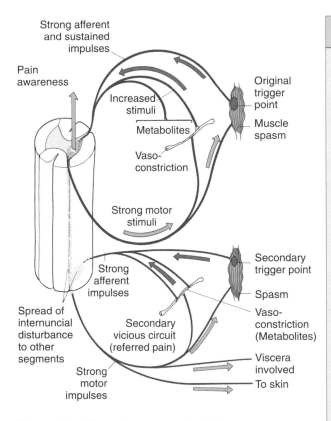

Figure 6.4 Schematic representation of the secondary spread of neurologically induced influences deriving from acute or chronic soft tissue dysfunction, and involving trigger point activity and/or spasm.

Box 6.2   Treating trigger points (Fig. 6. 5)
Leon Chaitow

Many methods exist for the obliteration of trigger points:
- These range from injection of pharmacological agents such as Novocaine or Xylocaine, to application of coolant sprays, ultrasound and acupuncture techniques (as described in this chapter by Dr Peter Baldry), and manual methods.
- Manual methods of trigger point treatment include ischaemic compression, positional release and various stretching approaches.
- Clinical experience and has shown that an absolute requirement for trigger point deactivation (apart from removal of the causes) involves the need to restore the muscle in which the trigger lies to its normal resting length. Failing the achievement of this goal, all methods of treating trigger points are likely to provide only short-term relief.
- Dr John Mennell (Mennell 1975) states that whatever the means used to 'block' the trigger activity,

---

Box 6.2 (Contd.)   Treating trigger points

and whatever the neuropathological routes involved, the critical factor in the restoration of pain-free normality is that the affected muscle should have its normal resting length restored by stretching. Mennell favours chilling the trigger area by vapocoolant or ice massage – an approach supported by both Travell and Simons, who now advocate muscle energy technique (postisometric relaxation) stretching as well.
- Once symptoms have been relieved, the muscle containing the trigger must be gently stretched to its normal resting length, or symptoms will return, irrespective of the technique used (chilling, pressure, injection, acupuncture, etc.).
- Such stretching should be *gradual* and *gentle* and the recommendation of Lewit (1991), and Travell (Travell & Simons 1992) is that muscle energy technique (MET), in which gentle isometric contractions followed by stretch are employed, is the method of choice. Lewit suggests that, in many instances, stretching in itself is adequate in deactivating trigger point activity.
CAUTION! In cases of fibromyalgia, stretching needs to be performed with the utmost care, as will be outlined in the manual treatment sections in Chapters 13.
- A combined sequence of treatment to achieve trigger point deactivation has been proposed, commencing with palpation/identification, followed by ischaemic compression, followed by adoption of a positional release posture (see bodywork treatment section, Ch. 13), followed by a stretching of the tissues housing the trigger point. The stretching in this sequence can follow a focused (to activate the fibres involved) isometric contraction. This sequence has been dubbed 'integrated neuromuscular inhibition technique' (INIT) (Chaitow 1994) (see p. 234).
- Dr Devin Starlanyl (Starlanyl 1994) advocates a combination of sine-wave ultrasound and electrostim, both diagnostically and for treatment of trigger points: 'Ultrasound with electrostim causes pain immediately over the TP, pinpointing the location as it breaks up the TP. ... Care must be taken to start gently, and allow the patient to decide the amount of pain tolerable. I use this treatment followed by gentle stretching. Breaking up the TP can cause fatigue and activation of aches for a day, followed by relief. ... I have also found ice is more effective in relieving spasticity and pain than heat if nerve entrapment is involved' (Starlanyl 1994). Clinical experience suggests that this advice is valid, whatever is done to a trigger point, especially in a patient with FMS: gentle approaches are best with stretching almost always necessary and, even if carefully applied, these lead to a 'reaction' for a day or so.
- The deactivation of myofascial trigger points offers one way of beginning to reduce the pain levels of patients with FMS.

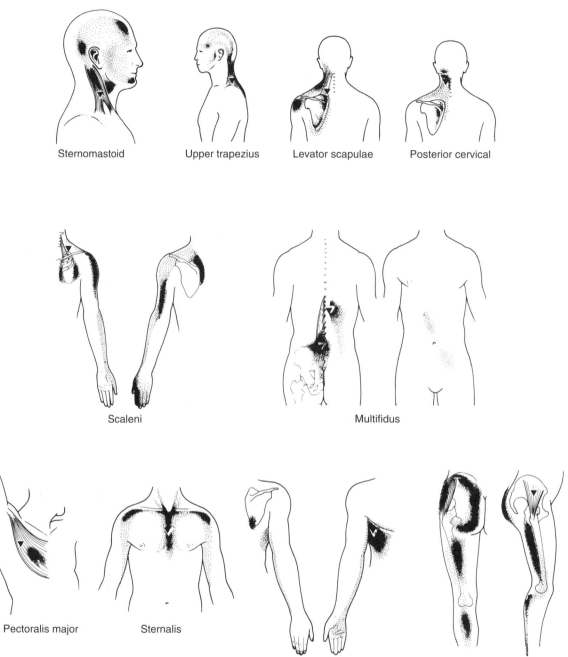

Sternomastoid

Upper trapezius

Levator scapulae

Posterior cervical

Scaleni

Multifidus

Pectoralis major

Sternalis

Serratus anterior

Gluteus minimus

Figure 6.5 Pain referral patterns from myofascial trigger points. ▲ = trigger point; shaded area = reference pain zone. (From Chaitow 1996, with permission)

REFERENCES

Baldry P E 1993 Acupuncture, trigger points and musculoskeletal pain, 2nd edn. Churchill Livingstone, Edinburgh, pp 91–103

Beal M 1983 Palpatory testing of somatic dysfunction in patients with cardiovascular disease. Journal of the American Osteopathic Association (July)

Bengtsson A, Henriksson K G, Jorfeldt L, Kadedal B, Lenmarken C, Lindstrom F 1986 Primary fibromyalgia: a clinical and laboratory study of 55 patients. Scandinavian Journal of Rheumatology 15: 340–347

Bennett R M 1986a Current issues concerning management of the fibrositis/fibromyalgia syndrome. American Journal of Medicine 81 (S3A): 15–18

Bennett R M 1986b Fibrositis: evolution of an enigma. Journal of Rheumatology 13(4): 676–678

Bennett R M 1990 Myofascial pain syndromes and the fibromyalgia syndrome. A comparative analysis. In: Fricton R, Awad E (eds) Advances in pain research and therapy. Raven Press, New York, vol. 17, pp 43–65

Bourne I A J 1984 Treatment of chronic back pain comparing corticosteroid–lignocaine injections with lignocaine alone. Practitioner 228: 333–338

Bowsher D 1990 Physiology and pathophysiology of pain. Journal of the British Medical Acupuncture Society 7: 17–20

Chaitow L 1994 Integrated neuromuscular inhibition technique in treatment of pain and trigger points. British Osteopathic Journal 13: 17–21

Chaitow L 1996 Modern Neuromuscular Techniques. Churchill Livingstone, Edinburgh

Churchill J M 1821 A treatise on acupuncturation, being a description of a surgical operation originally peculiar to the Japanese and Chinese, and by them denominated zin-king, now introduced into European practice, with directions for its performance, and cases illustrating its success. Simpkins & Marshall, London (German trans 1824, French trans 1825)

Churchill J M 1828 Cases illustrative of the immediate effects of acupuncturation in rheumatism, lumbago, sciatica, anomolous muscular diseases and in dropsy of the cellular tissue, selected from various sources and intended as an appendix to the author's treatise on the subject. Callow and Wilson, London

Deluze C, Bosia L, Zirgs A, Chantraine A, Vischer T L 1992 Electroacupuncture in fibromyalgia: results of a controlled trial. British Medical Journal 305: 1249–1252

Drewes A M, Andreason A, Poulsen L H 1993 Injection therapy for the treatment of chronic myofascial pain. A double-blind study comparing corticosteroid versus dicloferac injections. Journal of Musculoskeletal Pain 1(3/4): 289–294

Fibromyalgia Network 1995 Burckhardt R quoted in: Myofascial pain – diagnosis and treatment. Fibromyalgia Network October 1995: 10

Frost A 1986 Diclofenac versus lidocaine as injection therapy in myofascial pain. Scandinavian Journal of Rheumatology 15: 153–156

Frost P A, Jessen B, Siggaard-Andersen J 1980 A controlled double-blind comparison of mepivacaine injection versus saline injection for myofascial pain. Lancet 1: 499–501

Granges G, Littlejohn G 1993 Prevalence of myofascial pain syndrome in fibromyalgia syndrome and regional pain syndrome. Journal of Musculoskeletal Pain 1(2): 19–34

Gunn C C 1989 Treating myofascial pain. University of Washington, Seattle

Hong C 1996 Difference in pain relief after trigger point injections in myofascial pain patients with and without fibromyalgia. Archives of Physical Medicine and Rehabilitation 77(11): 1161–1166

Jaeger B, Skootsky S A 1987 Double-blind, controlled study of different myofascial trigger point injection techniques. Pain (4S): 292

Kellgren J H 1938 A preliminary account of referred pains arising from muscle. British Medical Journal 1: 325–327

Korr I 1970 Physiological basis of osteopathic medicine. Postgraduate Institute of Osteopathic Medicine and Surgery, New York

Korr I 1976 Spinal cord as organiser of disease process. Academy Applied Osteopathy Yearbook, 1976

Korr I (ed) 1977 Neurobiological mechanisms in manipulation. Plenum Press, New York

Lewit K 1979 The needle effect in the relief of myofascial pain. Pain 6: 83–90

Lewit K 1991 Manipulation in rehabilitation of the locomotor system. Butterworths, London

Lu G-D, Needham J 1980 Celestial lancets. Cambridge University Press, Cambridge, p 127

McCain G A 1994 Fibromyalgia and myofascial pain syndromes. In: Wall P D, Melzack R (eds) Textbook of pain, 3rd edn. Churchill Livingstone, Edinburgh, pp 475–493

Macdonald A J R, Macrae K D, Master B R, Rubin A P 1983 Superficial acupuncture in the relief of chronic low-back pain. Annals of the Royal College of Surgeons of England 65: 44–46

Margoles M S 1989 The concept of primary fibromyalgia (letter to the editor). Pain 36: 391

Mennell J 1975 The therapeutic use of cold. Journal of the American Osteopathic Association 74 (August)

Njoo K H, Van der Does E 1994 The occurrence and inter-rater reliability of myofascial trigger points in the quadratus lumborum and gluteus medius: a prospective study in non-specific low-back pain patients and controls in general practice. Pain 58: 317–323

Osler Sir William 1912 The principles and practice of medicine, 8th edn. Appleton, New York, p 1131

Simons D 1996 Clinical and etiological update of myofascial pain from trigger points. Journal of Musculoskeletal Pain 4(1/2): 93–121

Sola A E, Kuitert J H 1955 Myofascial trigger point pain in the neck and shoulder girdle. North West Medicine 54: 980–984

Sola A E, Williams R L 1956 Myofascial pain syndromes. Neurology 6: 91–95

Starnalyl D 1994 Comment. Journal of Musculoskeletal Pain 2(2): 141–142

Steindler A 1940 The interpretation of sciatic radiation and the syndrome of low-back pain. Journal of Bone and Joint Surgery 22: 28–34

Travell J 1957 Symposium on mechanism and management of pain syndromes. Proceedings of the Rudolph Virchow Medical Society 16: 128–136

Travell J, Rinzler S H 1952 The myofascial genesis of pain. Postgraduate Medicine 11: 425–434

Travell J, Simons D 1986 Myofascial pain and dysfunction. Williams and Wilkins, Baltimore, vol. 1

Travell J, Simons D 1992 Myofascial pain and dysfunction. Williams and Wilkins, Baltimore, vol. 2

Travell J, Simons D 1993 Myofascial pain and dysfunction. Williams and Wilkins, Baltimore, vol. 2

Wall P, Melzack R 1989 Textbook of pain. Churchill Livingstone, London

Waylonis G W 1977 Long term follow-up on patients with fibrositis treated with acupuncture. Ohio State Medical Journal 73: 299–302

Webber T D 1973 Diagnosis and modification of headache and shoulder, arm, hand syndromes. Journal of the American Osteopathic Association 72 (March)

Wolfe F, Smythe H A, Yunus M B et al 1990 The American College of Rheumatology criteria for the classification of fibromyalgia: report of the Multicenter Criteria Committee. Arthritis and Rheumatism 33: 160–172

Wolfe F, Simons D, Fricton J et al 1992 The fibromyalgia and myofascial pain syndromes: a preliminary study of tender points and trigger points in persons with fibromyalgia, myofascial pain syndrome and no disease. Journal of Rheumatology 19: 944–951

Yunus M 1993 Research in fibromyalgia and myofascial pain syndromes. Journal of Musculoskeletal Pain 1(1): 23–41

7

Interdisciplinary pain management in fibromyalgia

Paul J. Watson

There is growing consensus of opinion that chronic pain is a condition of such complexity that it can only be addressed by multidimensional assessment and treatment. Such an approach recognises that pain is not merely the end product of a passive transmission of nociceptive impulses from receptor organ to an area of interpretation; it is a dynamic process of perception and interpretation of a wide range of incoming stimuli, some of which are associated with actual or potential harm and some of which are benign but interpreted and described in terms of damage.

The ongoing pain from fibromyalgia is physically limiting and demoralising, leads to affective disorders and a reduction in social and personal contacts, and causes alteration in personal relationships, changes in social roles and increased reliance on healthcare and social services. The assessment of a patient with such a condition requires an evaluation of all these aspects of the condition.

THE PROBLEM OF THE MEDICAL MODEL IN FIBROMYALGIA

In the biomedical model, the patient's symptoms arise from abnormality of physiology and therefore an objective assessment of the physiology through objective testing for damage or malfunction will define the abnormality. Interventions are focused on the resolution of the problem; once repair has been effected, the symptoms will abate and normal function will be restored. The relationship between the objective tests, the severity of symptoms and the accompanying dysfunction should equate with each other. However, although there is a relationship between these factors it is at best very modest and there is evidence that relationships between the factors vary according to the duration of symptoms and individual subgroups within conditions (Waddell 1987, 1992; Turk et al 1996). In those people with chronic pain in particular, the identified abnormal pathology does not predict the accompanying degree of functional incapacity or psychological distress. The level of distress and disability is better explained by the individual's beliefs about the nature of his condition and by his ability to cope with the pain. Furthermore, persistent pain over a prolonged period is stressful and chronic stress may result in poor sleep, low mood and neuro-endocrine dysfunction, which in turn alter the perception of pain and affect the individual's ability to cope with that pain still further – a cycle leading to further distress and physical decline.

In fibromyalgia the absence of an obvious source of ongoing nociception or inflammation makes the application of a medical model inappropriate. With the exception of some studies into the management of sleep disorders by pharmacological interventions, medical interventions in fibromyalgia have been relatively unsuccessful (White & Harth 1996; Vancouver Fibromyalgia Consensus Group 1996). This has led to an opinion among many of those that care for those suffering from this condition that management should have a biopsychosocial perspective and be delivered by either a multidisciplinary team where members of different professions bring individual skills to the patient or by means of an *interdisciplinary* approach where generic behavioural management skills are common to all members of the team but where specific skills are presented by specialist professions (Masi & Yunus 1991, Burckhardt et al 1994, Bennett et al 1996, Vancouver Consensus group 1996). This type of programme should be patient orientated and return to patients a sense of control over their condition which is often lost in the round of medical consultations and passive therapies.

However, very few patients with chronic pain, which includes those with fibromyalgia, ever make it to chronic pain management clinics or programmes because of a lack of local service provision or financial constraints (Smith et al 1996, Feuerstein & Zastowny 1996). The requirement for skilled practitioners and the increase in demand for pain management programmes suggest that this scarce resource is likely to remain scarce: many practitioners will not have the luxury of referring patients to pain management programmes. It is hoped that these practitioners will find elements of this approach to help them in their own practise.

AIMS OF AN INTERDISCIPLINARY PAIN MANAGEMENT PROGRAMME

There exists a wide diversity in the content and delivery of pain management programmes (Flor et al 1992) which has dogged attempts to identify the elements most effective in bringing about a successful outcome. However, the principles and aims of these programmes remain the same. The Pain Society of Great Britain and Ireland (Pain Society 1997) clarified the overall aim of a pain management programme: 'The aim of a Pain Management programme is to reduce the disability and distress caused by chronic pain by teaching sufferers physical, psychological and practical techniques to improve their quality of life'. Note that the *relief* of pain is not a declared aim of pain management. Although reduction in the level of pain is a desirable outcome from pain management, the focus is on functional improvements.

COGNITIVE BEHAVIOURAL THERAPY

All modern pain management programmes are founded on the principles of cognitive behavioural therapy (CBT). CBT acknowledges that behavioural responses to illness are influenced by both positive and negative reinforcement, one of the tenets of operant behavioural theory. For example if an activity is painful, not engaging in activity may relieve pain in the short term. Such a response is respondent conditioning. If the individual in pain is observed by a solicitous spouse to be in pain when executing a task, the spouse might perform the task instead. Further demonstration of pain-associated behaviour will elicit help from the spouse even in the absence of pain: such is operant conditioning, and it may lead to the relinquishing of activities over time.

CBT also incorporates the view that both cognitive and affective factors influence behaviour. Whether a person re-engages in activity, even though it may cause an increase in pain initially, will be influenced by his perception of what the increase in pain means to him. If patients have an unshakeable belief that pain is an indication of increased harm and damage they are unlikely to relinquish resting as a way of coping. The CBT approach to the management of chronic pain accords well with the Melzack and Walls's (1965) description of the interpretation of pain in which pain and the resultant behaviour are a product of the interaction of nociception, its modulation by other efferent stimuli, and emotional, cognitive and motivational factors.

The objectives of such a programme are chiefly derived from Turk and colleagues (1983), Holzman and colleagues (1986) and Bradley (1996). These objectives (see Box 7.1) originally referred to the management of chronic pain in a behavioural context chiefly by psychologists and have been adapted here to incorporate the work of other professions.

The objectives are achieved through a number of essential components (Turk et al 1983, Bradley 1996, Keefe et al 1996). These are:

- Education
- Skills training
- Skills rehearsal and feedback
- Generalisation of skills taught to everyday situations and novel situations
- Strategies for maintenance and further improvement.

ASSESSMENT FOR PAIN MANAGEMENT

Pain management is a process not an event, and the initial assessment is the start of good patient management. All patients require a thorough assessment of their current status. This should include an assessment of current symptom severity, functional ability through self-report and functional testing, and psychological distress and quality of life evaluation. These form a baseline for planning specific treatments and some measures are repeated at the end of the programme for evaluation of outcome.

Fibromyalgia is a condition that may develop from a previous injury or coexist with other physical condition (e.g. myofascial pain, inflammatory arthritis) (Wolfe et al 1990, Rosen 1994, Wolfe et al 1995). It is therefore essential that any condition amenable to other therapies is identified and addressed. Just as adherents to the medical model may not address the psychosocial issues, the biopsychosocial practitioner must not forget the 'bio' or medical part of the equation. The pain management team has a duty to ensure that the patient's condition has been adequately

---

Box 7.1 Objectives of interdisciplinary pain management

- Assist patients in altering their belief that their problems are unmanageable and beyond their control
- Inform patients about their condition
- Assist patients to move from a passive to an active role in the management of their condition
- Enable patients to become active problem solvers to help them cope with their pain through the development of effective ways of responding to pain, emotion and the environment
- Help patients to monitor thought, emotions and behaviours, and identify how these are influenced by internal and external events
- Give patients a feeling of competence in the execution of positive strategies in the management of their condition
- Help patients to develop a positive attitude to exercise and personal health management
- Help patients to develop a programme of paced activity to reduce the effects of physical deconditioning
- Assist patients to develop coping strategies that can be developed once contact with the pain management team has ended

investigated and, where possible, that appropriate treatments have been used. Performing a full assessment should ensure the patient feels his condition is being taken seriously and fully investigated; this should give him confidence that things have not been missed. Only once these fears are resolved can the patient accept increasing function as an alternative to pain relief. A lack of satisfaction with their care and a perception that their condition is not being taken seriously is often cited as the reason why patients reject orthodox medicine in favour of alternative therapies (Dimmock et al 1997).

Possible exclusions

An assessment should aim to identify possible exclusions to participation in group pain management. These would include major psychiatric or psychological problems (psychotic patients, those with current major depressive illness) or major substance abuse including prescription drugs. These issues need to be addressed before the patient can usefully participate in rehabilitation. The presence of other significant medical problems may preclude participation in an active rehabilitation programme (e.g. major cardiorespiratory disease, severe structural deformity): these patients may be better dealt with on an individual basis.

Participation in ongoing litigation or the receipt of large sums in wages compensation is not a barrier to pain management provided that the patient is aware of the consequences of improved health on their financial position and can demonstrate that they are sufficiently motivated to change despite these consequences.

Barriers to progress

It is important that the assessment identifies barriers to progress which need to be addressed during the programme. Such barriers include:

- Distorted cognitions of the patient and the partner about the nature of their pain and disability
- Dysfunctional beliefs about pain and activity
- Negative expectation about the future

- Affective disorders that may contribute to the experience of pain (e.g. depression and anxiety)
- Patients perception of the control they have over the pain (Keefe et al 1996).

Assessing current activity

Current physical activity and social role and the patterns of activity are assessed. The patient's 'illness' and 'wellness' behaviours are assessed by questioning about the way in which patient and spouse currently behave when the patient is in pain. The amount of 'downtime' – time spent reclining or in inactivity – versus 'uptime' and the amount of time spent engaged in productive or meaningful activity are recorded. Some patients cope with pain by increasing their activity through walking or gentle exercise while others refrain from all exercise and resort to rest and consumption of medication. The pattern of activity can tell the team a lot about the patient's current ability to pace his activity. Activity levels in such patients can often be sporadic and contingent on the level of pain.

Once all the data is gathered, the team is in a position to determine whether the patient is liable to make progress. DiClementi and Proschaskas (1982) developed a 'stages of change' model which is useful to refer to here. In this model those who make successful changes in behaviour go through a number of stages. Those who do not see their current behaviour as a problem which needs to be addressed, or who are unwilling to accept responsibility for change, are described as pre-contemplative – they do not see the need for a change in their behaviour and have little concept of what they can do to change. Once a person sees the need for change he begins to weigh up the advantages, disadvantages and potential costs associated with that change: this is the stage of contemplation. Pre-contemplative individuals are unlikely to make progress in treatments that are designed to change behaviour. Those who are contemplating change need to be helped to move to the next stage of the model, towards preparation. Having identified the need for change, the patient then must start to make plans to change. Attendance on a programme is only one component of this: the patient must also plan to make change in the home and social environment.

Putting these plans into action is the next stage of change where behavioural change is enacted and goals are set. Movement may not be all one way. Patients often relapse into their old behaviours once faced by other stresses and other challenges, which in the case of fibromyalgia may be a flare up of the pain. Clinicians must enable the patient to have the knowledge and skills and develop strategies, not to slide back into old ways.

THE COMPONENTS OF AN INTERDISCIPLINARY PAIN MANAGEMENT PROGRAMME

Education

Education of the patient starts at the first consultation. Initial education in pain management should give the patient information that is required to help him make an informed decision about participating in a programme. It should offer the patient a credible rationale for engaging in pain management. On attendance at assessment for the first time, patients may believe that they are about to embark on another round of medical interventions similar to those they have experienced in the past. It may be quite a shock to find that they are being asked to accept an approach where 'curing' their pain is not to be the focus of treatment.

Both the patients and their partners need to be informed of the results of the initial assessment at a feedback interview. The aims and objectives, the level of commitment required, and the components of a pain management programme should all be made clear. It may not be possible to address all these issues at the initial assessment and many patients require a period of reflection and discussion with their partner and family, with additional information and a review appointment with a member of the pain management team, before they are in a position to make a choice about commencing pain management.

Education as a treatment intervention alone has been demonstrated to be effective in a number of studies into fibromyalgia: it has been used as a control condition for multidisciplinary programmes and has been demonstrated to give clear improvements in the patient group (Goossens et al 1996). However, there is a problem in determining what should go into an educational programme and when an educational programme becomes a cognitive intervention programme. Education is a cognitive event. It is the giving of information which, one hopes, will lead to some behavioural change and the application of that education to relevant situations. Good educational programmes in any walk of life require not only the giving of information from the teacher to the student but also the application and practice of that information with correction, evaluation, feedback and explanation. The descriptions of education only studies in the literature make it difficult to clarify to what extent the educational programmes were 'low grade' cognitive intervention programmes. By contrast, those educational programmes that concentrate on didactic information giving by a teacher cannot be considered to be truly 'educational'.

There is a general agreement on the content of educational components of pain management programmes. Information on the condition itself is thought essential:

- The key features of fibromyalgia
- The prognosis of the condition
- The role of sleep and information about coexisting conditions (e.g. irritable bowel syndrome and fatigue).

A simple guide to pain physiology is a good starting point, particularly when this is linked to the psychosocial influences on the perception of pain and the development of incapacity, including the role of mood and emotion on pain. This can be done through a simple explanation of the factors which 'open' and 'close' the pain gate. It is essential that the patient understands that a multiplicity of factors may influence our perception of pain and that this does not always mean that the condition is worsening.

Separating the link between hurting and harming is vital in fibromyalgia patients. Many will believe that ongoing pain is a symptom of ongoing damage and that an increase in pain is evidence of further damage. If they are to participate in rehabilitation to the full, fibromyalgia patients must be sure that increases in symptoms following mild exercise are a normal bodily response in a deconditioned system.

The way in which others respond to the way the pain patient feels, especially the responses of well-meaning partners and family, helps both patient and family identify reinforcers of incapacity. Ergonomic influences on pain include education and advice about safe lifting and working postures, the identification of good and poor posture, and adjusting work posture and work practices to allow efficiency of movement. The effects of deconditioning and the benefits of exercise and healthy lifestyles are also included.

Didactic teaching has a limited role in the delivery of education. It may be seen as patronising by some patients for a fit and pain-free professional to stand before them telling them what it is like to be in chronic pain. For this very good reason discussion groups and tutorial-based education drawing on the experiences of the group is more appropriate. The participation in the educational sessions of the partner (or at least one family member) is highly desirable.

Goal setting and pacing

Limited physical capacity and lowered pain tolerance restrict function in chronic pain patients. Engaging in activity may exacerbate the pain immediately or for some time after the activity has finished. Although the patient is educated to remain active despite the pain, it is necessary not to precipitate the pain to such an extent that activity has to be limited. Conversely, some patients avoid activity to such an extent that they do not progress and do not achieve improvement.

Pacing exercise has been described by Gil and colleagues (1988) as moderate activity–rest cycling. It is a strategy to enable patients to control exacerbations in pain by learning to regulate activity and, once a regime of paced activity is established, to gradually increase the activity level. The converse of this is the 'overactivity–pain–rest' cycle.

Chronic pain patients often report levels of activity that fluctuate dramatically over time. On questioning at initial assessment they report that they frequently persist at activities until they are prevented from carrying on by the resulting level of pain. This leads them to rest until the pain subsides or until frustration moves them to action, whereupon they then try again until defeated by the increase in pain. How many times have we met the patient who tells us that they do as much as they can on a good day only to suffer for it over the following days? Over time the periods of activity become shorter and those of rest lengthen, disability increases and the individual becomes more anxious and even fearful of activity. The patient may also misattribute the normal muscle aching and stiffness which follows unaccustomed exercise in normal individuals as further injury and damage.

The physiological effects of this are a gradual physical deconditioning of the patient through the avoidance of exercise characterised by reduced strength and aerobic capacity (Bennett et al 1989, Jacobsen et al 1991, Bengtsson et al 1994). Excessive increases in pain following excessive exercise and engendered by post-exertional pain in an unfit individual can also serve to increase excitation of pain receptors in an already sensitive pain system, presumably through secondary central sensitisation (Corderre at al 1993, Mense 1994, Henriksson & Mense 1994, Bennett 1996).

The purpose of goal setting is to regulate daily activities and to structure an increase in activity through the gradual pacing of activity. Activity is paced by timing it or by the introduction of quotas of exercise interspersed by periods of rest or change in activity (Fordyce 1976; Gil et al 1988; Keefe et al 1996).

Goals should be set in three separate domains:

1. Physical, which relates to the exercise programme the patient follows and sets the number of exercises to be performed or the duration of the exercise and the level of difficulty.

2. Functional/task relates to the achievement of functional tasks of everyday living such as housework or hobbies and tasks learned on the programme.

3. Social, where the patient is encouraged to set goals relating to the performance of activities in the wider social environment.

It is important that goals are personally relevant, interesting, measurable and achievable.

The concept of setting goals in pain management is supported by two influential pieces of psychological theory. Locke (1967) suggested that increased task performance was facilitated by the setting of specific, challenging but *attainable* goals. Demotivation and a sense of failure occur if the goals set are unattainable. Bandura (1977) formulated a concept of self-efficacy theory which has been very influential in pain management. In self-efficacy theory, increased performance occurs under two forms of expectation. These are:

- Efficacy expectations, or the belief that one has the personal ability to perform actions that will lead to specific outcomes
- Outcome expectations, or the belief that specific outcomes can be achieved as the result of specific behaviours.

Of these, efficacy expectations may be the most potent determinants of change in pain management. Previous research has demonstrated a close link between increased self-efficacy and good outcome from rehabilitation and pain management with respect to increased activity, increased positive coping and reduced pain behaviour (Bucklew et al 1994, Burckhardt et al 1994).

In the initial stages of the rehabilitation programme, patients may suffer from low self-efficacy. Increases in self-efficacy can be brought about in a number of ways:

1. By information from others, including professionals
2. Through vicarious learning from others
3. By personal experience and practice
4. By physiological arousal – so called 'psyching oneself up' to things.

Of all of these, personal experience and practice are the most influential. Increases in perceived self-efficacy in the performance of any task depend on the patient's perception of his own competence in the performance of that task. Failure to perform a task (total inability to perform an exercise) or incompetent performance of the task (failure to reach the required level of performance, e.g. required number of repetitions) lead to a fall in perceived self-efficacy. Achievement of a task or competence in a task will result in an increase in perceived self-efficacy and a willingness to explore other possibilities (more exercises or a more demanding task). Continued goal attainment will reinforce self-efficacy and lead to a perception of mastery over the task or problem (managing to exercise despite the pain). It is therefore important that goals are set which encourage success but are sufficiently challenging to assure progress.

The setting of goals should be a matter of negotiation between the patient and the therapist. The use of goal-setting charts is essential. Patients set a target for activities each week and record their achievements on the charts. Through this exercise they not only monitor their progress but become more accurate in setting attainable goals.

Physical exercise

The main focus of physical exercise is to redress the effects of prolonged deconditioning (the key aims are given in Box 7.2). Although the long-term effects of deconditioning, decreased fitness, increased weight, joint stiffness and weakness are readily acknowledged by most people with fibromyalgia, the key to compliance with and acceptance of the beneficial effects of exercise is a reduction in the fear of activity.

Exercise should have two major components:

- Stretching to increase soft tissue length and joint mobility
- Aerobic conditioning to increase fitness. Weight-resisted strengthening exercises, although not contraindicated, should be introduced with caution because of the likely effect of an increase in pain.

Stretching and range of motion exercises

It has already been stated that fibromyalgia may have started with an initial injury or condition, or occur with coexisting musculoskeletal problems. Although the pain is widespread, there may be areas where it is greatest. Stretching exercises need to be general to address the general loss of flexibility, and also specific to the individual's needs.

Motion through complete joint range is required to assist in the nutrition of the cartilage of synovial joints, as well as in the maintenance of the length and strength of the soft tissue of the joint, such as the joint capsule and ligaments. Repeated motion through a restricted range results in limitation of joint range through the shortening of such structures and an impoverishment of joint nutrition.

Low impact, full range, free exercises are an elementary component of a warm-up and warm-down programme in most exercise regimes and this is so in pain management programmes. They should be combined with stretching exercises to capitalise on increased range of motion.

There is a wide literature on the performance of stretching exercises and the physiological mechanisms will not be discussed here. There are two main schools of thought on stretching technique:

1. Static/sustained, where the muscle is taken to its limit and the stretch is maintained for at least 5–6 seconds (although many authors suggest longer)
2. Ballistic stretching where dynamic, rhythmic bouncing exercises are performed at the outer range of the muscle.

Exaggerated guarding and increased myostatic stretch reflexes have been identified in those with painful muscles (Corderre et al 1993, Mense 1994). Additionally, psychological factors have been demonstrated to be closely associated with abnormal patterns of muscle activity (Watson et al 1997). Such abnormalities of movement could potentially lead to ineffective stretching and, at worst, injury to the muscle, therefore the ballistic stretching technique is inadvisable. Combining

---

Box 7.2   Objectives of a physical activity programme

- Overcome the effects of deconditioning
- Challenge and reduce patients' fear of engaging in physical activity
- Reduce physical impairment and capitalise on recoverable function
- Increase physical activity in a safe and graded manner
- Help patients to accept responsibility for increasing their functional capacity
- Promote a positive view of physical activity in the self-management of health
- Introduce challenging functional activities to rehabilitation

---

muscle relaxation skills (discussed below) with stretching will increase the effectiveness of the stretch.

Stretching exercises should be performed daily and should form part of a warm-up and warm-down from aerobic exercise sessions. Initially patients may not be able to sustain a stretch for more than a few seconds. Goal setting should encompass increases in the length of time the stretch is maintained as well as the number of stretches performed. Introducing regular stretching into daily work and home routines, especially between different activities and after periods of static work (e.g. reading, typing) is extremely desirable.

Aerobic conditioning

Most of the studies on patients with fibromyalgia have concentrated on the role of aerobic conditioning as a way of improving their condition. Wigers and colleagues (1996) have described an intense aerobic conditioning regime for FMS patients (forty 45-minute sessions over 14 weeks) where patients self-monitored their pulse rates and were instructed to reach a target maximum of 60–70% of age-related heart rate maximum during the programme. Measures at completion of treatment demonstrated significant beneficial changes in pain distribution, dolorimetry scores, depression and physiological work capacity. However, only pain distribution remained significant at 4-year follow-up. Short-term changes in pain perception and report for exercise alone were also described by Martin and colleagues (1996) following an aerobic, flexibility and strength training programme but there were no changes in function or self-efficacy. Burckhardt et al (1994) also combined stretching exercises with aerobic conditioning to effect changes in self-efficacy and physical function in a group of female fibromyalgia sufferers.

Paced walking, stationary exercise cycle, stair walking, a stair climber and non-impact aerobic classes have all been suggested as ways of increasing physical fitness in chronic pain patients (McCain 1988, Bennet 1996, Martin et al 1996, Burckhardt et al 1994, Haldorsen et al 1998, Bennett et al 1996). The exercises should be performed at least three times each week for best effect. Where possible, patients should exercise to 60–70% of aerobic capacity or should pace themselves up to achieve this level of intensity if maximum advantage is to be gained.

Most exercise programmes have reported a reduction in compliance with exercise following programmes (Lewthwaite 1990, Proschaska & Marcus 1994). Wigers and colleagues found that 73% of patients failed to continue an exercise programme when followed up, although 83% felt they would have been better if they had done so. There is no record of whether patient-centred goal setting was part of this research. Compliance with exercise is more likely if the individual finds it interesting and rewarding. Exercising in a gym may not be suitable for all. Some may not have access to such facilities, others may not be motivated by this form of exercise. Developing activities that are patient and family orientated and can be integrated into the normal daily routine will help to improve adherence with exercise. Exercise should become part of life, not an intrusion into it.

Psychological management

Managing anger

By the time that many patients arrive in pain management they will be disabled and have poor social interaction; many express anger. However, this anger may not be overt. Anger develops from attribution of blame, the deviation of the behaviour of another person from an anticipated course or norm which results in an unexpected and undesirable consequence. It may manifest itself in aggression but may also be a passive/aggressive form of anger in which the anger is expressed in non-compliance or lack of engagement in the rehabilitation process (Fernandez & Turk 1995). It is useful for patients to be helped to examine why they have developed this anger and resentment, which is usually related to loss of function and status. In such a situation the anger must be given a release valve but concentrating on the anger is not fruitful and patients must be helped to turn their attention from what they have lost to what they currently have and the gains that they are striving for. In short, they must become future- rather than past-orientated.

In the course of their illness they may have been though a host of ineffective treatments and been given a lot of assurances about the efficacy of these treatments. In addition to this they may have encountered professionals who are, to say the least, sceptical of the diagnosis of fibromyalgia. It may have been suggested, or even stated baldly, that there is nothing wrong with them. Patients are often angry at the medical system and sometimes with good reason. In our own clinic a specific session, taken by a physician, is set aside to discuss the matter of previous medical care. The aim is to try and help the patient understand that many doctors and therapists, when confronted by a distressed patient in a lot of pain, respond emotionally too. They try interventions simply because they wish to help with the tools they have available (drugs, manipulation). Additionally, patients are encouraged to discuss their own treatment history with the medical staff.

Unfortunately the attitudes of some medical and paramedical professions experienced by some patients are very difficult to explain. The important point is that the patients are helped to draw a line under the experience and look towards what they can achieve for the future. In a few cases the anger is so intense that patients may require individual therapy before they are ready to move forwards.

Reducing pain behaviour

Pain behaviours are 'all outputs of the individual that a reasonable observer would characterise as suggesting pain' (Loeser & Fordyce 1983). Most commonly, these are verbal complaints, altered postures and movement, and deviation from normal behaviour (lying down, resting for long periods). Patients are relatively unaware of their demonstration of such behaviour and the effects that it has on other people. Pain behaviours are closely associated not only with pain intensity but also with fear of activity, low self-efficacy and psychological distress (Keefe & Block 1982, Waddell 1992, Bucklew et al 1994, Watson & Poulter 1997).

The most florid pain behaviour is demonstrated during exercise sessions. Operant behavioural theories suggest that the physiotherapist should ignore all pain behaviours and recognise only well behaviours and improved function (Fordyce 1976). This may not be as productive as is often claimed. Patients with fibromyalgia are frequently of the opinion that their condition has not been taken seriously in the past. Well behaviours and achievements should be acknowledged, but simply ignoring pain behaviour without explanation can be counter-productive. An explanation by the therapist that they understand that everyone in the group is in pain, that is why they are there, and it is not useful for them as the therapist to respond to every demonstration of pain from each person in the group – the therapist knows that things are tough but they will never ask the patients to do things that may result in injury. This can do a lot to head off any anger from those who may feel they are being ignored.

As has been mentioned above, family and partners often respond to pain behaviours in a solicitous manner and in doing so unwittingly reinforce the behaviour. This is rarely an overt manipulation by the patient. Asking the patients and the partners to identify the behaviours and their responses to them is useful way of demonstrating the interaction between the expectation of pain, beliefs about pain and their own reactions. Video recording the patients during standardised tasks is an established method of recording pain behaviours (Keefe & Block 1982, Watson & Poulter 1997), but video recording patients during the programme, especially when performing tasks and interacting with others, is also a useful way of confronting patients with their own pain behaviour.

Relaxation

Suffering chronic pain is a stressful experience and fibromyalgia patients often report feeling under stress from factors associated with the pain (poor family relations, guilt, anxiety) and have difficulty in truly relaxing despite feeling fatigued. In addition, people who have muscle pain may increase their muscle tension in response to pain and this may also contribute to pain (Flor & Turk 1989, Watson et al 1998). To help counter this, relaxation is included in many pain management programmes. These is little or no evidence that relaxation alone is useful in widespread muscle pain (Arena & Blanchard 1996) but is a useful adjunct to pain management.

Relaxation in pain management is learning to remain alert and in control while reducing muscle tension and developing a state of emotional calmness. By training in this skill the patients should be able to 'switch' into relaxation after a few minutes of application of the skills. There are a number of approaches to relaxation and patients may have to try more than one until they find the most effective. A combination of these techniques is favoured by many patients. Relaxation can also be augmented with the use of biofeedback but this will not be discussed here.

Progressive muscle relaxation was developed by Jacobsen (1929). In progressive muscle relaxation the patient learns to progressively relax major muscle groups systematically. The method utilises the sensation of tensing the muscles prior to 'letting go' of that tension to achieve relaxation. Through this and self-monitoring of muscle activity by training awareness of tension, patients are able to establish an improved kinaesthetic feedback. Through self-monitoring they become more aware of the situations that led to increased tension and can more effectively monitor and reduce it.

In relaxed imagery relaxation the patient imagines a peaceful and relaxing scene. This could be walking through a forest or lying on a beach. The purpose of this is to chose an image that patients can readily access and rehearse until they are able to bring the image to mind within a few minutes of beginning the relaxation. Imagery is idiosyncratic and each patient has to develop his own strategy with the help of the therapist.

Repeating relaxing phrases over and over is autogenic relaxation. Once again it is useful if patients develop their own phrases but there are lists of standardised phrases for patients to practise this technique (Blanchard & Andrasik 1985). The patient concentrates on the phrase and repeats it quietly to himself while developing a feeling of calmness.

Deep diaphragmatic breathing is one of the most useful techniques and one that is easily incorporated into the techniques above. Many chronic pain patients breathe rapidly and typically utilise primarily the upper chest during the breathing cycle. Using slow, controlled diaphragmatic breathing, the patient progressively reduces his breathing rate until he is breathing at a rate of about 6–8 breaths per minute. The effectiveness of relaxation or breathing control as a therapy in its own right is not established, and it is almost always used as an adjunct to other techniques, although it does give the patient a sense of control over his own body. It is important that patients feel this sense of control to give them a feeling of optimism that they can develop self-management strategies.

Whichever strategy the patients decide to adopt, they should practice relaxation at least twice per day. However, once patients identify those situations which increase stress and tension they require a relaxation strategy that can be used in everyday activities. Keefe et al (1996) suggest the development of a 'brief relaxation method' once the patient is able to achieve a relative state of relaxation. Initially these are performed in sitting and are developed to more demanding situations, eventually leading to their introduction during conversation.

Sleep management

Poor sleep quality is one of the hallmarks of fibromyalgia and is deeply implicated in the development and maintenance of muscle tenderness (Moldofsky 1993, Wolfe et al 1990). These have been managed medically by low dose tricyclic antidepressants, especially amitriptyline and nortriptyline. Advice on sleep management and good sleep hygiene is important to fibromyalgia sufferers. Patients are advised about avoidance of caffeine and alcohol, and about the importance of establishing a routine for good sleep. This can be combined with the skills learned in the relaxation training.

Rehearsal of coping skills

Patients have to identify situations which they find threatening and 'high-risk' where their ability to cope with the pain may be compromised. By identifying possible ways of dealing with stressful situations through role play and problem solving using video or written case studies patients can 'try out' strategies. This may prove difficult for patients as many may have become dependent on others during the development of their disability – a learned helplessness. Learning from other members of the group who have successfully coped with stressful events is an important learning experience. Similarly they can identify unsuccessful coping and how this might be better managed.

Patients find that the pain is less intrusive when they are occupied, distracted and in a positive frame of mind. Identifying those stressors that may compromise their coping strategies and the development of strategies for dealing with these is essential. It is not possible to address these factors here and the reader is directed to other books on the subject (Gatchel & Turk 1996, Phillips & Rachman 1996, Jamison 1996).

Persistent pain leads to the development of negative thoughts which are often self-defeating. Patients may believe that because they are not able to achieve as much as a 'normal' person they are of less worth. They generalise the inability to perform certain tasks into an inability to function in a wider social context. Catastrophic thinking styles evolve and in turn can lead to a feeling of helplessness and hopelessness (Flor et al 1993). These thoughts undermine the individual's confidence and result in depression, which in turn affects the perception of pain. Patients are made aware of this reaction and are encouraged to identify when they are making these bleak overgeneralisations, to replace them with more accurate statements, and to identify which thoughts lead to positive actions which help them manage their condition and which may lead to inactivity and depression. Patients focus on current achievements and progress towards goals rather than measuring their progress by past (prefibromyalgia) levels of activity and interaction.

Prolonged adoption of a reduced social role and the relinquishing of tasks to other family members result in changed roles and responsibilities. Patients may find it difficult to regain roles lost to other family members and may have to reassert themselves back into their former roles and to resume tasks. Assertiveness training may be required in some people to allow them to reclaim their role without risking confrontation. Assertiveness is a skill of particular importance in developing a good relationship with, and getting the best from, doctors and other health professionals.

Homework tasks are set for patients to reinforce learning. This is often in the form of case history examples: patients have to read these, identify such factors as barriers to change and strategies to overcome these, and prepare their responses for their next attendance on the programme. They are encouraged to work through them with their family members to help educate them about pain management. Homework also includes getting the patient to identify problems at home. These can be problems with functional tasks or, more challenging, problems with relationships. Homework assignments place the pain management process into a personal framework for the patient.

Relapse self-management

It is almost inevitable that fibromyalgia patients will, at some stage, experience a flare-up of their pain and a relapse in their condition. During the programme they should imagine situations that might make them prone to relapse. Fibromyalgia patients are just as liable to strains, pulled muscles and injuries as the rest of the population once they become active.

Relapse may not be entirely caused by an individual physical event. The build-up of daily stresses may produce challenges to patients' daily coping resources and their ability to manage their pain. Differentiating what is a new pain, associated with new pathology, and their usual fibromyalgia pain is essential. They need to be informed about drug usage during flare-ups and how to 'manage' their physician or other therapists to give them appropriate treatment for any new condition without compromising their own self-management strategies. The development of an 'emergency card' in collaboration with their family and partner can be useful in these situations. This is a written plan of how they will deal with increases in pain and/or new pathology. This includes developing criteria for visiting their physician, the taking of medication, relaxation, rest and pacing activity and returning to normal activity as soon as possible. This of course cannot cover all eventualities but helps the patient to retain a feeling of control.

From time to time practitioners may encounter patients who have completed pain management programmes but who may turn to them in times of increased pain, requiring help to manage the flare-up. Patients with fibromyalgia are just as prone to minor injury as the rest of us and probably more so if they become more active. It is essential that therapists who are not experienced in pain management, but to whom the patient might turn as a source of short-term symptomatic relief, do not unwittingly encourage patients back into a round of treatment interventions which threaten their sense of self-control and their self-management programme.

The first approach is to reassure the patient that the increase in pain is not a sign of a worsening of the condition or an inevitable decline, but that it is part of the natural variation in the pain pattern (as is almost invariably the case). An increase in pain should not be taken by the patient as failure or evidence of an inability to manage his own condition. It is a challenge to self-management not the end of it. Reassurance on these points and getting patients to identify how successful they have been thus far can help 'rescue' them at this stage. If new pathology is identified then the management of this must be incorporated into the patient's own self-management. Control for the management of the new problem should be developed with the patient where possible, and the benign nature of musculoskeletal pain must be communicated.

Although resolution of fibromyalgia symptoms has been reported (Granges et al 1994), it is disingenuous of practitioners to suggest to fibromyalgia patients that they are able to cure the condition through their (the practitioner's) own approach. If any specific treatment is clearly indicated (e.g. manipulation, mobilisations, trigger point therapy) it must be time-limited and should be presented to the patient as a short-term measure to assist him over the crisis and to support him in getting back on track in his self-management programme (Vancouver Fibromyalgia Consensus Group 1996). It is totally inappropriate to foster dependency through encouraging repeated consultations. This is very unlikely to be in the patient's best clinical or financial interest but it may serve the practitioner.

The practitioner should question patients about their self-management strategies, and particularly about their emergency relapse self-management programme if they developed one while on pain management. The focus of management is assisting the patient to implement this. Where possible, advice should be sought from the pain management programme that the patient attended, and the opportunity of joint management should be discussed. In any event, resumption of a graded exercise programme is to be encouraged early on, with appropriate attention to pacing and goal setting.

Most evidence points to the unfortunate fact that those with fibromyalgia will have it for a long time, and possibly for life. Although a greater understanding of the problem will hopefully provide better treatments in the future, currently we do not have a 'cure' for the problem. Management of the symptoms of fibromyalgia is not the same as rehabilitation and will not solve the wider issues of incapacity associated with this condition. All practitioners have a duty to assist patients to continue an independent lifestyle as much as possible. This should also mean a life free from further ineffective investigations and treatments. We must ensure that patients remain in control of their lives and of the management of their condition.

Box 7.3 Biochemistry, the mind and fibromyalgia syndrome (see also Figs. 4.5 and 4.6)
Leon Chaitow

In this chapter cognitive behaviour modification methods are detailed by Paul Watson, who has specialised in treating chronic pain in general and fibromyalgia in particular using these approaches. This section offers another viewpoint, that of Dr Jay A. Goldstein, who has mapped this controversial territory from his unique perspective (Goldstein 1996). (See also Box 7.4, which summarises other research findings.) Goldstein defines CFS/FMS as *neurosomatic* disorders, quoting Yunus (1994) on the fact that they are 'the commonest group of illnesses for which patients consult physicians'.

- Goldstein believes these disorders to emerge from biochemical imbalances within the neural network.

- He administers multiple medications to try to exert normalising effects, with claims of a high success rate.

- Neurosomatic disorders are illnesses which Goldstein suggests are caused by 'a complex interaction of genetic, developmental and environmental factors', often involving the possibility of early physical, sexual or psychological abuse (Fry 1993).

- Symptoms emerge as a result of 'impaired sensory information processing' by the neural network (including the brain). He clarifies this by saying, 'actually processing occurs properly, but "gating", the control of data input and output from processing centers, is dysfunctional'.

- Examples given are of light touch being painful, mild odours producing nausea, walking a short distance being exhausting, climbing stairs being like going up a mountain, reading something light causing cognitive impairment – all of which examples are true for many people with CFS/FMS.

- Some of the key biochemical aspects of this misprocessing (resulting from genetic, developmental and environmental factors, see below) include:
  a. insufficient glutamate, an exitatory amino acid, which leads to
  b. decreased levels of NE (norepinephrine which is responsible for enhancing the processing of sensory input). When low NE levels occur 'much sensory input will reach the cerebral cortex, some of it irrelevant', leading to misperception and distractibility in stimulus situations.
  c. When NE is low, substance P levels will be high, further lowering the threshold for 'irrelevant' stimuli reaching the brain (including pain messages).

- Goldstein is highly critical of psychological approaches to treatment of these conditions, apart from cognitive behaviour therapy (see this chapter), which he suggests 'may be more appropriate, since coping with the vicissitudes of these illnesses, which wax and wane unpredictably, is a major problem for most of those afflicted'.

- He claims that most major medical journals concerned with psychosomatic medicine rarely discuss neurobiology and 'apply the concept of somatization to virtually every topic between their covers'.

The four basic influences on neurosomatic illness are, he states:

1. Genetic susceptibility, which can be strong or weak. If strong, the individual will develop a neurosomatic illness almost inevitably, often in childhood. If only a weak tendency exists, other factors are needed to influence the trait (Hudson et al 1992).
2. If a child feels unsafe between birth and puberty hypervigilance may develop and interpretation of sensory input will alter. The neurochemical expression of this may lead to, 'elevated levels of SP [substance P] enabling him to attend to a wide range of stimuli, as well as transiently elevated cortisol with subsequent down-regulation of the HPA [hypothalamic–pituitary–adrenal] axis. Central NE [norepinephrine] levels would also be low, contributing to disautonomia as well as abnormalities in sensory processing in the circuit between the dorsolateral prefrontal cortex, thalamus and the hippocampus.'
3. Genetically predetermined susceptibility to viral infection affecting the neurons and glia: 'Persistent CNS viral infections could alter production of transmitters as well as cellular mechanisms'.
4. Increased susceptibility to environmental stressors due to reduction in neural plasticity (resulting from all or any of the causes listed in 1,2,and 3 above). This might include deficiency in glutamate of nitric oxide secretions which results in encoding new memory. 'Neural plasticity' capacity may be easily overtaxed in such individuals which, Goldstein suggests, is why neurosomatic patients often develop their problems after a degree of increased exposure to environmental stressors such as acute infection, sustained attention, exercise, immunization, emergence from anaesthesia, trauma, etc.

Goldstein also describes the limbic system and its dysregulation:

- The limbic system acts as a regulator (integrative processing) in the brain with effects on fatigue, pain, sleep, memory, attention, weight, appetite, libido, respiration, temperature, blood pressure, mood, immune and endocrine function.

- Limbic function dysregulation influences all or any of these functions and systems.

- Regulation of autonomic control of respiration derives from the limbic system; major abnormalities in breathing function (hyperventilation tendencies, irregularity in tidal volume, etc.) are noted in people with chronic fatigue syndrome, along with abnormal responses to exercise (including failure to find expected levels of cortisol increase, catecholamines, growth hormone and somatostatin, increased core temperature, etc.) (Gerra et al 1993, Goldstein & Daly 1993, Griep et al 1993, Munschauer 1991).

- Dysfunction of the limbic system can result from central or peripheral influences ('stress'). Sensory gating (the weight given to sensory inputs) has been shown to be less effectively inhibited in women than in men (Swerdlow et al 1993).

Box 7.3 (Contd.)   Biochemistry, the mind and fibromyalgia syndrome

• Many biochemical imbalances are involved in limbic dysfunction and no attempt will be made in this summary to comprehensively detail these; however, Goldstein lists viral and early developmental influences as possible triggers (see discussion of allostasis in Ch. 2, Fig. 2.3C).

• The trigeminal nerve, states Goldstein, modulates limbic regulation: 'The trigeminal nerve may produce expansion of the receptive field zones of wide dynamic range neurons and nociceptive-specific neurons under certain conditions, perhaps involving increased secretion of substance P, so that a greater number of neurons will be activated by stimulation of a receptive zone, causing innocuous stimuli to be perceived as painful' (Dubner 1992).

• Goldstein reports that nitric oxide, which is a primary vasodilator in the brain, has profound influences on glutamate secretion, and the neurotransmitters which influence short-term memory (Sandman et al 1993), anxiety (Jones et al 1994), dopamine release (Hanbauer et al 1992) (so affecting fatigue), descending pain inhibition processes, sleep induction, and even menstrual problems: 'Female patients with CFS/FMS usually have premenstrual exacerbations of their symptoms. Most of the symptoms of late luteal phase dysphoric disorder are similar to those of CFS, and it is likely that this disorder has a limbic aetiology similar to CFS/FMS' (Iadecola et al 1993).

Allostasis is a major feature of Goldstein's model. He reports that:

• Approximately 40% of FMS/CFS patients screened have been shown to have been physically, psychologically or sexually abused in childhood (Teicher et al 1993).

• By testing for brain electricity imbalances, using brain electricity activity mapping (BEAM) techniques, Goldstein has been able to demonstrate abnormalities in the left temporal area, a feature of people who have been physically, psychologically or sexually abused in childhood (as compared with nonabused controls).

• Major childhood stress, he reports, increases cortisol levels which can affect hippocampal function and structure (Sapolsky et al 1990, McEwan 1994).

• It seems that early experience and environmental stimuli interacting with undeveloped biological systems lead to altered homeostatic responses, 'for example exaggerated or insufficient HPA axis responses to defend a homeostatic state in a stressful situation could result in behavioural and neuro-immunoendocrine disorders in adulthood, particularly if stimuli that should be nonstressful were evaluated ... inappropriately by the prefrontal cortex' (Meaney et al 1994).

Sapolsky has studied this area of 'allostasis' (regulation of internal milieu through dynamic change in a number of hormonal and physical variables that are not in a steady state condition) and identifies as a primary feature a sense of lack of control. In studies of this topic,

CFS/FMS patients are found to predominantly attribute their symptoms to external factors (virus, etc.) while control subjects (depressives) usually experience inward attribution (Powell et al 1990). Sapolsky also identifies a sense of lack of predictability and various other stressors which influence the HPA axis and which are less 'balanced' in individuals with CFS/FMS; all these stressors involve 'marked absence of control, predictability, or outlets for frustration'.

Allostatic load, in contrast to homeostatic mechanisms which stabilise deviations in normal variables, is 'the price the body pays for containing the effects of arousing stimuli and the expectation of negative consequences' (Schulkin et al 1994). Chronic negative expectations and subsequent arousal seem to increase allostatic load. This is characterised by anxiety and anticipation of adversity leading to elevated stress hormone levels (Sterling et al 1981).

Goldstein attempts to explain the immensely complex biochemical and neural interactions which are involved in this scenario, embracing areas of the brain such as the amygdala, the prefrontal cortex, the lower brainstem, and other sites, as well as miriad secretions including hormones (including glucocorticoids), neurotransmitters, substance P, dopamine and nitric oxide. Finally, he states, prefrontal cortex function can be altered by numerous triggering agents in the predisposed individual (possibly involving genetic features or early trauma) including:

• 'viral infections that alter neuronal function'
• 'immunizations that deplete biogenic amines' (Gardier et al 1994)
• 'organophosphate or hydrocarbon exposure'
• 'head injury'
• 'childbirth'
• 'electromagnetic fields'
• 'sleep deprivation'
• 'general anaesthesia'
• 'stress' e.g. 'physical' such as marathon running, or 'mental or emotional'.

What Goldstein is reporting is an altered neurohumoral response in individuals whose defence and repair systems are predisposed to this happening, either because of inherited tendencies or because of early developmental (physical or psychological) insult(s), to which additional multiple stressors have been added. His solution is a biochemical (drug) modification of the imbalances he identifies as key features of this situation.

Alternative approaches might attempt to modify behaviour (see this chapter) or to alter other aspects of the complex disturbances, possibly using nutritional approaches. Goldstein has offered us insights and his own solutions.

Not everyone will necessarily accept these solutions but the illumination of the highly complicated mechanisms involved which he offers is to be commended.

Box 7.4 The mind and fibromyalgia syndrome: additional research findings
Leon Chaitow

Box 7.3. summarised the work of Dr Jay Goldstein, which points towards major biochemical disturbances involving key brain areas, with influences capable of producing all of the symptoms of CFS/FMS. In this summary of other research findings additional opinions are offered, with varying conclusions being drawn:

- Canadian research has examined the relationship between emotional factors, muscle activity, psychological stress and the occurrence of fibromyalgia and myofascial pain. The conclusion is that chronic muscular pain is not a life stress syndrome and has to be understood in terms of organic disorders which are aggravated by psychological factors. The psychological changes which occur as a *result* of severe, chronic, muscle pain, however, require appropriate psychological treatment (Merskey 1993).

- A Swedish study has evaluated the question, does a fibromyalgia personality exist? 155 women with FMS completed a questionnaire which analyses personality traits. The traits which were most obviously different in FMS women were a need for order and a low need for exhibition, autonomy and aggressive non-conformance. 'FMS patients are pedantic and have great needs for order, perfectionism, planning and cleanliness. There was no evidence of a greater tendency towards developing depression' (Johannsson 1993).

- Physical exercise (cardiovascular training) as well as low level antidepressant medication have both been shown to offer benefits to people with FMS. A study conducted in Finland evaluated the benefits of combined antidepressant medication and exercise therapy in treatment of FMS. The results indicated that a combined protocol was more beneficial than either the exercise or the medication alone. 'Although low levels of amitriptyline has only minor antidepressive effects, it may improve the quality of sleep and correct aberrations of serotonin in the brain stem. This may raise spirits, as does physical training, by causing post-exercise hypoalgesia through increased endogenous opioids in the brain. It is known that physical training is able to alleviate depression and to improve the quality of sleep' (Isomeri et al 1993).

- Dutch research attempted to determine whether a combined psychological and behavioural therapy protocol (psychomotor and marital counselling) was useful in treating fibromyalgia patients (50 treated, 50 untreated as controls). There was a high drop-out rate (33%) and although many patients reported improvements in their ability to deal with their disabilities the researchers could not confirm these reports: 'There was no significant differences compared to the non-treatment controls.' There was no reduction of pain or other physical complaints (de Voogd et al 1993).

- Don Goldenberg MD, professor of medicine at Tufts University School of Medicine, has reviewed the literature and concludes that: 'fibromyalgia is not a psychiatric illness. A subset of patients may have major depression and there is evidence that stress may play an important role in fibromyalgia. Depression may be a biologic marker for fibromyalgia in some families with a spectrum of "affective disorders" ' (Goldenberg 1994). Among the more specific conclusions Goldenberg includes the following:

1. Most patients with FMS do not have psychiatric illness
2. There is no correlation of the core FMS symptoms or treatment response with psychological factors
3. There may be a greater lifetime history and family history of depression in FMS compared with rheumatoid arthritis and normal controls
4. There may be greater levels of daily stress in FMS than in rheumatoid arthritis.

- Behaviour modification as a treatment option in FMS was evaluated at the school of medicine of the University of Missouri. The conclusion was that: 'behavioural theory can be used to understand some of the patterns associated with pain [and that] behavioural treatment suggestions and cognitive behavioural treatment programs provide options for improving the quality of life associated with fibromyalgia' (Buckelew 1994; and see this chapter).

- Mohammed Yunus MD, professor of medicine at the University of Illinois and a leading researcher into the care of fibromyalgia syndrome, is definite in his conclusion that, 'Presently available data indicate that FMS is not a psychiatric condition.' He notes that between 25% and 35% of FMS patients seen at rheumatology clinics have significant psychological problems but that the proportion of such patients seen in primary care settings is lower and that it is because of referral bias that a high number end up at specialist clinics. He is clear that psychological abnormalities are not necessary for the emergence of FMS; however, he cautions that some patients with psychological distress may be more difficult to manage in treating their pain and fatigue (Yunus 1994).

- Researchers compared the clinical and psychological features of patients with widespread chronic musculoskeletal pain (WCMP) and patients with fibromyalgia (FMS). The conclusions arrived at were that the clinical and psychological features of the two groups were similar and were also similar to patients with osteoarticular diseases. They believe that FMS should be considered an advanced clinical stage of a continuum of widespread musculoskeletal pain, and not a psychological condition (Moral et al 1997).

- There is much clinical support for the hypothesis that most depression and anxiety associated with FMS is a result rather than a cause of the condition (Mason et al 1991, and that fibromyalgia and depression may be caused by a common underlying set of factors (Kate 1997).

REFERENCES

Arena J G, Blanchard E B 1996 Biofeedback and relaxation therapy for chronic pain disorders. In: Gatchel R J, Turk D C (eds) Psychological approaches to pain management. Guildford Press, New York

Bandura A 1977 Self-efficacy: towards a unifying theory of behavioral change. Psychological Review 84: 191–215

Bengtsson A, Backman E, Lindblom B, Skogh T 1994 Long term follow-up of fibromyalgia patients: clinical symptoms, muscular function, laboratory tests – an eight year comparison study. Journal of Musculoskeletal Pain 2: 67–80

Bennett R M 1996 Multidisciplinary group treatment programmes to treat fibromyalgia patients. Rheumatic Diseases Clinics of North America 22(2): 351–367

Bennett R M, Clarke S R, Goldberg L et al 1989 Aerobic fitness in patients with fibrositis. A controlled study of respiratory gas exchange and ^{133}xenon clearance from exercising muscle. Arthritis and Rheumatism 32(10): 1113–1116

Bennett R M, Burkhardt C S, Clarke S R, O'Reilly C, Weins S N, Campbell S M 1996 Group treatment of fibromyalgia: a 6 month outpatient programme. Journal of Rheumatology 23: 521–528

Blanchard E B, Andrasik F 1985 Management of chronic headache: a psychological approach. Pergamon Press, New York

Bradley L A 1996 Cognitive therapy for chronic pain. In: Gatchel R J, Turk D C (eds) Psychological approaches to pain management. Guildford Press, New York, ch 6, pp 131–147

Buckelew S 1994 Behavioural interventions and fibromyalgia. Journal of Musculoskeletal Pain 2(3): 153–161

Bucklew S P, Parker J C, Keefe F J et al 1994 Self efficacy and pain behavior among subjects with fibromyalgia. Pain 59: 377–384

Burckhardt C S, Mannerkorpi K, Hedenberg L, Bjelle A 1994 A randomised, controlled trial of education and physical training for women with fibromyalgia. Journal of Rheumatology 21: 714–720

Corderre J T, Katz J, Vaccarino A I, Melzack R 1993 Contribution of central neuroplasticity to pathological pain: review of clinical and experimental evidence. Pain 52: 259–285

de Voogd J et al 1993 Treatment of fibromyalgia syndrome with psychomotor therapy and marital counselling. Journal of Musculoskeletal Pain 1(3/4): 273–281

DiClementi C C, Proschaskas J O 1982 Self change and therapy change of smoking behavior: a comparison of processes in cessation and maintenance. Addictive Behaviors 7: 133–144

Dimmock S, Troughton P R, Bird H A 1997 Factors predisposing to the resort to complementary therapies in patients with fibromyalgia. Clinical Rheumatology 15(5): 478–482

Dubner R 1992 Hyperalgesia and expanded receptive fields. Pain 48: 3–4

Fernandez E, Turk D C 1995 The scope and significance of anger in chronic pain. Pain 61: 165–175

Feuerstein M, Zastowny T R 1996 Occupational rehabilitation: multidisciplinary management of work related musculoskeletal pain and disability. In: Gatchel R J, Turk D C (eds) Psychological approaches to pain management. Guildford Press, New York, pp 458–585

Flor H, Turk C 1989 Psychophysiology of chronic pain: do chronic pain patients exhibit symptom-specific psychophysiological responses. Psychological Bulletin 105: 215–259

Flor H, Behle D, Birnbaumer N 1993 Assesment of pain related cognitions in chronic pain patients. Behavior Research and Therapy 31: 63–73

Flor H, Fydrich T, Turk D C 1992 Efficacy of multidisciplinary pain treatment centres: a meta analytic review. Pain 49: 221–230

Fordyce W E 1976 Behavioural methods for chronic pain and illness. CV Mosby, St Louis

Fry R 1993 Adult physical illness and childhood sexual abuse. Journal of Psychosomatic Research 37(2): 89–103

Gatchel R J, Turk D C (eds) Psychological approaches to pain management: a practitioner's handbook. Guildford Press, New York

Gerra G et al 1993 Noradrenergic and hormonal responses to physical exercise in adolescents. Neuropsychobiology 27(2): 65–71

Gill K M, Ross S L, Keefe F J 1988 Behavioural treatment of chronic pain: four pain management protocols. In: France R D, Krishnan K R R (eds) Chronic pain. American Psychiatric Press, Washington, pp 317–413

Goldenberg D 1994 Psychiatric illness and fibromyalgia. Journal of Musculoskeletal Pain 2(3): 41–49

Goldstein J, Daly J 1993 Neuroimmunoendocrine findings in CFS before and after exercise. Cited in: Chronic fatigue syndrome: the limbic hypothesis. Haworth Press, Binghampton, NY

Goossens M E, Rutten-van-Molken M P, Leidl R M, Bos S G, Vlaeyen J W, Teeken-Gruben N J 1996 Cognitive educational treatment of fibromyalgia: a randomised clinical trial. II. Economic evaluation. Journal of Rheumatology 23(7): 1246–1254

Granges G, Zilko P, Littlejohn G O 1994 Fibromyalgia syndrome – assessment of the severity of the condition 2 years after diagnosis. Journal of Rheumatology 21: 523–529

Griep E et al 1993 Altered reactivity of the hypothalamic–pituitary–adrenal axis in primary fibromyalgia syndrome. Journal of Rheumatolgy 20: 469–474

Haldorsson E M H, Kronholm K, Skounen J S, Ursin H 1998 Multimodal cognitive behavioural treatment of patients sicklisted for musculoskeletal pain: a randomised controlled study. Scandinavian Journal of Rheumatolgy 27: 16–25

Hanbauer I et al 1992 Role of nitric oxide in NMDA-evoked release of [^{3}H]dopamine from striatal slices. NeuroReports 3(5): 409–412

Hudson J et al 1992 Comorbidity of fibromyalgia with medical and psychiatric isorders. American Journal of Medicine 92(4): 363–367

Iadecola C et al 1993 Localization of NAPDH diaphorase in neurons in rostral ventral medulla: possible role of nitric oxide in central autonomic regulations and chemoreception. Brain Research 603: 173–179

Isomeri R, Mikkelson M, Latikka P, Kammonen K 1993 Effects of amitriptyline and cardiovascular fitness training on pain patients with primary fibromyalgia. Journal of Musculoskeletal Pain 1(3/4): 253–260

Jacobsen E 1929 Progressive relaxation. University of Chicago Press, Chicago

Jacobsen S, Wildshiodtz G, Danneskiold-Samsoe B 1991 Isokinetic and isometric muscle strength combined with transcutaneous electrical muscle stimulation in primary fibromyalgia. Journal of Rheumatology 18(9): 1390–1393

Jamison R N 1996 Mastering chronic pain: a professional's guide to behavioral treatment. Professional Resource Press, Sarasota, FA

Johannsson V 1993 Does a fibromyalgia personality exist? Journal of Musculoskeletal Pain 1(3/4): 245–252

Jones N, Loiacono R, Moller M, Beart P 1994 Diverse roles for nitric oxide in synaptic signalling after activation of NMDA release-regulating receptors. Neuropharmacology 33: 1351–1356

Kate R 1997 Fibromyalgia, depression and alcoholism. Clinical Bulletin of Myofascial Therapy 2(1): 84

Keefe F J, Block A R 1982 Development of an observational method for assessing pain behavior in chronic low back pain. Behavior Therapy 13: 363–375

Keefe F J, Beaupe P M, Gil K M 1996 Group therapy for patients with chronic pain. In: Gatchel R J, Turk D C (eds) Psychological approaches to pain management. Guildford Press, New York

Lewthwaite R 1990 Motivational considerations in physical therapy involvement. Physical Therapy 70(12): 808–819

Lock E A 1967 Towards a theory of task motivation incentives. Organisational Behavior and Human Performance 3: 157–189

Loeser J D, Fordyce W E 1983 Chronic pain. In: Carr J E, Dengerik H A (eds) Behavioural science in the practise of medicine. Elsevier, Amsterdam

McCain G A, Bell D A, Mai F M, Halliday P D 1988 A controlled syudy of the effects of a supervised cardiovascular fitness training program on the manifestations of primary fibromyalgia. Arthritis and Rheumatism 31: 1535–1542

McEwan B 1994 The plasticity of the hippocampus is the reason for its vulnerability. Seminal Neuroscience 6: 239–246

Martin L, Nutting A, Macintosh B R, Edsworthy S M, Butterwick D, Cook J 1996 An exercise program in the treatment of fibromyalgia. Journal of Rheumatology 23(6): 1050–1053

Masi R, Yunus M B 1991 Fibromyalgia – which is the best treatment? A personalized, comprehensive, ambulatory, patient-involved management programme. Baillères Clinical Rheumatology 4(2): 333–370

Mason J et al 1991 Fibromyalgia impact assessment form. Arthritis Care Resident 4: 523

Meaney M, Tannenbaum B, Francis D et al 1994 Early environmental programming of hypothalamic–pituitary–adrenal responses to stress. Seminal Neuroscience 6: 247–259 1994

Melzack R, Wall P D 1965 Pain mechanisms: a new theory. Science 50: 971–979

Mense S 1994 Referral of muscle pain: new aspects. American Pain Society Journal 3(1): 1–9

Merskey H 1993 Chronic muscular pain – a life stress syndrome? Journal of Musculoskeletal Pain 1(3/4): 61–69

Moldofsky H 1993 Fibromyalgia, sleep disorder and chronic fatigue syndrome. In: Block G R, Whelan J (eds) Chronic fatigue syndrome. Wiley, Chichester, pp 262–279

Moral R et al 1997 Bio-psychological features of patients with widespread chronic musculoskeletal pain in family medicine clinics. Family Practice 14(3): 242–248

Munschauer F, Mador M, Ahuja A, Jacobs L 1991 Selective paralysis of voluntary but not limbically influenced autonomic respirations. Archives of Neurology 48: 1190–1192

Pain Society 1997 Report of a working party of the Pain Society of Great Britain and Ireland: desirable criteria for pain management programmes. Pain Society, London

Philips H C, Rachman S 1996 The psychological management of chronic pain: a treatment manual, 2nd edn. Springer, New York

Powell R, Dolan R, Wessely S 1990 Attributions and self-esteem in depression and chronic fatigue syndromes. Journal of Pyschosomatic Research 14(6): 665–671

Proschaska J O, Marcus B H 1994 The transtheoretical model: applications to exercise. In: Dishman R K Advances in exercise adherence. Human Kinetics, New York, pp 161–180

Rosen N B 1994 Physical medicine and rehabilitation approaches to the management of myofascial pain and fibromyalgia. Baillères Clinical Rheumatology 8(4): 881–916

Sandman C, Barron J, Nackoul K, Goldstein J, Fidler F 1993 Memory deficits associated with chronic fatigue immune dysfunction syndrome (CFIDS). Biological Psychiatry 33: 618–623

Sapolsky R, Uno H, Rebert C, Finch C 1990 Hippocampal damage associated with prolonged glucocorticoid exposure in primates. Journal of Neuroscience 10: 2897–2902

Schulkin J, McEwan B, Gold P 1994 Allostasis, amygdala and anticipatory angst. Neuroscience Biobehavioural Review 18(3): 385–396

Smith B, Chambers W, Smith W 1996 Chronic pain: time for epidemiology. Journal of the Royal Society of Medicine 89: 181–183

Sterling P, Eyer J 1981 Allostasis: a new paradigm to explain arousal pathology. In: Fisher S, Reason H (eds) Handbook of life stress, cognition and health. John Wiley and Sons, New York

Swerdlow N, Auerbach P, Monroe S et al 1993 Men are more inhibited than women by weak prepulses. Biological Psychiatry 34:253–260

Teicher M, Glad G, Surrey J, Swett C 1993 Early childhood abuse and limbic system ratings in adult psychiatric outpatients. Journal of Neuropsychiatry and Clinical Neuroscience 5(3): 301–306

Turk D C, Michenbaum D H, Genest M 1983 Pain and behavioural medicine: a cognitive behavioural perspective. Guildford Press, New York

Turk D C, Okifuji A, Sinclair J D, Starz T W 1996 Pain, disability and physical functioning in subgroups of patients with fibromyalgia. Journal of Rheumatology 23(7): 1255–1262

Vancouver Fibromyalgia Consensus Group 1996 The fibromyalgia syndrome: a consensus report on fibromyalgia and disability. Journal of Rheumatology 23(7): 1237–1245

Waddell G 1987 A new clinical model for the treatment of low back pain. Spine 12: 632–644

Waddell G 1992 Biopsychosocial analysis of low back pain. Baillères Clinical Rheumatology 6(3): 523–557

Watson P J, Poulter M E 1997 The development of a functional task orientated measure of pain behaviour in chronic low back pain patients. Journal of Back and Musculoskeletal Rehabilitation 9: 57–59

Watson P J, Booker C K, Main C J 1997 Evidence for the role of psychological factors in abnormal paraspinal activity in patients with chronic low back pain. Journal of Musculoskeletal Pain 5(4): 41–55

Watson P J, Chen A C N, Booker C K, Main C J, Jones A K P 1998 Differential electromyographic response to experimental cold pressor test in chronic low back pain patients and normal controls. Journal of Musculoskeletal Pain 6(2): 51–64

White K P, Harth M 1996 An analytical review of 24 controlled trials for fibromyalgia syndrome (FMS). Pain 64: 211–219

Wigers S H, Stiles T C, Vogel P A 1996 Effects of aerobic exercise versus stress management treatment in fibromyalgia: a 4.5 year prospective study. Scandinavian Journal of Rheumatology 25: 77–86

Wolfe F, Smythe H A, Yunus M B et al 1990 The American College of Rheumatology 1990. Criteria for the classification of fibromyalgia: report of the multi-centre criteria committee. Arthritis and Rheumatism 33: 160–172

Wolfe F, Aarflot T, Brusgaard D, Henriksson K G et al 1995 Fibromyalgia and disability. Report of the Moss international working group on medico-legal aspects of chronic widespread musculoskeletal pain and fibromyalgia. Scandinavian Journal of Rheumatology 24: 112–118

Yunus M 1994a Psychological aspects of fibromyalgia syndrome. In: Masi A (ed) Fibromyalgia and myofascial pain syndromes. Ballière, London

Yunus M 1994b Psychological factors in fibromyalgia syndrome – an overview. Journal of Musculoskeletal Pain 2(1): 87–91

8

A medical perspective on fibromyalgia

Regina P. Gilliland

Fibromyalgia is not a neutral topic within the medical community. Physicians especially are not apathetic where this diagnosis is concerned, and usually belong to one of two groups. The first group includes those physicians who want nothing to do with fibromyalgia patients, and treat them only grudgingly. The second group includes those physicians who are active participants in the care of these patients. Although many physicians now at least believe in the existence of fibromyalgia, they often feel inadequately prepared to manage the complex issues associated with the condition. This is not surprising, since caring for these patients can be a daunting task. Most physicians are extremely knowledgeable and highly trained individuals, intimately familiar with, and capable of managing complex medical issues. So why do so many skilled physicians avoid dealing with fibromyalgia patients? Certainly, it is not for a dearth of excellent, credible, and readily available information. The answer lies partly in the reductionistic medical model taught in today's medical schools. Students study the human body from an unnatural perspective, as individual, independent organ systems. Furthermore, the diseases of these systems are investigated and treated as isolated units. In reality, the human body functions as a highly interrelated unit of communicating systems. The body is indivisible from the mind. Thus, the reductionistic model sees a container with fragmented, malfunctioning biologic parts, rather than a sick, distressed human being. Physicians have traded healing and caring for treating and managing and replaced attentive listening with sophisticated technology. We search for answers to our patients' complaints using the magic of technology rather than by taking a careful history and making a thorough examination. Fibromyalgia is not a disorder diagnosed by expensive medical technology, nor is it fixed with modern medical wizardry. The foundation of the healing of the fibromyalgia patient is a compassionate, caring physician (Lown 1996).

This chapter explores the art of healing and the paradigm shift that physicians must make in order to return to a doctor–patient relationship that promotes healing. An in-depth look at the initial history, physical examination and treatment discussion will provide today's physician with a step-by-step guide to developing a unique approach to caring successfully for the fibromyalgia patient. Finally, I have included a summary of the protocol that I have used successfully with fibromyalgia patients (see Box 8.1).

A RETURN TO THE ART OF HEALING

Physicians must accept a new paradigm if they are adequately to meet this challenge. The shift is towards medicine with a human face. According to Dr Bernard Lown, in his book *The Lost Art of Healing* (1996), this shift involves changing the approach from one of treating to one of healing. He makes the distinction that treating a patient involves a dysfunctional organ system, while healing involves a distressed human being. Today's physician must recognise that the art of healing is as important as a command of medical technology. Medical technology should complement the art of healing, never replace it (Lown 1996). The foundation of the art of healing is compassion. Information is readily available, but compassion is not so easily grasped. The virtue of compassion enables us to take seriously the suffering around us and makes us into physicians (Bennett 1993). The German physician Paracelsus, in the 16th century, stated that the qualifications of a physician should include 'intuition which is necessary to understand the patient, his body, his disease. He must have the

feel and touch which make it possible for him to be in sympathetic communication with the patient's spirit' (Lown 1996).

Along with compassion, the patient with fibromyalgia requires a physician who truly believes that the condition exists and who is skilled at listening. This establishes a bond of trust between physician and patient that nurtures the healing process (Lown 1996). The Greek physician Hippocrates, the 'father of medicine', almost 2500 years ago stated that 'some patients, though conscious that their position is perilous, recover their health simply through their contentment with the physician' (Lown 1996).

First, the fibromyalgia patient needs a physician who acknowledges that the condition is a true and documented illness. Unfortunately, many physicians refuse to recognise it as such. The American Medical Association recognised fibromyalgia as an illness and a major cause of disability in 1987 and in 1990 the American College of Rheumatology defined the diagnostic criteria; many studies have subsequently confirmed their conclusions. Ongoing research brings us closer to the complete elucidation of the clinical and therapeutic answers. A physician will be ineffective in helping patients overcome their misery if there is doubt to the validity of their symptoms and a denial of the existence of the illness (Starlanyl & Copeland 1996, Russell 1997).

Secondly, mastering effective listening involves all the senses, not just the ears. Effective listening is in itself therapeutic. Our aim in the brief interview process is to gather the medical facts and gain insight into the person inside the patient. Physicians must be aware that information necessary to solving the mystery of what ails the patient is not just verbal. It is also the unspoken word, the contradictory facial expressions, attitude, posture, gait, inappropriate twitch, clasping of the hands, and the absence of a spouse, or significant other. If not actively listening, the unspoken complaint will not be heard. It may take multiple visits to hear the whole story and piece together the entire picture before the healing process begins (Lown 1996).

Box 8.1   Protocol

- Take a detailed history
- Perform a thorough physical examination
- Discuss the diagnosis
  —Involve the spouse and family
  —Educate
- Discuss the treatment

1. Sleep
   a. Discuss normal sleep and abnormal sleep
   b. Keep a sleep diary for 2 weeks
   c. Sleep hygiene

2. Diet
   a. Eliminate caffeine from the diet slowly
   b. Stop all alcohol and tobacco
   c. Eliminate all refined sugar and white flour
   d. At least 64 ounces of water a day
   e. For 8–12 weeks limit carbohydrates to less than 60 grams a day
   f. Eat fresh fruits, vegetables, lean meats and fish, and drink skimmed milk
   g. Read food labels – know what is in the foods you eat
   h. Avoid bananas, carrots, corn, raisins, or popcorn
   i. Low carbohydrate foods to encourage: berries, citrus fruit, mangoes, papaya, peaches, cantaloupe, watermelon, leafy green vegetables, green beans, crooknecked squash, broccoli, cauliflower, cucumber, leeks, okra, garlic, and peppers
   j. Grains and cereals should be whole-grain only
   k. Consider liberalising the diet if the symptoms are improved after 3 months

3. Medication
   a. If narcotics are necessary for pain management, use them only for short periods of time
   b. Avoid steroids
   c. Most muscle relaxers are of limited benefit
   d. Trazodone, clonazepam, sertraline, and fluoxetine – good choices for restoring sleep maintenance disorders
   e. Zolpidem – good choice for sleep onset disorders
   f. Start all medications at low doses – have the patient cut the lowest dose available into quarters or halves for the first few doses, then titrate to the desired dose
   g. When medications are stabilised, review every 6 months

4. Education
   a. Include spouse, family, friends, and employers
   b. Use handouts, videos, and group classes
   c. Provide reference materials; include information on local support groups

- Follow-up office visits

1. Routine visits
   a. 2 weeks
   b. Every 4–8 weeks during acute rehabilitation
   c. At 1 and 3 months after completing the rehabilitation
   d. Thereafter, every 6 months

2. Non-routine visits
   a. As needed
   b. For flare-ups.

TAKING THE INITIAL HISTORY

It is absolutely essential that physicians listen very carefully and devote the time to document a detailed history. Today, of course, physicians are faced with time constraints, rising overhead costs, managed care, capitated rates, and declining revenues. Although it seems inconsistent, a meticulously taken history is truly a time saver. If incorrect assumptions are made – due to the absence of essential facts or a lack of insight into the patient's emotional life – the physician may pursue incorrect therapeutic options. Many patients are improperly diagnosed or denied beneficial treatments because of sloppy or incomplete histories. Furthermore, incorrect assumptions increase the risk of litigation, increase health costs, and increase frustration to the physician, due to recurrent visits and phone calls (Lown 1996).

Physicians should look for a few essential facts in the initial interview. You should hear the patient relate symptoms that meet the criteria for diagnosing fibromyalgia. The history, along with an appropriate examination, should confirm the correctness of the diagnosis. If the essential criteria are not present in the history, there should be a suspicion of other medical processes at work. In a carefully taken history, the patient usually tells the physician what is wrong and may even provide information on how best to manage the problems (Lown 1996).

Since there is a great apprehension of the unknown, begin the interview with a short explanation of what will transpire. This will help put patients at ease, facilitating their willingness to be honest and frank. The interview should be carried out in a comfortable room with the patient fully clothed. Encourage the patient to completely disclose his symptoms no matter how unusual or insignificant. Reassure the patient that you understand that some information may not make sense to him or may be of a sensitive nature. Be sure to emphasise that an incomplete or misleading history will only lead to potential harm (Lown 1996).

I acknowledge that we are limited by time when taking histories. We do not have all day to spend with one patient. Therefore, determine how much time will be devoted to the initial history, the examination, and the post-examination discussion. Begin by telling the patient how much time is available and when the physical examination will start. Remind the patient that a discussion of the findings and recommendations will follow the physical examination. Understanding the emotions involved, you will occasionally, and sometimes frequently, need to redirect the patient's focus.

For the history to be thorough, it should include most of the categories listed below:

- Pain
- Fatigue
- Coexisting conditions
- Medications
- Sleep
- Diet
- Exercise history
- Life history
- Allergies
- Functional history
- Perpetuating factors.

Do not rely on the chief complaint alone: this often leads physicians to focus treatment on a limited number of symptoms that happen to be the problem of the day, recent in onset and unreflective of the primary dysfunction (Lown 1996). Symptoms can change from day to day and may lead to symptom chasing if the physician is not careful. One thing to consider is that much of the information can be gathered by an experienced assistant in the office or through a carefully constructed questionnaire. The interview can then be tailored to obtain necessary information that is not yet recorded or needs elaboration. If you did not personally gather the information, review it prior to seeing the patient. As you interview the patient, restate a few of the most pertinent facts. It is important for the patient to know that you have thoroughly reviewed, and are fully aware of any information obtained by a questionnaire or assistant.

This outline is intended to be personalised for each individual patient. Understand that this is not an exhaustive list. The physician should question the patient about any areas that are pertinent to the healing process (Chaitow 1995, Clauw 1995, Russell 1997, Starlanyl & Copeland 1996).

THE INITIAL PHYSICAL EXAMINATION

With the interview complete, begin the physical examination. The physical examination should complement the history, confirm the diagnosis, and rule out other systemic diseases (Lown 1996, Starlanyl & Copeland 1996). Although the examination should not take as much time as the history, it should be thorough (I include a complete neurological, joint, and musculoskeletal evaluation).

When time runs short, it is easy to neglect all aspects of the examination except the tender point examination. This, together with your history, could give you a diagnosis but it might well be incomplete or inaccurate. If you take this approach you will perhaps overlook other coexisting illnesses. Your assumptions and your treatments will be incorrect, and both you and the patient will suffer.

Start the examination with the neurological system: this causes the least discomfort and requires the fewest position changes. Next, the joint evaluation should note any deformities, oedema or erythema, and the range of motion of the joint.

Your examination should evaluate gait, structural asymmetries, and the soft tissues – you can assess the patient's sitting posture while taking the history. Then assess the patient's gait. Is he able to ambulate without assistance? Are there gait deviations? How does the patient's body move during ambulation? Next, check for body asymmetry and for skeletal deformities and deficiencies. Inspect the soft tissues for tone, spasm, and tender points. Identify the presence of any taut bands, twitch responses, and trigger points which signal coexisting myofascial pain syndrome: this adds another dimension to the treatment. Record the tender points on a body drawing. This allows you to review and track the tender points over time. It also allows you to determine if the number and location of the tender points meet the physical criteria for the diagnosis of fibromyalgia.

With the history and physical examination complete, most of the important information is now collected, and you should be able to determine whether the patient has fibromyalgia. The recorded information may also lead the physician to suspect other coexisting diseases or syndromes. Laboratory tests and X-rays may clarify these concerns. There are a number of authors who review the recommended laboratory tests frequently used to screen fibromyalgia patients (Chaitow 1995, Teitelbaum 1995). There is no blood test or X-ray specific for fibromyalgia; these screening laboratory tests or X-rays are to establish the coexistence of other illnesses or conditions (Russell 1997).

DISCUSSING THE DIAGNOSIS AND TREATMENT

After the patient dresses, discuss the findings and recommendations. Consider that the typical fibromyalgia patient will be very fatigued. The entire initial evaluation can take several hours from the time the patient signs in at the front desk until they make their follow-up appointment and leave the office. Many patients experience concentration and memory problems which are worsened by their fatigue. These patients may not be able to follow your discussion and will remember very little of the conversation. This is why it is important to have a spouse or a family member included in the discussion. Even though the patient may be very tired, they typically want to know everything about fibromyalgia. Expect many questions and concerns regarding the diagnosis and treatment.

Patients often are sceptical that you so easily made the diagnosis when others could not. Your answers should be sensible and believable. These answers should contribute to the healing process you began at the interview and satisfy the patient's concern that a life-threatening disease has not been missed (Russell 1997).

Two basic areas to discuss at the initial visit are the diagnosis and treatment. First, discuss the diagnosis. The patient needs to know that he has fibromyalgia. It is important to give this mystery illness a name. Also, explain what fibromyalgia is and what it is not (Starlanyl & Copeland 1996). Since many of the patients are sceptical of the diagnosis, briefly review the diagnostic criteria that you used. This legitimises the diagnosis. Put the pieces together for the patient by explaining how his symptoms and physical findings meet the diagnostic criteria for fibromyalgia. It is prudent to inform the patient that currently there is no cure for fibromyalgia, but that, with proper rehabilitation and life-style changes, significant and lasting benefits can be achieved (Russell 1997). Discuss any concerns of coexisting diseases, whether you ordered any tests, and why.

Secondly, discuss how you treat fibromyalgia (an overview is sufficient). Provide any in-depth information in a handout and discuss this in more detail at the second visit. Four major topics should be covered: sleep, medication, diet, and rehabilitation (see suggested protocol, Box 8.1).

Sleep

Fibromyalgia patients experience a number of sleep problems. Quality sleep plays a vital role in good health and is essential to a sense of well-being. Poor sleep perpetuates and worsens the symptoms of fibromyalgia. It needs to be aggressively treated. Many patients do not understand what constitutes normal sleep or what the normal sleep requirements are, so a brief explanation is a good place to start. Ask the patient to complete a sleep diary over the next 2 weeks. The information should help clarify the abnormal sleep pattern and help determine the most appropriate interventions. Provide the patient with a list of the important elements of sleep hygiene (Searle 1994). Encourage the patient to practice good sleep hygiene.

Medication

Briefly explain the purpose of any medication that you prescribe. Give clear instructions on proper dosing schedules – for example whether the medicine can be taken with food, and any potential side-effects such as dry mouth or morning sedation. Remember that fibromyalgia patients are very sensitive to medication and side-effects are common. Therefore, always start new medications at low doses and slowly titrate the medication to the lowest effective dose. It may even be necessary to use a quarter of the lowest dose available. You can prevent complications and confusion about medication by providing written information to the patient. Do ask the patient to consult with you before starting any new medication or supplements. This avoids potentially harmful drug interactions.

Narcotics should be used judiciously. Narcotics have no place in the long-term treatment of fibromyalgia. In the absence of rheumatic disorders such as lupus, maintenance steroids are not indicated. A wide range of medications can be used in the treatment of fibromyalgia, including the following supplements (Chaitow 1995):

- Vitamins
- Minerals
- Amino acids
- Enzymes
- Fish oils
- Melatonin
- Herbals
- Antioxidants.

Diet

Changing the diet is one of the most challenging but essential aspects of the treatment. Many patients are resistant to dietary changes. Education is crucial to convincing the patient to make healthy dietary modifications.

Begin with a brief overview of the metabolic abnormalities present in fibromyalgia, including both the impairment of glycolysis and carbohydrate metabolism (Eisinger et al 1994). Many of the symptoms of fibromyalgia are worsened by a poor diet (Chaitow 1995, Starlanyl & Copeland 1996).

There are a number of popular diets to choose from and include in your treatment regime. However, many are as unhealthy as the patient's present diet. No two physicians agree on the same diet approach.

Regardless of the dietary approach you feel comfortable with, there is a consensus on several of the more important changes. First eliminate caffeine and alcohol from the diet. Give the patient guidelines for reducing caffeine intake and help set achievable goals. Never stop all caffeine intake at once. Caffeine withdrawal is very unpleasant – an increase in fatigue, anxiety, sleep disturbances, headaches, and pain are associated with removing caffeine from the diet too rapidly. The patient should avoid all alcohol for at least 3–6 months, after which alcohol intake should be limited to two drinks a day (Chaitow 1995, Starlanyl & Copeland 1996, Teitelbaum 1995). Next, if the patient smokes or uses other tobacco products, begin a programme of tobacco cessation immediately. Lastly, remove refined, processed, and chemical-laden foods from the diet. This includes sugar and white flour. Encourage increased consumption of fresh vegetables, fruit, and fish. Avoid high-calorie, high-fat junk foods which provide empty calories and lots of chemicals (Starlanyl & Copeland 1996).

Discuss realistic, achievable goals for the diet modifications. These dietary changes are part of a long-term life-style change that the patient must make to achieve optimum health. Physicians can learn more on effective diets for the fibromyalgia patient from two books now available, *The Zone* (Sears & Lawren 1995) and *Fibromyalgia and Muscle Pain* (Chaitow 1995).

REHABILITATION

The initial visit should conclude with a discussion of rehabilitation. Successful rehabilitation involves a team approach. The rehabilitation team includes a multidisciplinary team of professionals. It most commonly includes the physician, a medical psychologist, physical therapist, massage therapist, and exercise physiologist, all with expertise in the treatment of fibromyalgia and soft-tissue disorders. If at all possible, I recommend an osteopathic physician be included on the rehabilitation team. Osteopaths are trained in manual medicine and can be invaluable to the rehabilitation team.

Very rarely does a single modality give any lasting relief in fibromyalgia. The most effective approach combines bodywork, aerobic and movement exercise, aquatic therapy, and cognitive–behavioural modification. A brief description of the common approaches used by your rehabilitation team can be included in the educational information given to the patient at the end of the visit (Chaitow 1995).

Use patient-directed materials to provide more in-depth information. Accurate materials are available in a number of media forms (Russell 1997). If a particular topic or unique approach is not available, create a handout and include it with the other educational materials you give to the patient. Give all the educational materials to the patient in a *new patient packet*. The contents of each new patient packet should have the same basic information, but should be customised to the individual needs of the patient. The packet needs to include in-depth information on sleep, medication, diet and the rehabilitation approach you recommend. Include a list of resource materials such as books, newsletters and support groups.

This material should be reviewed by the patient and family at home. It may take several days of repetitively reading the material before the patient begins to understand the complexity of the diagnosis and the treatment. Improving the patient's health and well-being depends on thoroughly educating the patient and instilling the need for open communication.

I recommend that the physician – or an experienced assistant – recheck the patient in 1–2 weeks in order to review the handout material and answer questions. Encourage the spouse or family to attend this first follow-up visit with the physician. It is so important to involve the patient directly as you consider treatment options. During the first few visits, reinforce the importance of patients assuming responsibility for their health and wellness (Starlanyl & Copeland 1996).

SUGGESTIONS FOR FOLLOW-UP CARE

Your care for fibromyalgia patients should be as organised as possible. The previously discussed information will help get you started. Establish a logical schedule for follow-up visits to the physician's office or surgery. A systematic follow-up schedule allows for more efficient utilisation of your time, and for careful and purposeful modification of the programme to achieve the greatest benefit for the patient. This follow-up care is for review of the patient's medical status and review of aspects such as medication, sleep, and diet, and is in addition to visits the patient makes in his acute rehabilitation programme. If you will be providing regular treatment to the patient as part of this rehabilitation programme, for example counselling or bodywork, it may be unnecessary to set aside a separate follow-up appointment. This will certainly need to be tailored to each patient's needs and your particular practice.

Occasionally, there will be unanticipated needs and symptom exacerbation requiring a non-routine follow-up visit with you. There should be some purpose for each regularly scheduled follow-up visit. Each visit should direct the patient to the next destination in his journey towards the ultimate destination – wellness.

Do not automatically assume that every ache and pain is from fibromyalgia. New symptoms or functional problems should be carefully evaluated to determine if other treatable or life-threatening medical conditions exist. It also helps to have a well educated, caring staff. Not all the patient's problems or concerns need your direct attention. Many of the problems can be handled by the staff. The physician can easily become overloaded and quickly burn out (see Box 8.2). So, set limits early on with the patients. Inform them of your office hours, when prescriptions are refilled, when call-backs are done, and provide information regarding insurance and billing. Be direct with how much time will normally be devoted to each scheduled visit. Be sure you have the support needed to function efficiently and effectively. Delegate some of the educational responsibilities to the appropriate rehabilitation team members.

Be honest with your patients and require their honesty. Inform the patient of your expectations. Help set attainable goals that can be met by the next visit. Establish new goals at each visit.

If a patient is unwilling to follow a particular treatment recommendation, do not take it personally. Explain the potential consequences openly and honestly. You may be surprised to know that sometimes your patients will teach you more than you teach them. Be open to learning from your patients. Encourage the patient to share new information with you. Since most physicians are eager to stay abreast of the newest advances in medicine, why are they often resistant, or even hostile to a patient wanting to share information? There are probably a number of reasons, but are any of them very good reasons?

The rehabilitation team should direct treatment towards the ultimate goal – independent self-care. All treatments should be structured to impart knowledge and teach patients the skills necessary to manage independently from day to

---

Box 8.2 Physician burnout

Physicians of fibromyalgia patients have a real problem with burnout. With such a limited number of physicians treating fibromyalgia and such a large patient population, it is easy to become overloaded. The complex issues surrounding these patients demand a great deal of attention. The increased work leads to long, hectic days. Add unexpected issues and a few walk-ins, and you will often find yourself running late. Complaints escalate, and patient dissatisfaction diverts your attention to administrative rather than patient care issues. If left unchecked, this frustration will lead to burnout.

When patients are non-compliant, irresponsible, or unresponsive to treatment, you may feel responsible and perhaps pressured to find other more effective treatments. When patients are not improving they usually complain. Therefore, you spend additional time reassuring them while trying to maintain your regular schedule. Patients often expect excessive attention and forget that they are not your only patient. Occasionally their expectations are unrealistic – they expect miracles. Pressure for you to deliver becomes daunting.

I have experienced all this and found it essential that you confront the problems before they overwhelm you. Consider a few strategies to minimise the frustration and decrease the risk of burnout.

Your greatest defence is patient education. If you train your patients to recognise their flare-ups and to understand the variability of their symptoms, you will see fewer unnecessary office visits and phone calls.

Being organised is also crucial. Organise your records and educational materials. Develop forms for gathering information and provide patients with an office policy and procedures brochure that addresses their common

questions. This informs your patients of your operational procedures and rules. Ensure that your office is adequately staffed. Educate patients in your routine and methods. Also, train the staff to help with the paperwork, screen phone calls and help with patient education. They can relieve some stress by keeping you on time and on task.

Set limits and stick to them. Adhere to the allotted time for each office visit. Inform the patient of how much time is available, refocusing their discussion if necessary. Stick to your office hours for seeing patients – make exceptions only in emergencies. Require an appointment to be seen and discourage unscheduled visits. Only accept prescription refills during the specified time period. Limit your phone discussions to a reasonable amount of time. If more extensive discussion and problem solving are indicated, ask the patient to come to the office for reevaluation.

Develop a peer support system. The professionals on your rehabilitation team are usually experiencing many of the same stresses. It is helpful to have someone with whom you can discuss your frustrations. Avoid gaining excess weight, exercise regularly, and get plenty of sleep. For optimal functioning you must practice the basics of wellness that you recommend to your patients.

Periodically step away from the responsibilities and focus on something that is relaxing and pleasurable. Take regular vacations to relax and restore your body and mind. Your patients will survive without you, despite what they or you may think. Lastly, learn to say no. Know your limits and do not push beyond them. Your health and sense of well-being are crucial to a productive and satisfying practice.

day. As part of their self-care skills, the patient should be taught to manage any flare-ups, those times of extreme symptom exacerbation.

At the beginning of treatment, encourage the patient to keep a daily log or journal chronicling their symptoms, function, and activities. This can be an invaluable tool. The patient can and should refer to this journal to gain insight into the symptoms, perpetuators, stressors, and triggers. It can also be used to assist in problem solving, tracking treatment effects, and mood changes. The patient should devote a section of the journal to diet and medication. He should keep track of any changes, side-effects, and benefits. The journal also provides a source of information to identify behaviour patterns which may be symptom perpetuators (Starlanyl & Copeland 1996).

Learn all you can about sleep. Improving the quality of sleep is a major concern. Other symptoms are much more difficult to control and improve if the sleep disorders are not effectively treated. Remind patients to expect dream changes with medication to improve sleep. If the patient complains of vivid or occasionally disturbing dreams, reassure him that this can be expected and should resolve. The majority of patients will improve in 4–8 weeks, although a medication change may be necessary. If patients understand that this is not necessarily a side-effect but may be associated with sleep normalisation, you can usually eliminate the need to discontinue or avoid medication that is beneficial for restoring sleep.

Educate the patient in the difference between medication side-effects and the expected increase or change in symptoms that accompany many medication, nutritional supplement and dietary changes. Teach patients to listen to their bodies, and yourself to listen to patients (Lown 1996, Starlanyl & Copeland 1996).

SUMMARY

Many physicians are frustrated with caring for the fibromyalgia patient as a result of focusing on the illness and not the person. It is therefore imperative that physicians return to the concept of treating the whole person – mind and body – as an integrated system. This requires the expertise of a team of professionals working together to address patients' dysfunctional systems and the treatment needs of these patients. Improvement occurs when all the symptoms are addressed simultaneously in an environment that fosters healing and independence.

REFERENCES

Bennett W J 1993 The book of virtues. Simon and Schuster, New York
Chaitow L 1995 Fibromyalgia and muscle pain. Thorsons, London
Clauw D J 1995 Fibromyalgia: more than just a musculoskeletal disease. American Family Physician 52(3): 843–851
Eisinger J, Plantamura A, Ayavou T 1994 Glycolysis abnormalities in fibromyalgia. Journal of the American College of Nutrition 13(2): 144–148
Lown B 1996 The lost art of healing. Houghton Mifflin, Boston

Russell I J 1997 Fibromyalgia syndrome diagnosis, pathogenesis, and management. Physical Medicine and Rehabilitation Clinics of North America 8(1): 213–226
Searle 1994 Easy steps to help you sleep. Searle, USA
Sears B, Lawren B 1995 The zone. Harper Collins, New York
Starlanyl D, Copeland M E 1996 Fibromyalgia and chronic myofascial pain syndrome: a survivors manual. New Harbinger, Oakland
Teitelbaum J 1995 From fatigue to fantastic: a manual for moving beyond chronic fatigue and fibromyalgia. Deva Press, Annapolis

9

Physical medicine and a rehabilitation approach to treating fibromyalgia

Mark Pellegrino

BACKGROUND

Fibromyalgia is a common condition causing chronic muscle pain. Up to 4% of the general population have this problem and it is one of the most common diagnoses seen in ambulatory office settings (Wolfe 1993, Yunus et al 1981). Numerous medical professionals and specialists treat fibromyalgia; my own specialty, physical medicine and rehabilitation, is particularly skilled at diagnosing and treating chronic conditions such as fibromyalgia.

Physical medicine and rehabilitation emerged from two historical events about 50 years ago. The first was the polio epidemic which caused millions to suffer from acute pain and weakness and led to the 'physical medicine' component of the specialty. Physical medicine modalities (heat, electric stimulation, hydrotherapy, etc.) and exercises (stretches, strengthening, etc.) became important effective treatment approaches. The 'rehabilitation' component evolved from the Second World War. Improved medical trauma techniques on the field along with the widespread availability of penicillin led to an increased survival rate among injured soldiers. Consequently, the number of soldiers disabled by such problems as head injuries, spinal cord injuries, infections, and amputations also increased. Rehabilitation strategies developed in the USA to help these disabled veterans improve functional and vocational skills, and ultimately help them return to civilian society as productive workers.

The specialty of physical medicine and rehabilitation requires 4 years of training and emphasises the diagnosis and management of disorders that cause functional impairment. Specific philosophies of the specialty include utilising a multidisciplinary approach, identifying rehabilitation goals to improve function, and improving quality of life. The word *habile* from which rehabilitation is derived is Latin for 'to make able again', an embodiment of our unique treatment philosophy. In treatment of fibromyalgia, the physical medicine and rehabilitation philosophy is to empower the person with abilities to improve quality of life. Specific fibromyalgia treatment goals would include:

1. Decreasing pain even if pain is still present.
2. Improving function even if the person is still unable to do activities performed prior to developing fibromyalgia.
3. Teach the person a successful programme to self–manage fibromyalgia.

At present, fibromyalgia is not considered a curable disorder. However, it can be treated successfully and can go into remission with few symptoms even though examination may reveal persistent painful tender points.

EVALUATION OF THE FIBROMYALGIA PATIENT

History

The patient with fibromyalgia will complain of severe persistent muscle pain. When evaluating the fibromyalgia patient, there are key historical points to be noted. The International Association for the Study of Pain defines pain as an unpleasant sensory and emotional experience associated with actual or potential tissue damage (Merskey & Bogduk 1994). Pain is always subjective and unpleasant, by definition. Pain is difficult to measure, standardise, or reproduce because its perception is influenced by multiple factors such as personal beliefs, education, culture differences, learned experiences, and genetics.

Fibromyalgia is one condition that causes pain, and despite the unlimited variations possible for the condition, there are usually consistent features in the history of a fibromyalgia patient.

When taking a history of a patient with fibromyalgia, these key features should be noted:

1. Region of pain: generalised or localised? Associated headaches, jaw pain or other specific regions? Most people with fibromyalgia will complain of generalised pain, but may have regions that are more painful relative to the overall generalised pain.

2. Onset of pain: gradual over time, or sudden? Sometimes the pain onset is so gradual that patients cannot remember the beginning of the pain. Sometimes the pain began after a trauma that the patient can recall to the exact moment.

3. Aetiology from patient standpoint: trauma, infection, stress, hereditary? Over half the patients attribute their symptoms to some type of trauma or severe stress.

4. Duration: persistent chronic pain, new onset, intermittent flare-ups? Fibromyalgia is characterised by chronic pain which often flares up or becomes more severe.

5. Aggravating factors: weather changes, air conditioning draught, increased activity, decreased activity, stress? All of these factors can increase pain in fibromyalgia.

6. Improving factors: heat, massage, mild exercise, rest? These factors often relieve some of the pain in fibromyalgia.

7. Characteristics of pain: constant, sharp, radiating, paraesthesias, diffuse ache? Usually a person describes multiple types of pain when fibromyalgia is present.

8. How pain has interfered with life: difficulties with everyday activities of daily living (ADLs), difficulty with work-related activities, interfering with hobbies or recreational activities, interpersonal relationship difficulties? Most people with fibromyalgia will report some disruption of their abilities from the pain.

9. Previous treatments for pain: medicines, therapies, effective or not? Is a home programme being done? Even if a home programme is successful, patients with fibromyalgia will still experience flare-ups from time to time.

10. Patient's understanding and insight into the condition? Details and attention must be paid

to any psychologic factors such as depression, anxiety, and frustration, as well as common associated conditions of fibromyalgia (i.e. irritable bowel syndrome, fatigue, poor sleep) which may contribute to the patient's pain and may interfere with treatment and recovery, or require separate treatment approaches altogether.

11. Patient goals: are they realistic? Can a person continue working, or should a different job be considered? Do not assume the patient's main goal is to continue working; the patient may be seeking disability and may amplify symptoms.

A detailed history on the pain and other symptoms in fibromyalgia, with emphasis on how the pain affects the person's daily activities, is crucial in the overall rehabilitation evaluation. This information allows us to think about fibromyalgia as a possible diagnosis, and to plan individual goals for this patient.

I have come to appreciate several 'diagnostic statements' that patients with fibromyalgia make when reciting their history. Whenever any of the following statements are made one should think of fibromyalgia as the likely diagnosis:

'I hurt all over.'
'My pain moves around.'
'I feel like I've been run over by a truck.'

The history is only part of the overall clinical exam and, alone, is not sufficient to diagnose fibromyalgia. The physical examination must be carried out and must be consistent with fibromyalgia.

Physical examination

Examination of the fibromyalgia patient will reveal characteristic and reproducible signs, mainly tender points and abnormal muscle consistency. Characteristic well localised areas of pain with palpation are called tender points. Tender points are the key objective abnormality present in fibromyalgia. The American College of Rheumatology performed a landmark study establishing criteria for the diagnosis of fibromyalgia based on a consistent reproducible pattern of tender points (Wolfe et al 1990). The

criteria state that pain must be present for at least 3 months, must be widespread, and there must be at least 11 of 18 positive tender points in characteristic locations (Fig. 9.1).

This '11 of 18' criterion has been agreed upon for academic and research purposes to enable a consistent fibromyalgia 'gold standard'. In the clinical setting, however, fewer than 11 of 18 tender points may be present and still be consistent with the diagnosis of fibromyalgia (Wolfe 1994). Indeed, many patients with fibromyalgia have fewer than 11 tender points in the characteristic locations, but have typical symptoms and findings that enable the clinician to diagnose fibromyalgia. Many patients have regional pain and clustering of tender points consistent with a regional fibromyalgia (with fewer than 11 of 18 designated tender points). Many physicians believe that the condition of myofascial pain syndrome and regional fibromyalgia are synonymous terms. Myofascial pain syndrome has been described by Drs Travell & Simons (1983), and some feel it is a separate condition from fibromyalgia. My own view is that myofascial pain syndrome and fibromyalgia are more similar than dissimilar, and that myofascial pain syndrome is a subtype of the fibromyalgia 'spectrum'.

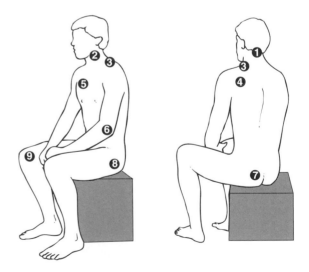

Figure 9.1 Characteristic 18 tender points located in 9 pairs (from Pellegrino 1997, reproduced with permission of Anadem Publishing, Columbus, OH).

Tender points are the key abnormalities upon examination of the fibromyalgia patient, but other findings may also be present. Trigger points are distinct areas of muscles or soft tissues which, when palpated, cause pain or paraesthesias to refer to a distant location (Fig. 9.2). The ability to reproduce the patient's complaints of paraesthesias by identifying trigger points on examination is helpful in ruling out other causes of paraesthesias such as radiculopathy or nerve entrapment.

Muscles in persons with fibromyalgia typically have an abnormal consistency that can be palpated. Using the pads of the thumbs or index fingers, an examiner can palpate muscle areas and feel 'lumps and bumps' (Fig. 9.3). Nodular and ropy textures are common descriptions of the abnormal muscle consistency. Unlike normal muscles which have a consistency of a firm gel, muscles in fibromyalgia have a different consistency described as 'nodular' or 'ropy'.

The physical examination may reveal pain behaviours common with chronic pain.

Examples of pain behaviours include slow deliberate movements, walking with an inconsistent limp, exaggerated flinching upon palpation, frequent facial grimacing, frequent sighing, and frequent indication of 'I can't' when asked to perform a certain movement or task (Keefe & Bloch 1982).

Chronic pain syndrome is an abnormal condition in which pain is no longer a symptom of acute injury, but in which pain and pain behaviour becomes a primary disease process (Sternbach 1990). Many individuals with fibromyalgia can ultimately develop chronic pain syndrome in which there are significant subjective and functional limitations and pain behavioural manifestations that are out of proportion to the physical examination findings. In my experience, the person with chronic pain syndrome does have true pain and often has coexisting fibromyalgia; both conditions can pose a challenge to the treating physician.

The physical examination of a person with fibromyalgia should not reveal the following abnormalities:

- True neurologic weakness
- Loss of reflexes
- Joint swelling, heat, or inflammation
- Atrophy or wasting of muscles
- Abnormal muscle tone.

If any of these physical findings are present, then a condition in addition to or other than

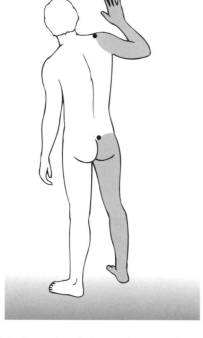

Figure 9.2 Examples of trigger points and referred paraesthesias (from Pellegrino 1997, reproduced with permission of Anadem Publishing, Columbus, OH).

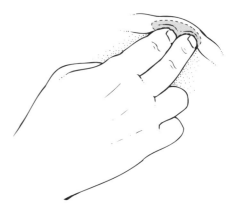

Figure 9.3 A fibromyalgia nodule can be palpated in the muscle (from Pellegrino 1997, reproduced with permission of Anadem Publishing, Columbus, OH)

fibromyalgia must be present. In fibromyalgia, the most important and meaningful finding is the painful tender points in characteristic locations

DIAGNOSTIC APPROACH TO FIBROMYALGIA

The diagnosis of fibromyalgia is fairly straightforward. There are very few conditions that cause widespread muscle pain with a chronic course characterised by waxing and waning of symptoms. Various conditions may mimic fibromyalgia, including polymyalgia rheumatica, connective tissue disease, hypothyroidism, myopathy, and osteoarthritis. But in most cases, these additional diagnostic considerations can be ruled out by a careful history and physical examination with documentation of the typical tender points.

Useful laboratory screening tests include erythrocyte sedimentation rate, serum creatinine kinase, complete blood count, thyroid function tests, and perhaps tests for rheumatoid factor and anti-nuclear antibody (Goldenberg 1987). Abnormal results could prompt further testing that could include X-rays, electrodiagnostic testing, or a muscle biopsy. In fibromyalgia, routine labs and tests are often normal, yet it is a common condition that can be easily diagnosed with a careful history and physical examination, as with most diagnoses in medicine.

TREATMENT OF FIBROMYALGIA

At the present time, there is no single treatment that eliminates the symptoms of fibromyalgia or cures the condition. However, various treatments can help individuals with fibromyalgia even if the condition does not disappear or become completely cured. Each person's treatment programme needs to be individualised, and what works for some may not work for others. Hopefully, the patient will find some treatments that are helpful in dealing with the pain and that will enable specific goals to be accomplished: decreasing pain to the lowest level, improving function, and teaching a successful programme to self-manage fibromyalgia.

My treatment philosophy is to use a multi-disciplinary approach to achieve two general goals:

1. Find out what works
2. Teach the person a successful home programme.

The patient needs to be an active member of the multidisciplinary team approach. There are numerous health professionals who treat fibromyalgia including doctors, chiropractors, physical therapists, occupational therapists, psychologists, massotherapists, nutritionists, vocational counsellors, dental specialists, and more. These health professionals can be valuable team members in a multidisciplinary approach to fibromyalgia, with the patient being the team 'captain'. Interventions that I frequently utilise are:

1. Education
2. Medications
3. Nutritional strategies
4. Therapies
5. Psychological strategies.

Each of these will now be described in more detail.

Education

Patients need to understand the nature of fibromyalgia and the chronic ongoing pain that it causes. However, it is important for patients to appreciate that fibromyalgia is not lifethreatening, deforming, or paralysing, and that it does not turn into an inflammatory condition. Many patients are relieved to know that there is indeed a name for their condition and their symptoms are validated. Patients with fibromyalgia can develop a realistic appreciation of their condition and its chronicity, but at the same time learn that improvements can occur even if the condition currently cannot be cured. I encourage all patients with fibromyalgia to learn everything they can about the condition and how it affects their everyday lives. I emphasise the importance of self-responsibility: learning to take control of fibromyalgia and striving to cope successfully with this condition each and every day (Pellegrino 1997).

Written resources

There are various books, brochures, newsletters, and articles to educate health professionals and patients about fibromyalgia. I provide patients with a handout listing various reference sources. A wealth of information is also available on the Internet, and many patients take advantage of this resource.

Support groups

A support group can be a valuable means for both education and treatment in fibromyalgia. Having the opportunity to share experiences with someone else who has the same condition can be a powerful therapeutic tool. Health professionals readily recognise that all of our modern medicines and treatments may not be enough, and a support group can provide a unique treatment dimension. Support groups usually meet on a monthly basis for a few hours with a mixture of education and support. Our support group has a group facilitator, and frequently our group has invited guest speakers on different topics related to fibromyalgia.

Families

Fibromyalgia not only involves the patient, but also the patient's significant others, including spouse, family members, and co-workers. Educating others who are affected by the diagnosis is an important treatment process as it helps the patient's family, friends and colleagues to understand the condition and learn to provide support and encouragement for the patient.

Medications

Prescription medicines can help control symptoms of fibromyalgia. Pain relief, improved sleep, and improved mood are goals that prescription medicines could help accomplish. There is no magical pill that will cure fibromyal-

gia, but many drugs can be effective in reducing pain and improving overall feelings of well-being. No one type of medicine works for everyone, and no one medicine causes 100% improvement. The prescribing physician and the patient need to experiment to find out what works best. Various categories of drugs used in the treatment of fibromyalgia include:

- Analgesics
- Non-steroidal anti-inflammatory drugs
- Antidepressant medicines (tricyclics and selective serotonin reuptake inhibitors)
- Muscle relaxants
- Sleep modifiers.

Carefully controlled studies have shown that low doses of tricyclic antidepressant medicines can benefit fibromyalgia patients (Carette et al 1986, Goldenberg et al 1986). Using a combination of a serotonin reuptake inhibitor during the day and a tricyclic at night-time can be effective (Goldenberg 1996).

CAUTION: All medicines have potential side-effects, and patients with fibromyalgia are often sensitive to medicines. The prescribing physician and the patient need to work closely together to monitor the benefits as opposed to the side-effects and determine if a particular medicine combination is effective.

My basic strategies for using prescription medicines include:

1. Narcotics/opiates can be used sparingly and responsibly for pain control.
2. Use the lowest effective dose of medicine and wean off medicines whenever possible, especially if the patient is at a 'stable baseline'.
3. Discontinue any medicine that is not effective.

No medicine will cure fibromyalgia, but they may help improve symptoms and make the patient more comfortable without side-effects.

Injections

Therapeutic injections are a way of administering medicine for pain management. The most common injections used in fibromyalgia are trigger point injections. I recommend trigger point injections be considered when a few areas (two to four) are causing most of the patient's 'severe pain'. These areas are determined by careful palpation. For an average trigger point, I generally use 2–3 cc of 1–2% Lidocaine. Sometimes a small amount of an intermediate acting corticosteroid can be added to decrease the irritant effect of the local anaesthetic and prolong the effect of the trigger point injection. Painful areas are accurately localised and injected 'bullseye' fashion. The patient will confirm the accurate localisation by reporting increased pain during the injection. Often the pain is referred to a distant location similar to the patient's subjective complaints of paraesthesias. The needle can be partially withdrawn and repeatedly reinserted in a peppering fashion, but I prefer to inject once 'bullseye' fashion and remove the needle, thus minimising the actual needle trauma to the muscle.

Trigger point injections can be helpful from a diagnostic standpoint (i.e. they decrease pain and numbness and confirm a tender/trigger point), and also helpful from a therapeutic standpoint (i.e. the benefits can last for weeks). I have found trigger point injections to be a useful adjunct that enables other treatments to work more effectively.

Other types of therapeutic injections have been tried in patients with fibromyalgia, including epidural steroid injections, selective nerve root blocks, joint injections, and proliferative injections (prolotherapy). As with prescribed oral medicines, therapeutic injections can be considered on an individual basis as part of a multidisciplinary treatment approach.

Nutritional therapy

Numerous studies have been published to describe various nutritional aspects of pain management. Medical professionals have long recognised the importance of diet in diseases such as diabetes, heart disease, gout, and osteoporosis. There has been increasing interest in the role that diet and nutrition play in a patient's overall health. Nutritional strategies can play an important role in the treatment of fibromyalgia. I believe there are some basic principles in trying to optimise nutrition in fibromyalgia.

- Eat at least three meals a day to help maintain proper energy for daily needs. Many people with fibromyalgia actually do better by eating six smaller meals a day, especially those who are bothered by irritable bowel syndrome.
- Emphasise a diet that is low in fat, low in refined sugars, high in natural fruits and vegetables, and relatively higher in protein.
- Avoid caffeine, nicotine, and alcohol as these all interfere with the body's ability to manufacture energy and proteins and carry out efficient biochemical reactions.
- Nutritional supplementation strategies which include a multivitamin, and magnesium and malic acid supplements. The combined effects of magnesium and malic acid were found to help decrease pain in fibromyalgia patients (Abraham & Flechas 1992, Russell et al 1994). (Specific nutritional approaches are discussed in Ch. 11 and 12)

Therapy programme

A therapy programme is an important part in the overall treatment of fibromyalgia. Different therapies may work better for different persons, and the goal is to determine what is the best therapy approach for any individual. Any therapy programme should consider the following: patient safety, relative ease of administration, affordable, and good efficacy. Additionally, a therapy programme should ultimately be one that can be self-administered.

Various components of a therapy programme include therapeutic modalities, manual therapy and adjustments, massotherapy, and exercise therapy. The combination of these various components is often effective, and different health professionals can be involved including physical therapists, massotherapists, chiropractors, exercise physiologists, etc. As with any treatment prescription, the patient's response, accomplishment of goals and changes or modifications should be monitored by the physician. Different components of a therapy programme will be reviewed at this time.

Therapeutic modalities

Therapeutic modalities include thermal agents and electrotherapy, cryotherapy or cold therapy, and superficial and deep heat.

- Cryotherapy is often used for acute soft tissue injuries with the goal of decreasing oedema and spasticity. It can also be helpful in more chronic pain of fibromyalgia by reducing pain and muscle tightness.
- Therapeutic heat consists of both superficial (hot packs, hydrotherapy, and paraffin), and deep heat (ultrasound, diathermy). It is often used for its analgesic effect, and deeper heating modalities can help decrease pain and improve flexibility of the soft tissues.
- Contrast baths use both heat and cold and can be helpful in patients with fibromyalgia who experience more neuropathic-type pain or reflex sympathetic dystrophy-type pain.
- Electrotherapy includes transcutaneous electric nerve stimulation (TENS), functional electrical stimulation, interferential therapy, and iontophoresis. The landmark study on the gate control theory published in 1965 led to the development of numerous electrotherapy modalities (Melzack & Wall 1965). Many patients with fibromyalgia respond favorably to electrotherapy.

Adjustments and manual therapy

Osteopathic physicians, chiropractic physicians, and manual therapists are trained to perform manipulations and adjustments. These techniques can mobilise joints, improve range of motion, relax muscles, and reduce muscle pain. All of these can benefit patients with fibromyalgia.

Massotherapy

Massage can help decrease pain in fibromyalgia by various mechanisms including relaxing muscles, improving circulation and oxygenation, removing waste build-up in the muscles, and increasing muscle flexibility. Various massage techniques include

- Stroking, which is the gliding of palms and fingers firmly over the muscles in a slow rhythmic movement
- Kneading is when the muscles are grasped between the fingers and thumb and slightly lifted and squeezed in a slow rhythmic sequence
- Friction massage penetrates deep into the muscle and uses slow circular movements with the tips of the fingers or thumbs.

Myofascial release, trigger point therapy, and craniosacral therapies are examples of specialised techniques to help relieve pain in fibromyalgia and other conditions causing pain.

Self–massages are a simple procedure that patients can learn easily to work on their own muscles to try to achieve pain reduction and relaxation. A spouse or a significant other can be trained how to perform therapeutic massage as well.

Exercise

Patients with fibromyalgia often experience increased pain after exertion due to a combination of tight muscles and being less aerobically fit overall (Bennett et al 1989). Fibromyalgia patients who attempt to begin an exercise programme often experience an increase in muscle pain which may discourage them from continuing to work on improving their level of fitness. I find that a prescribed, supervised exercise programme is helpful for fibromyalgia patients, and helps them achieve a gradual increase in overall physical fitness, flexibility, and functional ability (Pellegrino 1995).

The key features of a successful exercise programme are:

1. Emphasise stretching and flexibility exercises of all major muscle groups and focus on a warm-up period that consists of stretching only.

2. Regular performance of a low impact aerobic type programme which I call a 'light conditioning' programme. Such a programme can include walking, water aerobics, using an exercise bicycle, or performing a low impact aerobic programme.

3. Gradually progressing in an exercise programme as tolerated. The goal is to achieve improvement, but also to achieve a stable baseline.

4. Continue a regular exercise programme at least three times a week, even on days when there is increased pain.

5. Follow proper posture and body mechanics to minimise strain of the muscles and joints.

Not everyone with fibromyalgia can achieve a high level exercise programme. In some patients, performing a daily stretching and flexibility programme may be all that is tolerated, but this is still considered an exercise programme. Progressive stretching and exercises are best introduced after the acute pain of fibromyalgia subsides following the initial therapy programme.

An excellent and safe programme involves water/aquatic exercise. Exercising in the water has many benefits even for someone who cannot swim. Since most of the body weight is buoyed by the water, the gravity stress on the muscles and joints is reduced. The water should be kept at a comfortable temperature, usually around 88–90° F. Range of motion, flexibility, strengthening and aerobic exercises can all be done in the pool and can initially be supervised by a trained professional until individuals feel comfortable in following through with their own programme.

Benefits of exercise

There are many proven benefits from exercise: these include decreased pain, improved flexibility, improved strength, more energy, better sleep, better weight control, improved cardiovascular fitness, improved self-esteem and overall improved feeling of well-being. I believe that a regular stretching and exercise programme is ultimately a key in successfully managing fibromyalgia.

Psychological therapies

Many patients with fibromyalgia can develop associated psychological problems. These include decreased self-esteem, depression, anxiety, strained interpersonal relationships, and altered coping mechanisms. Psychological interventions need to be considered as part of the overall treatment programme for fibromyalgia.

Psychological treatments can include a variety of approaches such as psychotherapy, counselling, pain and stress management, biofeedback, relaxation, coping strategies, and other techniques. One-on-one psychological intervention and group therapy can be employed to help patients develop better coping mechanisms and improved outlook. Psychologists, psychiatrists, counsellors, social workers, clergy, and other qualified individuals can assist in helping patients cope with fibromyalgia and make necessary lifestyle adjustments to deal successfully with this chronic disorder.

THE BASELINE

A comprehensive rehabilitation approach in the treatment of fibromyalgia can help individuals achieve a realistic stable baseline level. A stable baseline is not the same as no pain, rather it is a level where there may still be pain but it is stable and not preventing the patient from performing desired functional tasks. The baseline level is different for everyone, but each person can eventually learn what his or her baseline state will be.

The baseline is not a perfect state. There are fluctuations of pain above and below the baseline; some days the patient will feel better and other days he or she will feel worse. Fibromyalgia flare-ups are common and are essentially part of fibromyalgia.

A comprehensive rehabilitation approach to fibromyalgia can help in reducing the pain to a lower, more functional level (i.e. a stable baseline). I emphasise patient self-responsibility in maintaining a stable baseline. A combination of stretches, home exercises, following proper posture, taking medicines as prescribed, using modalities such as heat, and continuing to educate oneself on fibromyalgia will enable a person successfully to manage the symptoms on his or her own. Despite the best efforts to maintain a stable home programme, flare-ups can still occur and may overwhelm the individual's coping technique. If such a flare-up occurs, the patient should follow up with the physician to consider specific prescribed treatments to reduce the flare-up to a lower level where the patient can manage the symptoms again on his or her own.

SUMMARY

Fibromyalgia presents a challenge to both patients and medical professionals, not only to recognise fibromyalgia, but to try to understand it and treat it successfully, and to minimise its impact on the individual and the community until a cure is found. Fibromyalgia is not life-threatening, but it can cause profound functional impairments and can ultimately lead to disability. Physicians who treat fibromyalgia can help individuals overcome the morbidity of fibromyalgia and improve the quality of life. Even if fibromyalgia cannot be cured at this time, it can certainly be treated and many people can lead useful, functional lives in spite of the fibromyalgia.

REFERENCES

Abraham G E, Flechas J D 1992 Management of fibromyalgia: rationale for the use of magnesium and malic acid. Journal of Nutritional Medicine 3: 49–59

Bennett R M, Clark S R, Goldberg G L et al 1989 Aerobic fitness in patients with fibrositis. A controlled study of respiratory gas exchange and ^{133}xenon clearance from exercising muscle. Arthritis and Rheumatism 32: 454–460

Carette S, McCain G A, Bell D A, Fam A G 1986 Evaluation of amitriptyline in primary fibrositis: a double-blind placebo controlled study. Arthritis and Rheumatism 29: 655–659

Goldenberg D L 1987 Fibromyalgia syndrome: an emerging but controversial condition. Journal of American Medical Association 257: 2782–2787

Goldenberg D L 1996 A randomized double-blind crossover trial of fluoxetine and amitriptyline in the treatment of fibromyalgia. Arthritis and Rheumatism 39: 1852–1859

Goldenberg D L, Feison D T, Dinerman H 1986 A randomized controlled trial of amitriptyline and naproxen in the treatment of patients with fibromyalgia. Arthritis and Rheumatism 29: 1371–1377

Keefe F J, Bloch A R 1982 Development of an observation method for assessing pain behaviour in chronic low back pain patients. Behaviour Therapies 13: 363–375

Melzack R, Wall P D 1965 Pain mechanism: a new theory. Science 150: 171–179

Mersky H, Bogduk N (eds) 1994 Classification of chronic pain: descriptions of chronic pain syndrome and definitions of pain terms, 2nd edn. Task Force on Taxonomy of the International Association for the Study of Pain. IASP Press, Seattle, pp 180–196

Pellegrino M J 1995 The fibromyalgia survivor. Anadem Publishing, Columbus, ch 3

Pellegrino M J 1997 Fibromyalgia: managing the pain, 2nd edn. Anadem Publishing, Columbus, ch 20

Russell R J, Michalek J E, Flechas J D, Abraham G E 1994 Treatment of fibromyalgia syndrome with Super Malic: a randomized double-blind placebo controlled crossover pilot study. Journal of Rheumatology 22: 953–958

Sternbach R A 1990 Psychophysiological pain syndromes. In: Bonica J J (ed) The management of pain. Lea and Febiger, Philadelphia

Travell J G, Simons D 1983 Myofascial pain and dysfunction: the trigger point manual. Williams and Wilkins, Baltimore

Wolfe F 1993 The epidemiology of fibromyalgia. Journal of Musculoskeletal Pain 1: 137–148

Wolfe F 1994 When to diagnose fibromyalgia. Rheumatology Disease Clinics of North America 20:485–501

Wolfe F, Smythe H A, Yunus M B et al 1990 The American College of Rheumatology 1990 criteria for the classification of fibromyalgia: report of the multicenter criteria committee. Arthritis and Rheumatism 33: 160–172

Yunus M B, Masi At, Calabro J J et al 1981 Primary fibromyalgia: clinical study of fifty patients with matched normal controls. Seminars in Arthritis and Rheumatology 11: 151–171

10

The metabolic rehabilitation of fibromyalgia patients

John C. Lowe and Gina Honeyman-Lowe

Recent evidence indicates that fibromyalgia (FMS) is a manifestation of impaired metabolism. In most cases, the cause appears to be inadequate thyroid hormone regulation of cell function. The inadequate regulation may result from a thyroid hormone deficiency or from cellular resistance to normal levels of thyroid hormone. The measurable features of FMS can be improved or relieved in most patients through therapy that is best termed 'metabolic rehabilitation'. The four components of our protocol are nutritional supplements, thyroid hormone, exercise to tolerance, and physical treatment. For some patients undergoing metabolic rehabilitation, FMS pain scores normalise only after soft tissue treatment and spinal manipulation control or eliminate noxious neural input from the musculoskeletal system to the central nervous system. Treatment decisions are data-driven. During a patient's treatment, FMS status is assessed at 1- to 2-week intervals using five measures. These scores are posted to line graphs that provide a visual depiction of changes in the patient's status (see Figs 10.1 to 10.5 below). The patient's treatment is altered as necessary to cause the lines in the graphs to move over time in directions indicating improved status.

INTRODUCTION

Recent studies of patients with FMS provide strong evidence for three conclusions:

1. FMS is a condition of metabolic insufficiency in select tissues.
2. In most cases, the insufficiency is a result of hypothyroidism or cellular resistance to thyroid hormone.

3. Treatments that cause or encourage a sustained increase in metabolism are effective in improving or relieving FMS symptoms (see also Box 10.1).

In view of these, does the bodyworker doing soft tissue treatment have a role to play in the care of FMS patients? Definitely. For most patients, soft tissue treatment provides palliative relief during the process of metabolic rehabilitation. More importantly, the use of soft tissue treatment is necessary in many cases if patients are to fully recover from the most distinguishing symptom of FMS: chronic widespread pain. We describe the modifications in technique that are advisable for treating most FMS patients.

FMS AS A MANIFESTATION OF HYPOTHYROIDISM OR CELLULAR RESISTANCE TO THYROID HORMONE

The clinical features of FMS and hypothyroidism are virtually the same (Wilson & Walton 1959, Fessel 1968, Bland & Frymoyer 1970, Golding 1970, Hochberg et al 1976, Beetham 1979, Wilke et al 1981, Delamere et al 1982, Sonkin 1985, Awad personal communication 1990, Lowe 1995). The 13 most common FMS symptoms (pain, fatigue, stiffness, headaches, sleep disturbance, bowel disturbance, depression, poor memory and concentration, anxiety, cold intolerance, numbness and tingling, dry tissues, and difficulty exercising) are also common symptoms of hypothyroidism. Moreover, every objectively verified abnormality in FMS can be explained by inadequate thyroid hormone regulation of cell function (Lowe 1998, 1999). These include the low serotonin (Russell et al 1992) and high substance P (Vaerøy et al 1988) levels that may mediate the chronic widespread pain and pressure sensitivity of FMS patients. Inadequate thyroid hormone regulation can plausibly explain both low serotonin secretion and high substance P levels (Frankhyzen & Muller 1983, Yellin 1997). We discuss these abnormalities in detail below.

Hypothyroidism in FMS

There is an extraordinarily high incidence of hypothyroidism in FMS patients. The incidence of primary hypothyroidism (thyroid hormone deficiency due to impaired thyroid gland function) in the general US population is about 1%

Box 10.1 The hypometabolism hypothesis of fibromyalgia

Scientific studies and years of related clinical experiences have led to several conclusions about the pathogenesis of FMS and its treatment:

- In most cases, FMS is caused by, or related to, inadequate thyroid hormone regulation of cell function. The inadequate regulation results from one of two phenomena: (1) thyroid hormone deficiency, or (2) partial cellular resistance to the hormone.

- Other factors may also induce and sustain symptoms that lead to a diagnosis of FMS if those factors impede the metabolism of the tissues from which FMS symptoms and signs arise. Such factors include B complex vitamin deficiencies, the use of beta-receptor blocking drugs, and deconditioning. Whereas one such factor may not be enough to induce FMS symptoms, combinations of factors may be sufficient (Lowe 1999, Lowe 1998).

- The metabolism-impeding factors responsible for FMS must be controlled or eliminated before a patient can significantly improve. When FMS results from inadequate thyroid hormone regulation, thyroid hormone is indispensable if the patient is to improve or recover.

- For most patients, nutritional supplements are also essential. They synergistically interact with thyroid hormone to cause a sustained increase in metabolism (Lowe 1997b). As thyroid hormone accelerates metabolism, the body's requirement for nutrients – especially B complex vitamins – increases. Not taking vitamin supplements may result in vitamin deficiency or cardiomyopathy (Travell & Simons 1983). Taking supplements can avert such adverse effects and facilitate a thyroid hormone-induced increase in metabolism.

- For all patients, exercise to tolerance is necessary. Exercise enables patients to capitalise on the increased metabolic capacity provided by thyroid hormone and nutritional supplements (Lowe 1997b). Resistance exercises contribute to the increase in metabolism by increasing lean tissue mass, which has a higher metabolic rate than fat tissue (Pratley et al 1994). Aerobic exercise contributes by increasing the metabolic rate of the lean tissues (Shinkai et al 1994).

(Hershman 1980). The incidence of primary hypothyroidism among FMS patients has been reported as 10% (Eisinger et al 1992, Gerwin 1995), 10.5% (Lowe 1997a), 12% (Shiroky et al 1993), and 13.0% (Lowe et al 1998b). The incidence of central hypothyroidism (thyroid hormone deficiency due to hypothalamic or pituitary dysfunction) in the population at large is about 0.00021% (Hershman 1980). We found an incidence among FMS patients of 52.6% (Lowe 1997a) and 43.5% (Lowe et al 1998b). Ferraccioli and colleagues (1990) and Neeck & Riedel (1992) reported similarly high incidences of central hypothyroidism among FMS patients. Thus, the incidence of primary hypothyroidism among FMS patients may be some 10 times higher than in the population at large, and the incidence of central hypothyroidism some 250 000 times higher.

Euthyroid hypometabolism in FMS (partial cellular resistance to thyroid hormone)

We found that 36.8% (Lowe 1997a) and 43.5% (Lowe et al 1998b) of FMS patients were euthyroid (had normal laboratory thyroid function test results). What could cause hypothyroid-like symptoms in these patients? Any factor that impedes the same metabolic pathways as those impeded by thyroid hormone deficiency. Examples of such factors are folic acid deficiency and beta-adrenergic blocking drugs. But our studies and clinical experiences indicate that euthyroid FMS is most often a result of cellular resistance to thyroid hormone. Symptoms and objective abnormalities resulting from cellular resistance are virtually the same as those resulting from thyroid hormone deficiency.

Only one cause of thyroid hormone resistance, mutations in the c-erbAβ gene on chromosome 3, has been proven (Refetoff et al 1993) to date. It is possible that such mutations underlie the hypothyroid-like symptoms and objective findings in euthyroid FMS patients (Lowe et al 1997d). At this time, we conclude that a patient has cellular resistance to thyroid hormone when several conditions are met. When the patient:

1. Is euthyroid before beginning to use thyroid hormone

2. Recovers from hypothyroid-like FMS symptoms and signs with 'supraphysiologic' (higher than normal) dosages of T_3, the metabolically active thyroid hormone

3. After beginning treatment, has an 'abnormally' high blood T_3 level

4. Has no tissue overstimulation (thyrotoxicosis) due to the high T_3 levels, according to the results of ECGs, and laboratory and bone density tests.

We find this pattern in virtually all our euthyroid patients who benefit from metabolic rehabilitation. And according to these criteria, we have documented the presence of thyroid hormone resistance in FMS patients in several double-blind, placebo-controlled, crossover studies (Lowe et al 1997a, 1997b, 1997c). It appears, then, that the hypothyroid-like FMS symptoms and signs of many – and perhaps most – euthyroid FMS patients are a result of cellular resistance to thyroid hormone (Lowe 1998, 1999).

That FMS in most patients is a result of inadequate thyroid hormone regulation is further supported by an important study completed in 1998 (Lowe et al 1998a). *Its results are the first to demonstrate long-term effectiveness of an FMS treatment.* The study was a 1- to 5-year follow-up comparing patients treated with metabolic therapy to untreated patients. Twenty FMS patients who underwent metabolic treatment were matched with 20 FMS patients who did not. Patients were matched by sex, thyroid status, and the time since their initial evaluations. All patients were initially evaluated 1 to 5 years before the follow-up study began. In each group, 10 patients (50%) had been classified as euthyroid, 6 (30%) as primary hypothyroid, and 4 (20%) as central hypothyroid. Before 20 of the patients began treatment, there was no statistical difference on any measure between them and the 20 patients who were to have no treatment. At follow-up, analyses showed that treated patients had decreased their use of antidepressants and NSAIDS; untreated patients had increased their intake of antidepressants and anxiolytics. Comparison of baseline measures with follow-up measures for each group showed that treated patients improved on all FMS measures;

untreated patients improved on none. The conclusion is that at 1- to 5-year follow-up, the FMS status of euthyroid and hypothyroid patients who underwent metabolic therapy significantly improved compared to matched, untreated FMS patients. The continuation of improved FMS status in treated patients for 1–5 years effectively rules out two possible mechanisms of improvement: a placebo effect, and a tendency to improve over time (regression toward the mean).

The available evidence indicates that the most likely mechanism is inadequate thyroid hormone regulation of cell function. This is caused by a deficiency of thyroid hormone or by partial cellular resistance to thyroid hormone (Lowe 1999).

POSSIBLE CAUSES OF INADEQUATE THYROID HORMONE REGULATION

To what do we attribute the inadequate thyroid hormone regulation in FMS? Hypothyroidism in adults results most frequently from autoimmune thyroiditis, but it often occurs following radiation exposure, surgical removal of part of the thyroid gland, or pituitary failure (Oertel & LiVolsi 1991). For some FMS patients, contamination with dioxin or PCBs may be the source of interference with normal thyroid hormone regulation. These environmental contaminants are nearly ubiquitous in our environment and are abundantly present in human breast milk, fat, and blood (McKinney & Pedersen 1987). The contaminants cause the liver to eliminate thyroid hormone at an abnormally rapid rate (Van den Berg et al 1988). They also displace thyroid hormone from the protein (transthyretin) that transports it into the brain, possibly reducing the concentration of the hormone in the brain (Lans et al 1993). PCBs and dioxin also appear to interfere with the binding of thyroid hormone to its receptors on genes. This interference alters transcription patterns and produces hypothyroid-like effects (McKinney & Pedersen 1987).

ASSESSMENT

We describe below the steps we take to diagnose FMS, monitor for changing status, and treat

patients. Our initial assessment of a patient includes paper and pencil tests, a history, physical examination, an ECG, and thyroid function tests. We use a modified tender point exam and assessment of pain distribution and symptoms that provide greater precision and quantification than the 1990 ACR method (see Box 10.2). Also, the modifications enable us to make decisions in patient care that are more evidence-based (Lowe 1999).

Paper and pencil tests

Our patients complete several forms at their initial visit and at subsequent evaluations:

FibroQuest Questionnaire

This provides us with historical and current information about the patient. We use the responses as a jumping off point for discussion of the patient's complaints. The questionnaire contains visual analog scales for the 13 most common FMS symptoms (pain, fatigue, stiffness, headaches, disturbed sleep, depression, disturbed bowel function, cognitive disturbance, anxiety, paraesthesias, coldness, dry mucous membranes, exercise intolerance, and dysmenorrhea). We total the ratings of symptom severity, divide by 14, and post the mean score on a graph similar to that in Fig. 10.2.

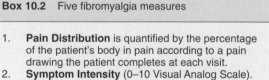

Box 10.2	Five fibromyalgia measures

1. **Pain Distribution** is quantified by the percentage of the patient's body in pain according to a pain drawing the patient completes at each visit.
2. **Symptom Intensity** (0–10 Visual Analog Scale). One VAS for each of the 14 associated symptoms is marked by the patient. A 14th VAS is for the patient's estimate of pain intensity. The average of the 14 scores is posted to a graph.
3. **Tender Point Sensitivity** (the pressure/pain threshold) at each of the 18 tender points is measured with an algometer (calibrated force gauge). The average for the points is calculated.
4. Functional capacity is assessed through the **Fibromyalgia Impact Questionnaire**.
5. Depression is quantified with the **Zung's Self-Rating Depression Scale**, which grades the presence and degree of depression.

At subsequent evaluations, the patient completes the FibroQuest Symptoms Survey. This survey form contains only visual analog scales for the 14 FMS symptoms. The patient estimates the severity of each symptom by marking the appropriate scale. We calculate the mean severity of the 14 symptoms and again post it to graph 1. This running graph provides a visual depiction of changes in symptom intensity. We use the information from this graph and the other four graphs we mention below to make decisions about the patient's management, such as dosage adjustments (Fig. 10.2).

Pain distribution body form

This form contains drawings that show the front, back, and both sides of the body. The patient shades in where he or she has had aching, pain, soreness, tenderness, or paraesthesias since the last evaluation. The patient must be precise in depicting the distribution of the pain. To score these forms, we place a transparent template (that divides the body into 36 areas) over the patient's drawing. The pain distribution is the percentage of the 36 body divisions that contain pain. The percentage is placed on a graph similar to that in Fig. 10.3.

Fibromyalgia Impact Questionnaire

The patient completes this form which measures the impact the patient's condition is having on his or her functional abilities (Fig. 10.4).

Zung's Depression Inventory

This form allows the clinician to classify the patient according to presence and severity of depression (Fig. 10.5).

Patients fill out all four forms at each reevaluation. The single score from each and the mean of the pressure/pain thresholds of the 18 tender points (see below) are posted to separate line graphs. Figures 10.1 to 10.5 show line graphs for the five measures. The graphs show the changes in FMS measures during metabolic rehabilitation of a euthyroid FMS patient reported by

Honeyman (1997). We typically do reevaluations at 1- to 2-week intervals. The graphed data allow us to assess the patient's status in relation to previous evaluations. (Usually, all measures change together in a direction of 'improvement', 'no improvement', or 'worse'.) This permits us to make data-based decisions about changes in the patient's treatment regimen. Through working with the patient and his or her treatment regimen, we manipulate the trend of the lines in the graphs until they reach and stay within the normal range. The patient's subjective status usually corresponds closely to what the trend lines indicate.

Examination

We perform the following each time a patient visits:

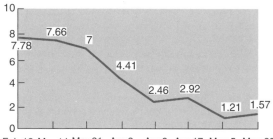

Figure 10.1 The mean intensity of 14 FMS symptoms, determined from the 0–10 visual analog scales of the FibroQuest form. At each evaluation, the mean intensity is calculated and posted to the line graph.

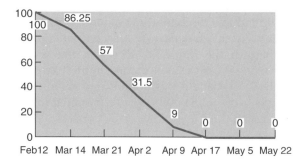

Figure 10.2 Pain distribution. Scores show the percentage of 36 body divisions containing pain at each evaluation (determined by the patient's pain drawing). At each evaluation, the percentage was posted to the graph.

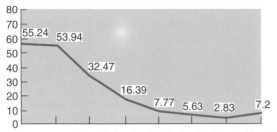

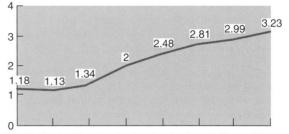

Figure 10.3 Fibromyalgia Impact Questionnaire (FIQ). Scores indicate the patient's level of impaired function. At each evaluation, the total score for the FIQ was posted to the graph. The line shows the trend of changing scores.

Figure 10.5 Tender point sensitivity. At each evaluation, the mean of the pressure/pain thresholds of the 18 FMS tender points (measured with an algometer) was calculated and posted to the graph.

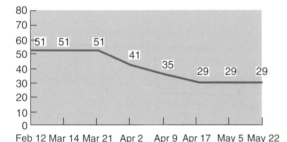

Figure 10.4 Zung's Self-Rating Depression Scale. At each evaluation, the score for Zung's was posted to the graph. Key: ≥70, severe depression: 60–69, moderate depression; 50–59, mild depression; < 50, normal.

Algometer (pressure/pain gauge) exam of tender points

We examine the 18 tender points. We use the same form the patient has shaded to record at each point the pressure in kg/cm^2 at which the algometer tip induces discomfort (an algometer is a calibrated force gauge). We teach patients to distinguish the threshold at which the slowly increasing pressure takes on the slightest noxious quality. We post the mean of the algometer measurements of the 18 points to a graph similar to that in Fig. 10.1.

Achilles reflex

The relaxation phase of the Achilles reflex is abnormally slow in most FMS patients before they begin taking thyroid hormone.

The speed of the relaxation phase is a measure of the status of muscle energy metabolism in the calf muscles. When energy metabolism is low in the calf muscles, they take longer to muster enough energy to fuel separation of the actin and myosin filaments so that the muscle fibers can lengthen. When subnormal muscle energy metabolism is corrected with thyroid hormone, the contraction and relaxation phases of the reflex occur at an equal, brisk speed. Progressive changes in the reflex are a convenient barometer of increasing muscle metabolism in the FMS patient taking thyroid hormone.

Pulse rate and blood pressure

Most FMS patients have low blood pressure, and their pulse rates are usually slow to normal. Recently, some researchers have come to refer to low blood pressure in FMS patients by terms such as 'neurogenic hypotension'. Our model accounts for this, in that the failure of thyroid hormone to regulate transcription allows an increased α-adrenergic receptor count in cells that regulate blood pressure adjustments. This appears to reduce cardiac contractility sufficiently to result in low peripheral blood pressure. Thyroid hormone therapy virtually always normalizes the heart rate and contractility, and usually normalizes the blood pressure.

3. Other tests

We perform an ECG and thyroid function testing at baseline, and we repeat the ECG at various intervals.

ECG

We do a baseline ECG and repeat the test at intervals. The heart is particularly sensitive to exogenous thyroid hormone. For some patients, changes in the ECG are sensitive signs of treatment response. For example, some patient's initially have low voltage ECGs. The PR, QRS, or QT interval may be of maximum normal width or greater. As the thyroid hormone dosage reaches an amount that increases the beta-adrenergic receptor density on heart muscle cell membranes, the intervals usually shorten. The amplitude of the deflections also increase. The most common change, however, is an increase in heart rate, which does not require an ECG to assess. If there is any question whether the patient is having an adverse cardiac effect from exogenous thyroid hormone, we perform another ECG. In an occasional patient, increased heart rate and contractility may amplify underlying cardiac abnormalities. If this occurs, we adjust the patient's thyroid hormone dosage to ensure safety. We also have the patient consult a cardiologist for an evaluation.

Thyroid function testing

Before beginning a patient's treatment, we determine his or her thyroid status. Primary hypothyroidism (thyroid hormone deficiency due to thyroid gland dysfunction) in most patients can be determined with a standard thyroid profile containing a T_4, T_3 uptake, free T_4 index, and TSH. In untreated primary hypothyroidism, the TSH is elevated. (TSH is the pituitary hormone that stimulates the thyroid gland to release thyroid hormone.) This diagnosis is tentative unless the patient has had a thyroidectomy, antithyroid drug therapy, or evidence of antithyroid antibodies. Even in the absence of these in FMS patients, however, a trial of thyroid hormone therapy is warranted.

Euthyroidism (normal function of the hypothalamic–pituitary–thyroid gland axis) and central hypothyroidism (thyroid hormone deficiency due to pituitary or hypothalamic dysfunction) can be identified most conveniently with a TRH stimulation test. [4](TRH is the hypothalamic

hormone that stimulates the pituitary gland to release TSH.) In this test, a blood sample is taken to measure the basal TSH level. TRH is injected and 30 minutes later another blood sample is taken to measure the TSH level again. The clinician subtracts the baseline TSH level from the 30-minute level to derive the TSH response to TRH. A result between 8.5 and 20.0 $\mu U/ml$ is consistent with normal thyroid function. A result below 8.5 $\mu U/ml$ is consistent with pituitary hypothyroidism. A result above 20.0 $\mu U/ml$ is consistent with central hypothyroidism (an exaggerated TSH response to TRH does not distinguish between pituitary and hypothalamic hypothyroidism). The diagnosis is tentative unless there is evidence of other pituitary or hypothalamic hormone abnormalities (from assays), pituitary or hypothalamic structural abnormalities (from imaging), or mutations of the TRH or TSH gene (from nucleotide sequencing).

Because thyroid hormone dosage should be adjusted based on tissue responses, there is no value in reordering the standard thyroid profile after the initial one. The two assumptions that the basal serum TSH level correlates with tissue metabolic status and can be used to predict tissue thyrotoxicity cannot be justified scientifically, and the test should not be ordered for this purpose (Lowe 1999).

TREATMENT

Our treatment protocol primarily involves four components: the use of nutritional supplements, thyroid hormone, exercise to tolerance, and physical treatment.

Nutritional supplementation

In Box 10.3 we have listed the minimum nutritional supplements we require patients to take.

We explicitly instruct patients not to depend on nutritional products that contain only the RDAs. The RDAs provide only 50% more of each nutrient than the amount calculated to prevent abject deficiency disease. Dosages that increase the chances of optimal health are considerably greater.

Box 10.3 Minimum recommended nutritional supplements

Supplement	Dosage per day
B complex	50–100 mg of most
Vitamin C	2000–10 000 mg
Calcium	2000 mg
Magnesium	1000 mg
Multi-minerals*	
Vitamin E complex	800 IU
Beta carotene	30–90 mg

*Not possible to give a general recommendation here

Amounts of the B complex vitamins in products are usually in proper ratio to one another. This makes it convenient to use vitamin B_1 as a guide to dosage. The product would best contain at least 50 mg of vitamin B_1 per tablet, and the patient should take one tablet twice per day. It is important that the patient spread vitamin C intake through the day, taking 1000–3000 mg a minimum of twice daily, but ideally more often. The patient may have to develop tolerance to higher dosages of vitamin C by working up from smaller dosages.

In addition to the antioxidants vitamin C, beta carotene, and vitamin E, the patient should make sure that the mineral formulation contains the antioxidant selenium. The mineral formulation should also contain as wide an array as possible of mineral and trace elements.

Thyroid hormone

Use of supplemental thyroid hormone is central to our treatment regimen. We base the choice of T_4 or T_3 on the outcome of thyroid function testing, and we adjust patient dosages according to specific indications of tissue response at each dosage. As part of their treatment regimen, patients must make lifestyle changes. The changes enable them to maximise the benefits of their increased metabolic capacity. This is essential to the protocol, and they must make the changes as early as possible. Failing to do so is likely to compromise their level of improvement.

Effective treatment of FMS for most patients critically depends on three steps:

1. Selecting the proper form of thyroid hormone
2. Properly titrating the dosage
3. Inducing patients to engage in activities or lifestyle changes that capitalise on the increased metabolic capacity the thyroid hormone gives them.

1. Proper form of thyroid hormone

The euthyroid patient begins treatment with T_3 (usually Cytomel tablets). As a general rule, the patient with either primary or central hypothyroidism begins treatment with T_4. If the patient does not respond to T_4 after a fair trial (a small percentage do not), he or she switches to T_3. The prescribing physician also provides each patient with 20 mg propranolol tablets (which block the effects of thyroid hormone mediated by beta-adrenergic receptors) to use only in case of overstimulation that is bothersome or threatening.

2. Properly titrating dosage

With most FMS patients, 75 µg of T_3 or 0.15 mg of T_4 is a good starting point. We increase patient dosages at 1- to 2-week intervals with T_3 and 3- to 4-week intervals with T_4. Dosage increases at these intervals are 12.5–25 µg of T_3 and 0.05–0.075 mg of T4. We can increase patient dosages of T_3 more aggressively than dosages of T_4. This is because the effects of T_3 have a faster onset (with increased dosages) and offset (with decreased dosages). Finding the effective T_4 dosage usually requires more patience, as the effects of an increase may not be apparent for a couple of weeks. For some patients it may take a month or longer. Cookbook guidance is of limited help in properly adjusting dosages. Only experience with patients will teach the clinician how to properly adjust a patient's dosage.

An ECG before each dosage adjustment can assure patient safety in terms of cardiac function. This is of foremost concern. Most patients experience overstimulation as tremors, rapid heart rate, or excess body heat. These effects do not usually signal dangerous overstimulation, although some patients may be bothered by them. If a rapid or 'pounding' heart with minimal exertion is the predominant symptom indicating over-stimulation, the patient should have an ECG. The clinician should make sure that the sinus rhythm is normal, that the ST segment is not elevated, and that the QT interval is not abnormally short.

Middle-aged and elderly patients who are severely deconditioned should begin thyroid hormone at a very low dosage and increase it very gradually at greater intervals than recommended above. At the same time, they must engage in cardiovascular conditioning activities to tolerance, progressively increasing the intensity. They should also take nutrients scientifically shown to protect the human cardiovascular system.

There are four important considerations in adjusting the patient's dosage of thyroid hormone.

1. Patients with compromised cardiac function. If the patient has compromised heart function, the initial dosage should be low enough to avoid aggravating the heart condition. The starting dose may be 12.5 µg of T_3 or 0.025 mg of T4. If the patient tolerates this dosage well, the dosage can in most cases be increased by 12.5 µg of T_3 every 2–3 weeks, or by 0.0125 mg of T_4 once per month.

Before allowing these patients to increase their dosages, an ECG should be performed to confirm that no adverse cardiac effects have occurred from the previous increase. If adverse effects have occurred, the patient should reduce the dosage sufficiently to assure safety. It may be advisable for the patient to take 20–60 mg of propranolol (for 24–48 hours with T_3 and 1–2 weeks with T_4). These patients should also have a thorough cardiac evaluation.

2. Osteoporosis. If a patient has osteoporosis, we order a baseline bone density study and repeat the study at intervals. The patient should also use mineral supplements (including 1–2 g calcium), 'bone-jerking' types of exercises calibrated to tolerance, and possibly female sex hormone replacement if post-menopausal. We have found that in general, the bone mineral density of female patients who have improved or recovered with metabolic rehabilitation increases

somewhat over time. This probably results from their increased levels of physical activity.

New studies show that for most women, taking thyroid hormone does not significantly reduce bone density as long as the dosage is not excessive for them (and this may have nothing to do with the TSH level). Those at greatest risk are reported to be post-menopausal women not taking sex hormone supplements (Lowe 1999). Testing has shown that most of our FMS patients have not had adverse effects from the use of exogenous thyroid hormone.

3. Dosage adjustments made on the basis of peripheral measures. It is critical that the patient's thyroid hormone dosage *not* be adjusted based on an 'ideal' mid-range TSH level. Many clinicians mistakenly believe that the TSH level correlates with tissue metabolic rate. The TSH level and metabolic rate are out of synchrony in many, and perhaps most, patients. We have found no studies documenting a correlation between the two.

Fibromyalgia patients improve when their dosage is adjusted based on 'peripheral' or 'indirect' measures of metabolic status. These measures, such as the Achilles reflex, serum cholesterol, and increased voltage of the ECG, are more directly related to tissue metabolic status than is the TSH level. Also, we have spent considerable time discerning whether an FMS patient's subjective recovery and increased functional abilities correlate with improvement on the five FMS measures. They typically do, although not in all cases. Certainly, though, these measures are a better guide than the TSH level in making dosage adjustments.

We adjust dosage based on changes in the pencil and paper test results and the outcome of the exam findings at the reevaluations following the last dosage change. If these measures do not indicate that metabolism has increased sufficiently, the patient's dosage is increased. How much the dosage should be increased depends on the patient. For the patient with compromised cardiac function or osteoporosis, the precautions mentioned in the previous two sections should be observed. It may be necessary to increase a patient's dosage only after safety testing. Increases should be small enough and at intervals wide enough to assure patient safety.

4. Objective of dosage adjustments. The objective of dosage adjustments is maximum improvement on all measures of FMS status. Typically, improvement in the measures corresponds to the patient subjectively feeling improved. There may be a lag, however, between objective and subjective improvement, either one preceding the other in some cases. A minority of patients improve solely through the use of thyroid hormone. But complete recovery usually requires that a patient make lifestyle and medication changes as well. We detail these in the section below.

3. Lifestyle and medication changes most patients must make

Most FMS patients who improve only minimally or not at all with metabolic rehabilitation have failed to make lifestyle changes that are necessary parts of the regimen. Most often, these patients fail to engage in regular toning and aerobic exercise to tolerance or to take nutritional supplements. These components of the regimen are indispensable to a favorable outcome. Because of this, we refer patients who find it difficult to make these changes to a physical trainer and/or a nutritionist. Patients who find it difficult to swallow tablets and capsules can take nutritional supplements in liquid form or as wafers that dissolve in the mouth.

Fortunately, many long-suffering FMS patients, in their quest for relief, have already acquired a high quality, wholesome diet supplemented by almost every vitamin, mineral, and trace element. Many have also adopted other measures considered to induce and sustain health. In our experience, these patients have the highest probability of therapeutic success.

Some patients are not able to muster the drive to exercise because of their use of muscle relaxing, sedative, or narcotic medications. These drugs may have previously made life tolerable. However, for virtually all patients, use of these drugs during participation in metabolic rehabilitation sabotages the patient's improvement or recovery. This occurs mainly by the drugs' decreasing the patient's wherewithal for taking part in exercise to tolerance.

Other medications that may interfere with metabolic rehabilitation are tricyclic antidepressants (such as amitriptyline and cyclobenzaprine). These alone may cause tachycardia and ischaemic heart disease. Thyroid hormone typically increases the heart rate as it increases the density of beta-adrenergic receptors on cardiac muscle. In some patients, the use of both thyroid hormone and tricyclic antidepressants and causes a greater increase in heart rate than either medication alone. Patients should therefore stop tricyclic drugs before or soon after beginning to take thyroid hormone.

Patients must also stop beta-blocking medications. Beta-blocking drugs nullify the adrenergic effects of thyroid hormone, and it is these effects that mediate most of the metabolism acceleration from thyroid hormone.

Physical treatment

For most FMS patients as they undergo metabolic rehabilitation, pain scores improve to some degree even without physical treatment. But for many patients, pain measures will indicate maximum pain relief only after the patients undergo effective soft tissue treatment and spinal manipulation. In most cases, the soft tissue treatment must loosen hypertonic muscle and fascial adhesions, and it must desensitise myofascial trigger points. Less often, soft tissue treatment, manipulation, or physiotherapy are needed to resolve chronic musculoskeletal conditions that are sources of noxious neural input to the CNS. Among the most common of such conditions are chronic shoulder and spinal joint dysfunction. When soft tissue treatment is effective, the FMS patient's pain scores usually proceed further toward normal.

Soft tissue treatment

Some patients who respond well to metabolic therapy but who do not have physical treatment are left with regional musculoskeletal pain they may misinterpret as persisting FMS. Patients may continue to calculate this regional pain into their visual analog scales in the FibroQuest Symptom Survey. As a result, when they shade in parts of the body drawing where they have pain, the percentage of their body containing pain may not accurately reflect the benefit they have derived from the metabolic therapy.

Also, inadequate thyroid hormone regulation can cause an energy deficit in muscles. This can mediate energy deficiency contractures that sustain trigger point activity (see Box 10.4). The cycle of reduced blood flow and low threshold nerve endings in the taut bands of muscle housing the trigger points may persist even after a patient's general metabolism becomes normal. Soft tissue techniques may be necessary to inactivate these trigger points and help return the

involved muscle to a normal state. Inactivating the trigger points usually results in improvement in FMS measures, especially pain measures.

It is important that soft tissue treatment be strategically used so as not to exacerbate the patient's pain (see Box 10.5). The most important considerations are that the FMS patient's fascial mechanoreceptors may be hyper-responsive, and her central nervous system pain-modulating system may be impaired. The practitioner should apply soft tissue techniques gently. The goal is to increase circulation through the involved muscle regions while being careful not to increase noxious signal output from the mechanoreceptors.

As the FMS patient progresses through metabolic rehabilitation, more forceful techniques may be applied without adverse effects. Until

---

Box 10.4   Hypometabolism as a factor in the perpetuation of myofascial trigger points

Travell & Simons (1983) wrote of hypometabolism as an endocrine factor that can perpetuate myofascial trigger points (TPs). And in fact they stated that, in some patients, the irritability of TPs is a sensitive indicator of inadequate thyroid function. According to Travell & Simons, clinicians often mention patients with myofascial pain syndrome who also have untreated low thyroid function. In general, these patients are not treated with thyroid hormone for two reasons:

1. Their hypothyroid symptoms are mild
2. Their thyroid hormone blood levels are only low normal or borderline low.

Travell & Simons wrote that hypometabolic patients are more susceptible to myofascial TPs. Specific myofascial therapy usually provides the patients with only temporary relief. But the increased irritability of their muscles and their resistance to physical treatment are improved when they begin using supplemental thyroid hormone, especially T_3. Travell & Simons noted that in contrast to the hypometabolic patient, the hyperthyroid patient (who is, of course, hypermetabolic) rarely has active myofascial trigger points. This observation is consistent with our clinical experiences.

According to Travell & Simons, some hypometabolic patients with normal circulating thyroid hormone levels may still have irritable myofascial TPs. It appears that in these patients thyroid hormone fails to exert a normal effect on metabolism at the level of the patient's muscle cells. Simons contacted me (JCL) in 1994 after he read a paper (Lowe et al 1994) in which, with colleagues, I reported the cases of four patients with TPs and FMS.

The patients all improved or recovered with high dosages of T_3, combined with nutritional supplements and exercise to tolerance (D. G. Simons, personal communication 1994). We proposed in the paper that the patients required high dosages of T_3 because their cells were partially resistant to thyroid hormone. As a possible mechanism of the resistance, we cited the discovery some 6 years before of mutations in the c-*erb*Aβ gene (Refetoff et al 1993). This gene codes for the most common type of thyroid hormone receptor, and mutations in the gene cause mutant T_3 receptors that bind poorly to the hormone. After reading of the discovery, Simons told me that some 10 years before, he had made observations similar to those that we reported in the paper. He had observed that patients with treatment-resistant TPs were responsive to treatment after their hypometabolism was relieved by T_3. At the time, he had searched the published medical literature for a possible mechanism for the patients' improvement. Failing to find relevant studies, he complied with the wishes of some conventional endocrinologists that he abandon the use of T_3 therapy. Now, based on the new research findings, we have some justification for the discriminative use of thyroid hormone therapy for apparently hypometabolic patients. These patients have normal thyroid hormone levels but are resistant to appropriately applied physical treatment methods for myofascial TPs. We have confirmed our clinical observations in a small number of studies. Our need now is to build on these studies so that we learn more about using this hormone approach with hypometabolic patients who are resistant to the physical treatment of TPs.

Box 10.5 Pointers on bodywork techniques for treating patients with fibromyalgia

- Be flexible in positioning for maximum patient comfort.

- Your FMS patient's CNS is impaired in its ability to modulate down incoming sensory signals from mechanoreceptor afferents. Therefore, temper technique and pressure so that the patient's threshold for pain is not exceeded.

- Do not use pressure sufficient to induce a catecholamine release (instead of crossfrictioning, for example, stretching and ultrasound would best be used.)

- Aim to relieve the patient's pain. Understand, however, that until the patient's metabolic status is improved, manual therapies may be capable of providing only slight, and perhaps brief, pain relief.

---

then, however, the practitioner should keep one qualification in mind:

⚠ CAUTION: Except for cross-frictioning, the FMS patient is likely to benefit from any soft tissue technique the practitioner customarily uses with patients who do not have FMS. But with most FMS patients, the practitioner must use less mechanical force than with non-FMS patients. How much the force should be reduced depends upon how excessively sensitive to pressure the individual patient is. A useful method is to instruct the patient to verbally indicate how much discomfort the pressure is causing, on a scale from 0–10. With the typical FMS patient, post-treatment discomfort can be avoided by keeping the discomfort level during treatment between 1 and 5 (Lowe & Honeyman-Lowe 1998).

Spinal manipulation

Most patients benefit from spinal manipulation much as they do from soft tissue treatment. Manipulation relieves segmental facilitation. Facilitation lowers resistance to transmission of nociceptive signals from the periphery into the brain stem and brain through the spinothalamic tracts. It also lowers the threshold for activation of preganglionic sympathetic neurons and alpha motor neurons of an involved segment, possibly inducing peripheral vasoconstriction and shortening muscle fibers of the motor unit. Two controlled studies have shown that spinal manipulation (combined with paraspinal soft tissue manipulation) increased the 'global well-being' of FMS patients (Backstrom & Rubin 1992).

REFERENCES

Awad, E A Personal communication. April 6, 1992

Backstrom G, Rubin B R 1992 When muscle pain won't go away. Taylor Publishing Company, Dallas

Beetham WP Jr 1979 Diagnosis and management of fibrositis syndrome and psychogenic rheumatism. Medical Clinics of North America 63: 433–439

Bland J H, Frymoyer J W 1970 Rheumatic syndromes of myxedema. New England Journal of Medicine 282: 1171–1174

Delamere J P, Scott D L, Felix-Davies D D 1982 Thyroid dysfunction and rheumatic diseases. Journal of the Royal Society of Medicine 75: 102

Eisinger J, Arroyo P H, Calendini C, Rinaldi J P, Combes R, Fontaine G 1992 Anomalies biologiques au cours des fibromyalgies: III. Explorations endocriniennes. Lyon Méditerranée Médicine 28: 858–860

Ferraccioli G, Cavalieri F, Salaffi F et al 1990 Neuroendocrinologic findings in primary fibromyalgia (soft tissue chronic pain syndrome) and in other chronic rheumatic conditions (rheumatoid arthritis, low back pain). Journal of Rheumatology 17: 869–873

Fessel W J 1968 Myopathy of hypothyroidism. Annals of Rheumatic Disease 27: 590–596

Frankhyzen A, Muller A 1983 In vitro studies on the inhibition of serotonin release through α–adrenoreceptor activity in various regions of the rat CNS. Abstract of 5th Catecholamine Symposium, 137

Gerwin R 1995 A study of 96 subjects examined both for fibromyalgia and myofascial pain. Journal of Musculoskeletal Pain 3(S1): 121

Golding D N 1970 Hypothyroidism presenting with musculoskeletal symptoms. Annals of Rheumatic Disease 29: 10–41

Hershman J M 1980 Hypothalamic and pituitary hypothyroidism. In: Bastenie P A, Bonnyns M, VanHaelst L (eds) Progress in the diagnosis and treatment of hypothyroid conditions. Excerpta Medica, Amsterdam

Hochberg M C, Koppes G M, Edwards C Q, Barnes H V, Arnett F C Jr 1976 Hypothyroidism presenting as a polymyositis-like syndrome: report of two cases. Arthritis Rheumatism 19: 1363–1366

Honeyman G S 1997 Metabolic therapy for hypothyroid and

euthyroid fibromyalgia: two case reports. Clinical Bulletin of Myofascial Therapy 2(4): 19–49

Lans M C, Klasson-Wehler E, Willemsen M, Meussen E, Safe S, Bouwer A 1993 Structure-dependent, competitive interaction of hydroxy-polychlorobiphenyls, -dibenzo-*p*-dioxins and -dibenzofurans with human transthyretin. Chemico-Biological Interactions 88(1): 7–21

Lowe J C 1995 T_3-induced recovery from fibromyalgia by a hypothyroid patient resistant to T_4 and desiccated thyroid. Journal of Myofascial Therapy 1(4): 26–31

Lowe J C 1997a Thyroid status of 38 fibromyalgia patients: implications for the etiology of fibromyalgia. Clinical Bulletin of Myofascial Therapy 2(1): 36–41

Lowe J C 1997b Home page, web site: <www.drlowe.com>

Lowe J C 1998 Speeding up to normal: metabolic solutions to fibromyalgia. Hawthorne BioMedical Press, Houston

Lowe J C 1999 The metabolic treatment of fibromyalgia. McDowell Publishing Company, Tulsa

Lowe J C, Honeyman-Lowe G 1998 Facilitating the decrease in fibromyalgic pain during metabolic rehabilitation: an essential role for soft tissue therapies. Journal of Bodywork and Movement Therapies 2(4): 1–9

Lowe J C, Eichelberger J, Manso G, Peterson K 1994 Improvement in euthyroid fibromyalgia patients treated with T_3 (tri-iodothyronine). Journal of Myofascial Therapy 1(2): 16–29

Lowe J C, Garrison R L, Reichman A J, Yellin J, Thompson M, Kaufman D 1997a Effectiveness and safety of T_3 (triiodothyronine) therapy for euthyroid fibromyalgia: a double-blind placebo-controlled response-driven crossover study. Clinical Bulletin of Myofascial Therapy 2(2/3): 31–58

Lowe J C, Reichman A J, Yellin J 1997b The process of change during T_3 treatment for euthyroid fibromyalgia: a double-blind placebo-controlled crossover study. Clinical Bulletin of Myofascial Therapy 2(2/3): 91–124

Lowe J C, Garrison R L, Reichman A J, Yellin J 1997c Triiodothyronine (T_3) treatment of euthyroid fibromyalgia: a small-n replication of a double-blind placebo-controlled crossover study. Clinical Bulletin of Myofascial Therapy 2(4):71–88

Lowe J C, Cullum M, Graf L Jr, Yellin J 1997d Mutations in the c–*erb*Aβ_1 gene: do they underlie euthyroid fibromyalgia? Medical Hypotheses 48(2)Feb: 125–135

Lowe J C, Reichman A J, Yellin J 1998a A case-control study of metabolic therapy for fibromyalgia: long-term follow-up comparison of treated and untreated patients. Clinical Bulletin of Myofascial Therapy 3(1): 65–79

Lowe J C, Reichman A J, Honeyman G S, Yellin J 1998b Thyroid status of fibromyalgia patients. Clinical Bulletin of Myofascial Therapy 3(1): 47–53

McKinney J D, Pedersen L G 1987 Do residue levels of polychlorinated biphenyls (PCBs) in human blood produce mild hypothyroidism? Journal of Theoretical Biology 129: 231–241

Neeck G, Riedel W 1992 Thyroid function in patients with fibromyalgia syndrome. Journal of Rheumatology 19: 1120–1122

Oertel J E, LiVolsi V A 1991 Pathology of thyroid diseases. In: Braverman L E, Utiger R D (eds) Werner and Ingbar's The thyroid: a fundamental and clinical text, 6th edn., New York, J B Lippincott, New York, pp 601–644

Pratley R, Nicklas B, Rubin M 1994 Strength training increases resting metabolic rate and norepinephrine levels in healthy 50–65-year-old men. Journal of Applied Physiology 76(1): 133–137

Refetoff S, Weiss R E, Usala S J 1993 The syndromes of resistance to thyroid hormone. Endocrine Reviews 14: 348–399

Russell I J, Michalek J E, Vipraio J A, Fletcher E M, Javors M A, Bowden C A 1992 Platelet 3H-imipramine uptake receptor density and serum serotonin levels in patients with fibromyalgia/fibrositis syndromes. Journal of Rheumatology 19: 104–109

Shinkai S, Watanabe S, Kurokawa Y, Torii J, Asai H, Shephard R J 1994 Effects of 12 weeks of aerobic exercise plus dietary restriction on body composition, resting energy expenditure, and aerobic fitness in mildly obese middle-aged women. European Journal of Applied Physiology and Occupational Physiology 68(3): 258–265

Shiroky J B, Cohen M, Ballachey M-L, Neville C 1993 Thyroid dysfunction in rheumatoid arthritis: a controlled prospective survey. Annals of Rheumatic Diseases 52: 454–456

Simons D G Personal communication 1994

Sonkin L S 1985 Endocrine disorders and muscle dysfunction. In: Gelb B (ed) Clinical management of head, neck, and TMJ pain and dysfunction. W B Saunders, Philadelpha

Travell J G, Simons D G 1983 Myofascial pain and dysfunction: the trigger point manual. Williams and Wilkins, Baltimore, vol 1

Vaerøy H, Helle R, Øystein F, Kåss E, Terenius L 1988 Elevated CSF levels of substance P and high incidence of Raynaud phenomenon in patients with fibromyalgia: new features for diagnosis. Pain 32: 21–26

Van den Berg K J, Zurcher C, Brouwer A 1988 Effects of 3,4,3',4'-tetrachlorobiphenyl on thyroid function and histology in marmoset monkeys. Toxicology and Applied Pharmacology 41: 77–86

Wilke S W, Sheeler L R, Makarowski W S 1981 Hypothyroidism with presenting symptoms of fibrositis. Journal of Rheumatology 8: 627–630

Wilson J, Walton J N 1959 Some muscular manifestations of hypothyroidism. Journal of Neurology, Neurosurgery, and Psychiatry 22: 320–324

Yellin J 1997 Why is substance P high in fibromyalgia? Clinical Bulletin of Myofascial Therapy 2(2/3): 23–30

11

Integration: what seems to be helping?

• In Chapter 6 Peter Baldry gives an explanation for the potential of acupuncture in treating the pain of fibromyalgiqa syndrome (and myofascial pain syndrome).
• In Chapter 7 Paul Watson describes the potential benefits of cognitive behaviour therapy.
• In Chapter 8 Regina Gilliland provides her insights into current medical treatment of fibromyalgia syndrome, including aspects of complementary approaches to chronic fatigue syndrome and fibromyalgia syndrome.
• In Chapter 9 Mark Pellegrino describes his rehabilitation approach to fibromyalgia syndrome, and here too there is an integrated selection of methods, derived from both orthodox and unconventional sources at work (some of these are described in greater detail in Chapter 12).
• In Chapter 10 John Lowe and Gina Honeyman-Lowe describe their research into thyroid treatment (combined with bodywork) in fibromyalgia syndrome care.

In all these approaches, the overlap between mainstream and complementary/alternative health care is evident.

The vast majority of people suffering these ill-defined and multi-symptomatic conditions turn at least partially to sources outside of mainstream medicine for help, and an increasing number of specialists are utilising one or other – or a combination – of such methods in their treatment and rehabilitation protocols.

This chapter reviews those methods, orthodox and alternative, for which claims are made of benefit for patients with FMS/CFS. Following on from this, Chapter 12 examines additional approaches for which some evidence exists of potential benefit in relation to the associated conditions which often accompany FMS. In Chapter 13 bodywork options are outlined and evaluated.

The methods to be discussed in this chapter include:

- Aerobic exercise
- Acupuncture (see also Ch. 6)
- Chiropractic
- Combined group therapy
- Homeopathy
- Hypnotherapy
- Massage therapy
- Medication
- Nutritional supplementation
- Osteopathy
- Probiotics.

In the end, an integrated protocol which meets the individual needs of the patient should be selected from what is of proven value. It is only by selecting therapeutic choices on evidence-based approaches that a way forward will emerge in handling the devastation which chronic fatigue and fibromyalgia syndromes can cause to people's lives.

PATIENT ADVICE AND ADHERENCE ISSUES

Individuals should be encouraged to listen to their bodies; they should do no more than they feel is appropriate, in order to avoid potentially severe set-backs in progress when they exceed their current capabilities. It is vital that the whole process (whether this involves dietary change, exercise, use of hydrotherapy or anything else which is meant to be self-applied) is very carefully explained, as compliance (adherence) is not high when novel routines or methods are suggested unless they are well understood. This means that any procedures should be explained in terms which make sense to patients and their carer(s). Written or printed notes – ideally illustrated – help greatly to support and encourage adherence to verbal instructions, especially if simply translated instances of successful trials can be included as examples of potential benefit. Instructions, both verbal and written, need to answer in advance questions such as:

- Why is this being suggested?
- How often, how much?
- How can it help?
- What evidence is there of benefit?
- What reactions might be expected?
- What should I do if there is a reaction?
- Can I call or contact you if I feel unwell after exercise (or other self-applied treatment)?

It is useful to explain that *all* treatment makes a demand for a response (or several responses) on the part of the body and that a 'reaction' (something feels different) is normal and expected and is not necessarily a cause for alarm – but that it is OK to make contact for reassurance. It may be useful to offer a reminder that symptoms are not always bad and that change in a condition towards normal may occur in a fluctuating manner, with minor set-backs along the way.

Use of figures such as Figure 2.2 (see Ch. 2) can be helpful to explain to patients, in simple terms, that there are many stressors being coped with and that progress is more likely to come when some of the 'load' is lightened, especially if particular functions (digestion, respiratory, circulation, etc.) are working better.

A basic understanding of homeostasis (see Figs 2.3a, 2.3b, 2.3c in Ch.2) is also helpful ('broken bones mend, cuts heal, colds get better – all examples of how your body always tries to heal itself'), with particular emphasis on explaining processes at work in FMS or CFS. The breathing connection, for example, is dramatically illustrative of a common function with potential for influencing many symptoms common to FMS/CFS (see Fig. 3.3 in Ch.3).

WHAT SEEMS TO BE HELPING?

Research by Dr Don Goldenberg involving a 3-year observation of the natural history of 39 patients with FMS showed that over this time frame 60% complained of continuing symptoms despite virtually constant medication to control the symptoms. Remissions were rare and short-lived.

Goldenberg (1993) has shown that the following methods all produce benefits in treatment of FMS:

- Cardiovascular fitness training (McCain et al 1988)
- EMG-biofeedback (Ferraccioli et al 1989)
- Hypnotherapy (Bengtsson et al 1988)
- Regional sympathetic blockade (Felson & Goldenberg 1986)
- Cognitive–behavioural therapy (Goldenberg 1991).

Block (1993) discusses the waxing and waning nature of the symptoms of FMS, and reports that about 20% of patients with 'generalised rheumatism' achieve remissions which can last for a long time; he believes that therapy should be aimed at alleviating the symptoms where possible and helping patients to cope better.

Research (Wolfe 1986) in a selected patient group reported the results given in Table 11.1.

Clearly all the forms of treatment listed in Table 11.1 helped some patients; however, those groups of patients in this survey who tried exercise, rest, relaxation, physical treatment and chiropractic were the only ones where more people benefited than did not benefit. In the groups using the antidepressant medication there were more patients left feeling that they did not benefit than those feeling that they did; the same was found in the exercise group.

Now we cannot analyse just what exercise or physical therapy was employed, or the benefits,

if any, of methods not included in the survey – and so the best we can do from this survey is to learn that everything helps someone, and some methods help some people more than others. What also emerges from this review is that some orthodox medical approaches, as well as some unorthodox ones, seem to offer hope and relief.

CAUTION: Because examination of a particular method is included in this review (in this, previous and following chapters), it should not be taken as a recommendation for its use. This discussion is an exercise in reporting what is being claimed in what appear to be responsible publications, by a wide range of therapists and practitioners; however, there is no absolute 'quality control' or ability adequately to compare the accuracy of the reports on which these discussions are based.

AEROBIC EXERCISE (McCain 1986)

Cardiovascular exercise is stated to be helpful in rehabilitation from FMS.

The guidelines most commonly given involve the patient performing active aerobic exercise three times weekly (some say four times) for at least 20 (some say 15) minutes, during which time they are required to achieve between 60 and 85% of their maximum predicted heart rate. The methods of exercise best suited to FMS patients

Table 11.1 Results of research in a selected patient group (Wolfe 1986).

Treatment	% who tried treatment	% no improvement	% improvement
Exercise*	86.8	31.8	40.9
Relaxation*	84.2	21.8	46.8
Rest*	97.3	15.1	65.7
Vacation	76.3	53.4	29.3
Pain-killing drugs	88.2	46.3	31.3
Narcotics	61.5	45.8	45.8
Steroid injections	52.6	45.0	35.0
Tranquillisers	28.6	28.6	23.8
Antidepressants	51.5	51.5	36.3
Amitriptyline (bedtime low dose)	51.0	56.6	30.2
Physical therapy*	37.5	31.5	37.5
Chiropractic*	48.7	16.2	45.9

*Methods highlighted by an asterisk indicate treatments where more patients reported benefit than those reporting feeling worse

are said to be cycling (static cycle), walking or swimming.

Appropriate warm-up and warm-down periods are suggested, and a slow incremental programme is needed to reach the prescribed length and frequency of exercising. The release of hormone-like substances (endogenous endorphins) during aerobic exercise is thought to offer the means whereby pain relief and well-being are enhanced, along with the obvious increased self-esteem and psychological boost which comes with increased fitness.

A study involving 34 patients with fibromyalgia had some of the patients perform aerobic exercise (cycle exercise which was designed to achieve a heart rate of 150 per minute) or flexibility exercises (achieving no more than 115 beats per minute) three times a week for 20 weeks. At the end of this period those patients doing the aerobic routines achieved far greater reduction in pain than the flexibility group.

People with CFS (ME) may be unable to do any exercise at all in some stages of their illness.

Research

A Swedish study compared groups of FMS patients who, over a 6-week period, were given (six 1-hour) educational lectures about their condition and how to manage it, with a group who attended these same lectures but who also received (six 1-hour) sessions of physical training (Burckhardt et al 1994). A further group (used to compare the effect of doing something with doing nothing in similar patients) were untreated during this entire study but received treatment after it was over. The results (86 patients completed the study) showed that both the lecture and the lecture plus exercise groups showed a positive impact on their quality of life as well as their pain levels. However, it was those who performed the active exercises that were shown to maintain the benefits more effectively long-term. 87% reported that they were exercising at least three times weekly for 20 minutes or more. Around 70% were practising relaxation techniques. A number had been able to return to work as a result of the programme.

In another study the benefits of exercise (fitness, flexibility and strengthening) programmes were compared with relaxation exercises in a group of 60 FMS patients over a 6-week period at the medical school of the University of Calgary, Canada. Both groups of patients (those doing active exercise, and those doing relaxation) met three times a week for 6 weeks to carry out their routines under supervision. At the start, both groups had the same amount of pain, stiffness, etc. Of the 30 people starting the exercises, 18 completed the course, along with 20 (of the 30) in the relaxation group. Both groups showed an improvement in the number and sensitivity of tender points but those doing the active training exercises were much improved compared with the relaxation group. What this study shows is that a number of people (around a third) fall out of such programmes for one reason or another. Those that complete their assignments usually benefit, and exercising appropriately seems to be very beneficial in FMS (Martin et al 1996).

CAUTION: As previously mentioned, cautions regarding possible reactions to any treatment should be particularly carefully observed where exercise is being suggested. Exercise routines should be introduced with extreme caution and patience in individuals with FMS, and even more so with CFS.

ACUPUNCTURE

Acupuncture in general has an excellent track record in treatment of pain (see Ch. 6). One of the leading experts in use of acupuncture in pain relief, Dr P. Baldry, after asserting categorically that acupuncture is certainly the treatment of choice for dealing with myofascial pain syndrome or trigger point problems, states: 'The pain in FMS – which would seem to be due to some as yet unidentified noxious substance in the circulation giving rise to neural hyperactivity at tender points and trigger points – takes a protracted course and it is only possible by means of acupuncture to suppress this neural hyperactivity for short periods' (Baldry 1993). Baldry believes that it is necessary to repeat treatment every 2–3 weeks for months or even years, which he regards as unsatisfactory, 'but nevertheless some patients insist that it improves the quality of their lives'. Relief from pain for weeks on end and an enhanced quality of life would seem quite a desirable objective, perhaps helping ease the pain burden while more fundamental approaches are dealing with constitutional and causative issues.

Electro-acupuncture

A Swiss research team in Geneva has examined the effectiveness of electro-acupuncture in treating FMS in 70 patients (54 women) who all met the American College of Rheumatology criteria for FMS. They received either sham acupuncture ('wrong' points used) or the real thing. Various methods were used for patients to record their level of symptom activity and the amount of medication they used before and after treatment. Sleep quality, morning stiffness and pain were all monitored.

The electro-acupuncture treatment was administered over a 3-week period. Only the doctor giving the treatment knew whether or not the needles were being placed correctly and whether the amount and type of electrical current being passed through the needles was correct. Seven out of the eight measurements showed that only the acupuncture group and not the placebo (dummy acupuncture) group had benefits (as in all such studies a few minor improvements are always noted in the dummy or placebo group but these were only slight). The acupuncture group, after treatment, required far more pressure on tender points to produce pain while use of pain-killing medication was virtually halved, as was these patients' assessment of regional pain levels. There was also a significant improvement in quality of sleep. The length of time morning stiffness was experienced only improved a small amount. Around 25% of the treated group did not improve significantly; all the others showed a remarkable amount of improvement, with some having almost complete relief of all symptoms. The duration of the improvement was noted to be 'several weeks' in most patients, which seems to be in line with Dr

Baldry's observation of it being necessary to repeat treatment every few weeks (DeLuze et al 1992).

Dry needling and myofascial trigger points (Sandford Kiser et al 1983)

In a study, 46% of those people with myofascial pain syndrome found that 'dry needling' (see Ch. 6) offered them the longest lasting relief of symptoms compared with other forms of treatment they had received. 69% required less medication for some time afterwards.

CAUTION: Acupuncture should only be applied by suitably trained practitioners or therapists. There is evidence that following acupuncture a degree of 'soreness and discomfort' at the needle sites is experienced by individuals suffering FMS, and they should be cautioned to expect this. Anyone who is afraid of acupuncture should not be 'persuaded' into trying it.

CHIROPRACTIC

Chiropractic is one of the alternative approaches most used by patients with fibromyalgia. In one review it was reported that almost 50% of FMS patients attend for chiropractic treatment, with 46% of these reporting a moderate to a great degree of improvement (Wolfe 1986).

Significantly, in their review of chiropractic efficacy in treatment of FMS, Blunt and colleagues suggest that chiropractic management would be associated with additional potentially useful methods, including soft tissue massage and 'spray and stretch' (Blunt et al 1997). To what extent, in any given case, the soft tissue approaches alone produce the major benefits is certainly open to debate. They highlight various mechanisms which might be involved:

- Pain inhibition may be achieved in the following ways:
    - spinal mobility following manipulation tends to decrease central transmission of pain from adjacent structures (Gatterman et al 1990)
    - endogenous opioids may also be released following manipulation (Irving 1981)

— pressure pain thresholds of cervical paraspinal musculature increases following manipulation.

• Paraspinal muscles relax due to stretching of apophyseal joint capsules, reflexly inhibiting motor neuron pools which may be facilitated and so be responsible for increased tone. Intrafusal fibres are stretched during manipulation, helping restore balanced afferent/efferent impulses in the proprioceptive system of the joint and local musculature (Korr 1975, Shambaugh 1987).

• Articular adhesions may be reduced or broken in chronic cases (Kirkaldy-Willis et al 1984).

• Range of motion should increase (Lewit 1985).

In a pilot study (a randomised crossover pilot trial), a group of Canadian chiropractors (Blunt et al 1997) selected 21 rheumatology patients with FMS, aged between 25 and 70 years. Ten patients received treatment 3–5 times per week for 4 weeks. During this time the remainder (the controls) received no treatment, but received it in the following 4-week period (only nine were involved by this stage, as two patients had dropped out). Treatment consisted of:

• Soft tissue massage using a counterirritant cream
• Soft tissue stretching with and without fluoromethane as a chilling agent (used especially in early stages and on the scalene muscles)
• Spinal manipulation (minimal amplitude, low velocity) applied to joints with a 'hard' end-feel
• Education, involving provision of information of aggravating factors, sleep habits, body mechanics, understanding the aetiology of FMS.

The study confirms the benefit in pain modulation and functional status in FMS patients of carefully applied manipulative methods incorporating both osseous and soft tissue methods. Studies which compare joint manipulation with soft tissue approaches would help to clarify their relative benefits. There is no evidence that the underlying condition is assisted by these methods, although they clearly have an important role to play in management (as is strongly suggested by Dr Lowe in Chapter 10).

COMBINED (GROUP) TREATMENT
(Bennett et al 1996)

Research at the department of medicine of Oregon Health Sciences University in the USA evaluated the impact of 6 months (1 hour per week) of group treatment involving lectures and group sessions of active fitness training, stress reduction, relaxation, behaviour modification and flexibility (stretching exercises). A questionnaire was used to evaluate the impact of FMS on people's lives and their total tender point score was also measured regularly. Also measured were levels of fitness (how far could they walk in 6 minutes?), depression scores, quality of life scores, etc. Between 15 and 25 patients turned up regularly and their condition was monitored for 2 years after the end of the 6 months of the trial. Over a 4-year period, 170 patients took part in the study, with 104 completing the full 6 months during their time on the programme. The findings were as follows:

• After 6 months on this combined group programme, 70% of those completing it had reduced their number of tender points to fewer than 11
• There was a 25% improvement in the impact of fibromyalgia on their lives
• After 2 years, 33 patients who were questioned and examined showed continued improvement
• Approximately 30 people who never entered the programme were followed, for comparison with those in the active group. These non-active FMS patients showed no improvement over the same period.

HOMEOPATHY

Several studies have looked at the effects of a specific homoeopathic remedy, Rhus Tox, in treating FMS and 'fibrositis' – with quite different results.

There is a need to understand the basis of homoepathic prescribing in order to make sense of the different results in trials of this substance. Homoeopathic remedies comprise minute quantities of substances which in larger amounts would produce symptoms very similar to, or identical with, the symptoms being experienced. Once the substance has been 'proved' – by many human trials – it is then used in an extremely diluted form to treat the symptoms of the condition in people whose temperament and personality, as well as numerous other characteristics, fit the picture of the people most affected by the medication during its trials. When a remedy is selected in classical homeopathy, therefore, it is not just the symptoms which are taken into account but a 'constitutional profile' of the person affected. This means that while two people might have the same named condition – say asthma – they might require different remedies if they had different personalities, likes and dislikes, and were affected by different factors.

Although treatment of painful rheumatic conditions by homeopathy often involves the use of Rhus Tox, it is considered not to be suitable for all people with such conditions, but only for those with the profile of the medicine.

The ideal person for using Rhus Tox is:

• Restless, continually changing position, having a great deal of apprehension, especially at night, and finds it difficult to stay in bed; the head will feel heavy, and the jaw may be noisy, creaking, with TMJ pain.
• The tongue tends to be coated except for a red triangular area near the tip, and there is frequently a bitter taste in the mouth and a desire for milky drinks; there is often a drowsy feeling after eating.
• There may be a nagging dry cough and a sense of palpitation, most noticeable when sitting still. The back tends be stiff and normally feels better for moving about; limbs are stiff and any exposure to cold makes the skin feel sensitive or painful.
• Cold, wet weather makes symptoms worse, as does sleep and resting.
• What helps most, as far as symptoms are concerned, is warm, dry weather, movement, rubbing the uncomfortable areas, warm applications and stretching.

The remedy is Rhus Tox in the 6C potency.

Trials (Fisher et al 1989, Gemmell et al 1991)

In Britain, a study found that using the 6C dilution of Rhus Tox was effective in moderating the symptoms of patients with FMS, whereas in a trial in Australia involving just three patients who fitted all the criteria, including the profile for Rhus tox, there was no benefit when a 6X dilution was used.

The difference between 6X and 6C may seem unimportant, but the dilution difference is enormous. To make a 1C dilution, one part of the substance is vigorously mixed with 99 parts of ethanol (an alcohol used to preserve the substance). To make 2C dilution, one drop of the first mix is placed with another 99 drops of ethanol and the process is repeated. By the time you get to 6C the dilution is minute, and this is what was used in the first – successful – study mentioned. Paradoxically this is called a 'high' potency and is considered more powerful and faster acting in terms of triggering a healing response than a low potency. 'X' potencies are low: one drop of the substance to 9 drops of ethanol are needed to make 1X, with the process being repeated five more times to make 6X, as used in the second – unsuccessful – trial discussed above.

Since there is absolutely no chance of side-effects with homeopathy, there is little to be lost in trying the 6C dilution.

CAUTION: There are no contraindications to homoeopathic medication.

HYPNOTHERAPY (Haanen et al 1991)

In controlled trials it has been found that hypnotherapy helps more than physical therapy in those patients who do not seem to respond well to most other forms of treatment. Pain is reduced, fatigue and stiffness on waking are improved, and general feeling of well-being is greater.

CAUTION: Only fully qualified hypnotherapists should employ these techniques.

MASSAGE THERAPY

Research from the Touch Research Institute, University of Miami Medical School, indicate benefits from appropriate forms of massage in treatment of FMS (Sunshine et al 1996).

While many FMS patients frequently request deep work, this is contraindicated, based on what is known of the mechanisms involved in FMS. The most useful manual methods seem to involve non-specific wellness massage and lymphatic drainage plus finely targeted specific interventions using aspects of soft tissue manipulation, most specifically positional release and vibrational methods (see Osteopathy, below, and Ch. 13).

The removal or deactivation of myofascial trigger points and other local dysfunction by minimally invasive methods, combined with homeostatic enhancing approaches (nutrition, relaxation methods, hydrotherapy, etc.) would seem to be additionally useful applications of massage therapy.

CAUTION: Massage requires skill and patience, and only fully qualified massage therapists who understand the risks regarding excessively deep treatment or overtreatment in conditions such as FMS should be referred to. FMS patients often 'demand' deep tissue treatment for painful muscles, despite the fact that this is inappropriate (for reasons explained in earlier chapters, and in Ch. 12). Massage therapists specialising in chronic fatigue and FMS patients would be aware of this.

MEDICATION

• The most widespread treatment approach to FMS involves the use of various pharmacological agents and it is useful to evaluate the results of studies as to their efficacy. Tricyclic antidepressant medication increases the amount of serotonin in the central nervous system and increases the delta-wave sleep stage; it is found consistently to improve the symptoms of fibromyalgia, though not by acting as an antidepressant and not in all patients treated.

• Studies involving various forms of antidepressant medication tend to support use of amitriptyline (25–50 mg daily), with pain scores, stiffness, sleep and fatigue all improving on average, but by no means in all patients (Carette et al 1986).

• In one study, 77% of FMS patients receiving amitriptyline reported general improvement after 5 weeks as against only 43% of those receiving placebo medication. Side-effects from the antidepressant were, however, measurable, with a selection of drowsiness, confusion, seizure, agitation, nightmares, blurred vision, hallucinations, uneven heartbeat, gastrointestinal upsets, low blood pressure, constipation, urinary retention, impotence and mouth dryness all being observed or reported (Goldenberg et al 1986).

• When combined with osteopathic manipulative methods (mainly soft tissue techniques – see below), antidepressant medication offered greater relief (Rubin et al 1990).

• A study by Carette & Bell (1994) showed that amitriptyline was no more effective than placebo and that Flexyril caused widespread adverse effects in 98% of those taking it, with these being so severe in 13% that they had to cease taking it. Only 12% showed mild improvement in FMS symptoms (Carette & Bell 1994).

• A study involving the use of systemic corticosteroids (prednisone 15 mg daily) showed that there were no measurable improvements, and since side-effects with such medication are usual, this approach is clearly not desirable. In fact, if such medication were to produce an improvement it would be sensible to question whether fibromyalgia was indeed the correct diagnosis – some other rheumatic condition is more likely to improve symptomatically with the use of corticosteroids (Clark et al 1985).

• When muscle relaxants were tested in FMS patients, most were found to be useless, but cyclobenzaprine was found to improve pain levels, sleep and tender point count (10–40 mg daily, given at night to prevent daytime drowsiness); this is thought to be because it has a chemical similarity to amitripyline (Campbell et al 1985).

• Goldenberg conducted a double-blind, placebo controlled, crossover study involving 19 FMS patients in which a combination of drugs were evaluated. The results (reported in Fibromyalgia Network 1996) indicated that a combination of 20 mg Prozac in the morning and 25 mg Elavil in the evening produced the best results – reducing pain and enhancing sleep.

Benefits were noted within 3 weeks of starting. However, the report concludes, 'Goldenberg could not offer reassurance as to how long this positive improvement would last (Fibromyalgia Network 1996).

• Many other drugs are currently being researched and tried in treatment of FMS, ranging from antiviral agents to substances which modulate the immune system. Various cocktails of antidepressant and sedative medications are being tried out as well. Even aspirin has been tested and is said to be mildly useful!

CAUTION: There exists a range of herbal and nutrient-based alternatives to the sort of pharmacological agents discussed above (St John's wort for example, see below) and although these are potentially 'safer' than prescription drugs it is suggested that only practitioners who have had training in this area, or who have had appropriate postgraduate experience and training (medical physicians, medical herbalists, naturopaths, homeopaths, osteopathic physicians, chiropractors, etc.) should prescribe nutrients or herbal products which have the potential to modify depression or anxiety states.

NUTRITIONAL SUPPLEMENTATION

The information in this section on nutrition as a factor in fibromyalgia treatment is largely derived from information generously provided by one of the world's leading researchers into nutritional influences on illness, Melvyn Werbach MD, of Tarzana, California, whose texts *Nutritional Influences on Illness* and *Nutritional Influences on Mental Illness*, and his authoritative and comprehensive CD-Rom (Werbach 1998), offer clinicians and researchers invaluable resources. A summary of nutritional supplementation research as it applies to fibromyalgia (or 'muscular rheumatism', or non-articular rheumatism) is listed below (Werbach 1998).

Please note the cautions within and at the end of this section.

Thiamine

• The nutritional status of thiamine may be impaired in fibromyalgia (Eisinger et al 1992a,

Eisinger & Ayavou 1990) and this may be associated with magnesium deficiency since thiamine dependent enzymes require adequate magnesium (Eisinger et al 1994).

• Supplementation (via intramuscular injection) has been shown to be helpful in treating FMS in a French study in which 21 patients were supplemented with 50 mg thiamine pyrophosphate intramuscularly three times a week for 6 weeks: 20 of the patients (95%) showed good results. These results were compared with just five of 13 FMS patients benefiting who received 100 mg intramuscular thiamine hydrochloride three times weekly for 6 weeks. This indicates that deficiency of thiamine was not the problem but a defect in thiamine metabolism (Eisinger et al 1988, Eisinger 1987).

Magnesium

• A number of symptoms associated with FMS, including muscle pain, fatigue, sleep disturbance and anxiety, may result from magnesium deficiency (Romano & Stiller 1994).

• Many researchers believe that FMS may involve chronic hypoxia, predominantly caused by enhanced gluconeogenesis associated with muscle protein breakdown and deficiency of oxygen and other substances needed for ATP (energy) synthesis. Magnesium deficiency would result in such an inefficient respiratory chain (Abraham & Flechas 1992).

• When 100 patients with FMS were compared with osteoarthritic patients and what are regarded as normal levels, it was found that erythrocyte levels in FMS patients were on average lower, with the implication that magnesium status was low (Romano & Stiller 1994). In some studies, red-blood cell levels of magnesium were found to be low in FMS patients (Eisinger et al 1988), whereas in other studies (Eisinger & Ayavou 1990, Prescott et al 1992) no differences were found in red-cell magnesium concentrations when patients with FMS were compared with age- and sex-matched normal controls.

Selenium

• A number of studies suggest that selenium deficiency may be associated with muscle pain (van Rij et al 1979).

- Serum levels of selenium may be low in people with chronic muscular pain conditions (James et al 1985).
- Supplementation of selenium may be beneficial (100 μg daily as selenomethionine). In one New Zealand (where selenium levels in the soil are very low) trial (experimental double-blind study), nearly 60% of those with 'fibromuscular rheumatism' supplemented, benefited after 12 weeks (Robinson et al 1981).
- When selenium (140 μg sodium selenite) was supplemented together with vitamin E (100 mg daily α-tocopherol) in people with disabling muscular pain, marked benefits in pain reduction were achieved, especially in those patients who displayed an increase in glutathione peroxidase following supplementation (75% of those treated) (Jameson et al 1985).

Arginine

- Generalised pain and fatigue induced by growth hormone and serotonin depletion may be treated with arginine (or ornithine) supplementation (Eisinger et al 1992b). Up to 4 g arginine (or 2 g ornithine) are taken both morning and evening, away from meal times.

CAUTION: If arginine or ornithine are taken, it should be for a period of 2–3 months only, with a similar rest period before starting again. This is suggested to prevent imbalances in the amino acid content in the body from developing.

- Growth hormone stimulators should never be taken (unless under supervision) by anyone who has not completed their growth phase.
- Skin may become coarse if excessive growth hormone is released.
- A supplement of antioxidants (vitamins A, C, E, selenium) is suggested as a useful accompaniment to taking these amino acids.

Malic acid

- This is both derived from food sources (especially apples) and synthesised in the citric acid cycle, and plays an important role in generating mitochondrial ATP under both aerobic and hypoxic conditions. Supplementation, together with magnesium, may be beneficial.

- Not all trials have proved positive: for example, an experimental double-blind crossover study involving 24 patients with primary fibromyalgia who randomly received magnesium malate (Super Malic) 3 tablets twice daily (containing a total of 300 mg magnesium as magnesium hydroxide and 1200 mg malic acid) or placebo, each for 4 weeks, with a 2-week washout period in between, produced no evidence of benefit. The results of those patients taking magnesium malate were not significantly better than those taking the placebo, as assessed by pain, tenderness, and functional and psychological measures. Side-effects were limited to loose stools (Russell et al 1995).
- On the other hand, benefits were noted during an experimental study involving 16 patients with primary fibromyalgia who completed a 6-month open trial of magnesium malate (Super Malic, each containing 50 mg magnesium as magnesium hydroxide and 200 mg malic acid) in which the dose of magnesium malate was gradually increased to a mean of 8.8 tablets daily (range 4–14 tablets daily). Significant improvements were seen in pain and tenderness after 2 months but there were no improvements in functional or psychological measures. Side-effects were limited to loose stools (Russell et al 1995).
- In another single-blind experimental study, 15 patients with primary fibromyalgia were treated for an average of 8 weeks with 2–600 mg magnesium and 12–2400 mg malate. Pain scores dropped steadily during the trial and went up again within 24 hours of placebo being used instead of the malic acid/magnesium (Abraham & Flechas 1992).

S-adenosyl-L-methionine (SAMe)

- Supplementation of this may be beneficial in fibromyalgia, starting with an initial dosage of 600–1200 mg daily. If GI symptoms occur, the dosage should be reduced by half, then gradually increased again as tolerated. It may take several months for SAMe to achieve its full therapeutic effect (SAMe 1997).
- In an experimental study, 47 patients received 200 mg of intramuscular SAMe daily plus 400 mg

SAMe orally twice daily. After 6 weeks of SAMe supplementation, tenderness was significantly reduced, as were scores for depression and anxiety. It was well tolerated with few side-effects (Grassetto & Varotto 1994).

• In another experimental study, 30 patients with primary fibromyalgia received either SAMe or transcutaneous electrical nerve stimulation (TENS). After 6 weeks, those patients receiving SAMe demonstrated a significantly decreased number of tender points, felt better generally and had lower scores in depression and anxiety assessment. Patients in the TENS group only had significant reductions in anxiety levels with no significant pain reduction or alteration in depression levels (Benedetto et al 1993).

• In an experimental double-blind study, 44 patients with fibromyalgia received 800 mg SAMe daily for 6 weeks. Improvements were seen for clinical disease activity (p=0.04), pain experienced during the last week (p=0.002), fatigue (p=0.02), morning stiffness (p=0.03) and mood evaluated by Face Scale (p=0.006) in the actively treated group compared to placebo. The tender point score, isokinetic muscle strength, mood evaluated by Beck Depression Inventory and side-effects did not differ in the two treatment groups (Jacobsen et al 1991).

• In a short-term crossover trial, 17 patients with primary fibromyalgia, 11 of whom had a substantial depression, were treated with SAMe and placebo. The number of trigger points plus painful anatomic sites decreased after SAMe (p<0.02) but not after placebo. In addition, scores in various depression rating evaluations decreased significantly after SAMe but not after placebo (Tavoni et al 1987).

L-tryptophan

• Plasma/serum levels may be reduced in patients with fibromyalgia (Yunus et al 1992).

 CAUTION: The amino acid tryptophan is no longer available over the counter after a contaminated batch from Japan caused severe toxic reactions. 5-HTP (5-hydroxy-L-tryptophan), a tryptophan-like substance derived from an African bean, is now available and clinical experience suggests it is useful in sleep enhancement.

5-hydroxy-L-tryptophan (available in health food stores and pharmacies)

• Supplementation may be beneficial. In an experimental study, 50 patients with primary fibromyalgia syndrome received 5-hydroxy-L-tryptophan 100 mg three times daily. After 90 days, the number of tender points, anxiety, pain intensity, quality of sleep, and fatigue all showed significant improvement (p<0.001). 15/50 (30%) reported side-effects, but only one patient needed to be withdrawn. There were no abnormalities due to the treatment in laboratory testing (Puttini & Caruso 1992).

• In an experimental double-blind study, 50 patients with primary fibromyalgia syndrome randomly received either 5-hydroxy-L-tryptophan 100 mg three times daily or placebo. After 30 days there were significant declines in the number of tender points and in the intensity of subjective pain, and significant improvements in morning stiffness, sleep patterns, anxiety and fatigue compared to placebo. Only mild and transient side-effects were reported (Caruso et al 1990).

Hydrolytic enzymes

• Administration may be beneficial after some weeks or months. In an experimental double-blind multicentre study, 424 patients with non-articular rheumatism received either a mixture of trypsin, chymotrypsin, lipase, amylase, pancreatin, papain and bromelain or placebo. Significant symptom improvement was noted in the enzyme group. Side-effects were rare and minimal (Uffelmann et al 1990).

• In an experimental study, 1004 patients with rheumatic disability (407 with arthrosis, 238 with arthritis, 155 with soft tissue rheumatism and 204 with multiple rheumatoid diagnoses), seen by 141 practising physicians and specialists, received treatment with an enzyme mixture (trypsin, chymotrypsin, amylase, lipase, pancreatin, bromelain and papain). Clinical findings were rated on a 0–3 scale for pain at rest, pain upon weight-bearing, pain on pressure, morning stiffness, and functional impairment. 67% of the total group had a good to excellent response (p=0.05). Improvement was noted in 76% of patients with arthrosis, 86% of those with arthritis, *90% of those with soft tissue rheumatism*, and 76% of those with multiple diagnoses. The shorter the duration of illness, the better the results. Over 99% of patients and doctors reported that enzyme therapy caused virtually no side-effects (Horger et al 1988).

CAUTION:

• Supplements should be taken according to recommended dosages only – more is not necessarily better and some nutrients can be toxic.

• When recommending any of these supplements to someone who has a tendency to allergy or food intolerance/sensitivity it is wise to introduce just one at a time and to evaluate for reactions for some days before commencing any other supplement or therapeutic change. 'One at a time' is a rule which should be used for ALL changes in lifestyle, diet, medication, therapeutic intervention in individuals whose coping and adaptation mechanisms are already stretched and struggling. It is as well to keep in mind the example of allostasis, in which normal homeostatic responses are exaggerated or deficient, and to therefore ask for only one change at a time, however innocuous it may seem.

OSTEOPATHY

Osteopathic medicine, from which both SCS (Strain/Counterstrain – a form of 'positional release') and muscle energy technique (MET) derive (see Ch. 13), has conducted many studies involving FMS, including:

• Doctors at Chicago College of Osteopathic Medicine (led by A. Stotz and R. Keppler) measured the effects of osteopathic manipulative therapy (OMT, which includes SCS and MET) on the intensity of pain felt in the diagnostic tender points in 18 patients who met all the criteria for FMS. Each had six visits/treatments and it was found over a 1-year period that 12 of the patients responded well in that their tender points

became less sensitive (14% reduction in intensity as against a 34% increase in the six patients who did not respond well). Most of the patients – the responders and the non-responders to OMT – showed (using thermographic imaging) that their tender points were more symmetrically spread after the course than before. Activities of daily living were significantly improved, and general pain symptoms decreased overall (Stoltz 1993).

• Doctors at Texas College of Osteopathic Medicine selected three groups of FMS patients, one of which received OMT, another had OMT plus self-teaching (learning about the condition and self-help measures), and a third group received only moist-heat treatment. The group with the least reported pain after 6 months of care was that receiving OMT, although some benefit was noted in the self-teaching group (Jiminez et al 1993).

• Another group of doctors from Texas College of Osteopathic Medicine tested the difference in results involving 37 patients with FMS of using:

a. drugs only (ibuprofen, alprazolam)
b. OMT plus medication
c. a dummy medication (placebo) plus OMT
d. a placebo only.

The results showed that drug therapy alone resulted in significantly less tenderness being reported than did drugs and manipulation, or the use of placebo and OMT, or placebo alone. Patients receiving placebo plus manipulation reported significantly less fatigue than the other groups. The group receiving medication and OMT showed the greatest improvement in their quality of life (Rubin et al 1990).

• At Kirksville, Missouri College of Osteopathic Medicine, 19 patients with all the criteria of FMS were treated once a week for 4 weeks using OMT. 84.2% showed improved sleep patterns, 94.7% reported less pain and most patients had fewer tender points on palpation (Rubin et al 1990).

CAUTION: Unless osteopathic practitioners/physicians have experience of FMS, it is suggested that they avoid 'normal' degrees of force and pressure in treating such conditions, or that they refer to colleagues with appropriate experience. Cranial osteopathic treatment can be helpful, since it is both extremely gentle and of particular value in such conditions.

PROBIOTIC STRATEGIES

If the digestive system's flora are dysfunctional due to any of a number of reasons, including steroid medication, antibiotics or a high fat/high sugar diet, bowel dysbiosis may result. Irritable bowel problems, yeast and undesirable bacterial overgrowth are just some of the possible precursors of major systemic dysfunction involving toxicity, deficiency and liver and/or kidney overload (Sneath 1986) (see also Figs 3.4 and 11.1).

Use of probiotics – freeze-dried 'friendly' bacteria – has been shown to be one way of encouraging 'reflorastation' of the gut, as long as those practices which are mitigating against healthy bowel status are also addressed.

The friendly bacteria (Rasic 1990)

Before we examine the benefits these bacteria offer, and the health problems which can develop if they are damaged, we should briefly meet them individually:

Bifidobacterium bifidum. These friendly bacteria inhabit the intestines, with a greater presence in the large intestine (the colon) than in the small intestine. They also live in the vagina. Their major roles are:

- Preventing colonisation by hostile microorganisms by competing with them for attachment sites and nutrients
- Preventing yeasts from colonising the territories which they inhabit
- Helping to maintain the right levels of acidity in the digestive tract to allow for good digestion
- Preventing substances such as nitrates from being transformed into toxic nitrites in our intestines
- Manufacturing some of the B-vitamins
- Helping detoxify the liver.

Streptococcus thermophilus. This is a transient (non-resident) bacterium of the human intestine which, together with Lactobacillus bul-

garicus, is a yogurt culture, also found in some cheeses. It performs a number of useful roles, e.g.:

- Some strains produce natural antibiotic substances
- They enhance the ability to digest milk and its products by producing the enzyme lactase which is absent or deficient in almost half the adults on earth, and in many children, especially if they are of Asian, African or Mediterranean genetic stock
- Because they produce lactic acid (this is the only streptococcus to produce lactic acid, which it makes in even greater quantities than L. bulgaricus), they help to create an environment which encourages colonisation by the bifidobacteria (they are therefore known as 'bifidogenic' bacteria) and L. acidophilus, as well as helping to prevent colonisation by undesirable microorganisms.

Streptococcus faecium. This is a natural resident of the human intestine. It is found in human faeces as well as on some plants and insects:

- They are used as a part of the manufacture of cheeses (in some dairies, but not in all)
- Their potential benefit to humans remains a possibility but not a certainty
- They manufacture lactic acid from carbohydrates and so enhance the environment for colonising friendly bacteria.

Lactobacillus acidophilus. This natural inhabitant of the intestines also lives in the mouth and vagina. Its main site of occupation is the small intestine. They:

- Prevent colonisation by hostile microorganisms such as yeasts by competing with them for attachment sites and nutrients
- Produce lactic acid (out of carbohydrates) which helps maintain the correct environment for digestion by suppressing hostile organisms (other bacteria and yeasts)
- Improve the digestion of lactose (milk sugar) by producing the enzyme lactase
- Assist in digestion and absorption of essential nutrients from food
- Destroy invading bacteria (not all strains of L. acidophilus can do this)

- Slow down and control yeast invasions such as *Candida albicans.*

Bifidobacterium longum. This is a natural inhabitant of the human intestines and vagina. It is found in larger numbers in the large intestine than in the small intestine. Together with other bifidobacteria, this is the dominant organism of breast-fed infants (making up 99% of the microflora). In adolescence and adult life the bifidobacteria are still the dominant organism of the large intestine (when health is good). Main benefits include:

- Preventing colonisation by hostile microorganisms by competing with them for attachment sites and nutrients
- Production of lactic and acetic acids which inhibit invading bacteria
- Helping in weight gain in infants by retention of nitrogen
- Preventing harmful nitrites being formed from nitrates in the digestive tract
- Manufacturing B-vitamins
- Assisting in liver detoxification.

Bifidobacterium infantis. This is a natural inhabitant of the human infant's digestive tract (as well as the vagina, in small quantities). Its presence is far greater in the gut of breast-fed infants compared with bottle-fed infants. Among its main benefits are:

- Preventing colonisation by hostile microorganisms by competing with them for attachment sites and nutrients
- Production of lactic and acetic acids which inhibit invading bacteria
- Helping in weight gain in infants by retention of nitrogen
- Preventing harmful nitrites being formed from nitrates in the digestive tract
- Manufacturing B-vitamins.

Lactobacillus bulgaricus. This extremely useful friendly bacterium is not a resident of the human body, but a 'transient'. Once it enters the body through food (yogurt for example) it remains for several weeks before being passed, but while in the body it performs useful tasks. It performs a number of useful roles, such as:

- Some strains produce natural antibiotic substances
- Some strains have been shown to have anti-cancer properties
- These bacteria enhance the ability to digest milk and its products by producing the enzyme lactase which is absent or deficient in almost half the adults on earth, and in many children, especially if they are of Asian, African or Mediterranean genetic stock
- Because they produce lactic acid (as do all bacteria which have as the first part of their name 'lactobacillus') they help to create an environment which encourages colonisation by the bifidobacteria (they are therefore known as 'bifidogenic' bacteria) and *L. acidophilus,* as well as helping to prevent colonisation by undesirable microorganisms.

Other lactobacilli. Additional (useful) lactobacilli found in the digestive tract include:

- *L. casei* – a transient bacterium of the intestine
- *L. plantarum* – a transient bacterium of the intestine
- *L. brevis* – a transient bacterium of the intestine
- *L. salivarius* – a natural resident of the mouth and digestive tract
- *L. delbrueckii* – a transient bacterium of the intestine
- *L. caucasicus* (known as *L. kefir*).

List of benefits

List of benefits offered by friendly bacteria – *when they are healthy* (Dubos & Schaedler 1962, Gilliland et al 1985, Gilliland & Speck 1977):

- They improve the ability to digest milk products by producing the enzyme lactase
- They aid digestive function overall and improve the ability to digest and absorb nutrients from food
- They improve bowel function. When they are not healthy, bowel transit time (how long it takes food to be processed and wastes eliminated) is far slower

- Some strains (see individual characteristics above) can destroy invading bacteria by producing natural antibiotic products
- Some strains have anti-tumour effects
- By acting to detoxify the intestines (preventing amine formation for example) they help to prevent the formation of cancer-causing chemicals
- They reduce the levels of cholesterol in the system, so reducing the dangers which excess cholesterol poses to the health of the heart and circulatory system
- Some strains assist in recycling oestrogen which helps overall hormone balance as well as reducing menopausal symptoms
- They manufacture some of the B-vitamins including B_3, B_6, folic acid and biotin
- They maintain control over potentially hostile yeasts such as *Candida albicans*
- They produce lactic acid which enhances the digestibility of foods as well as improving the environment for themselves and making it hostile for invading organisms (for example they protect against most of the organisms which produce food poisoning).

These are the main benefits which the friendly bacteria offer when they are in good health. And we cannot live in a reasonable state of health ourselves unless the flora of the body – the friendly bacteria – are in good health. We therefore need to know what makes them healthy and what upsets them (see Fig. 11.1).

What disturbs the friendly bacteria in adults?
(Friend & Shahani 1984, Donovan 1986, Grutte et al 1980, Savage 1987, Speck 1975)

- Many drugs; the most obvious drugs which damage the natural flora are antibiotics, steroids (cortisone and prednisone for example) and chemotherapy drugs
- Anything at all which causes a gastric (stomach) upset, whether this is 'stress', smoking, or undesirable food combinations, or anything else
- Anything which alters the normal function of

the bowel, either slowing it down (constipation) or speeding it up (colitis, diarrhoea, etc.)
- Anything which reduces the levels of normal digestive acids in the stomach, which decline with age anyway (as they also do with zinc deficiency)
- Pernicious anaemia (which is associated with lowered stomach acid levels)
- A toxic state of the bowel, as occurs with chronic constipation for example
- A high fat diet
- A high sugar diet
- Smoking
- Excess alcohol
- Emotional stress
- Environmental pollutants (pesticides, petrochemicals, heavy metals such as lead, mercury, cadmium, etc.)
- Damage to the internal lining of the intestines, such as occurs in colitis, regional enteritis, diverticulitis and Crohn's disease
- Exposure to radiation (including X-rays)
- Liver disease, such as cirrhosis
- Immune deficiency – produced by infection (e.g. AIDS) or drugs (e.g. as used in transplant surgery to reduce chances of rejection)
- Most chronic disease.

Famed medical researcher Rene Dubos maintains that the most important elements which upset the friendly bacteria are the food the person eats, their stress levels and the drugs (antibiotics, etc.) they use (Dubos & Schaedler 1962).

List of diseases associated with damaged bowel flora (Simon & Gorbach 1981)

CAUTION: This is only a partial list since almost all conditions of the human body may have some aspect of bowel dysfunction as an associated factor.

- All allergic conditions which are associated with foods may have as a cause a reduced bowel flora efficiency for several reasons. If the bowel mucosa is irritated it can be 'leaky' and allow passage through it, to the bloodstream, of substances which will provoke an allergic reaction.

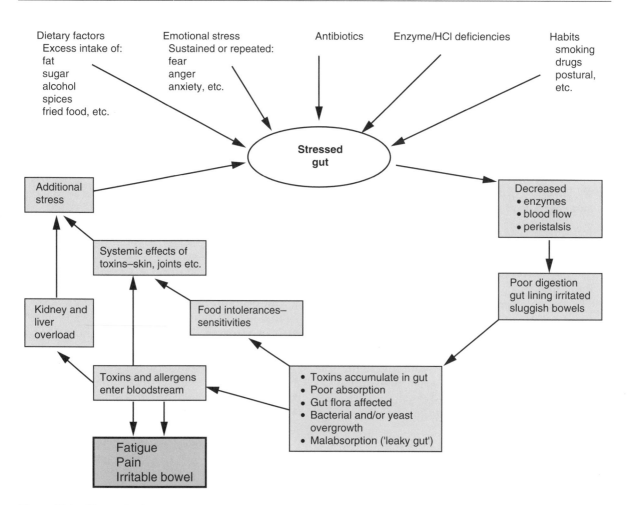

Figure 11.1 Stressed gut.

The 'leaky gut' can be helped by probiotic supplementation, as well as by other nutritional, medical and herbal strategies. Allergy can also be aggravated by the production of excessive amounts of histamine which some bacteria can produce when the flora is unbalanced (see notes above on individual characteristics).

• Autoimmune diseases such as rheumatoid arthritis, lupus and ankylosing spondylitis, in which particular associated bacteria are excessively present (for example *Proteus* in rheumatoid arthritis, *Klebsiella* in ankylosing spondylitis). All these bacteria can be controlled by the normal flora when they are in good health.

• Bladder infections become more likely when the normal bowel flora are damaged or operating inefficiently for any of the reasons listed above.

• High cholesterol levels. We make most of our own cholesterol, with only about 15% coming from the diet. Cholesterol is not just one substance but comes in 'good' and 'bad' (and 'very bad') forms. The friendly bacteria act to salvage and recycle good (high density) cholesterol which would otherwise be excreted through the bowels. The heart and cardiovascular system are therefore protected if the friendly bacteria are in good health.

• Irritable bowel problems (IBS) are commonly associated with bowel flora damage which has led to yeast or bacterial overgrowth in territories usually occupied by the friendly bacteria.

• *Candida albicans* overgrowth, which can produce IBS, also produces oral and vaginal thrush. It has been shown that treating the local outbreak of yeast infection (mouth for example) without also dealing with what is happening in the bowel will not control the situation for more than a short time. *Candida* is also linked to the development of the 'leaky gut' situation mentioned above (Cracchiolo 1997).

• Chronic fatigue syndrome (CFS) has been shown to be directly associated, in many cases, with a history of bowel dysbiosis and/or candidiasis – both of which are linked to a weakened state of the normal bowel flora (Stalanyl & Copeland 1996).

• Food poisoning becomes more likely when the normal flora is damaged, since the majority of food poisoning organisms can be easily controlled by *L. acidophilus* and/or the bifidobacteria when they are operating normally.

• Menopausal problems. Not just hot flashes but potentially dangerous problems such as osteoporosis are minimised by the salvaging and recycling by the friendly bacteria of oestrogen which would otherwise be excreted.

• Migraine headaches can be triggered by excessive amounts of the chemical tyramine which some bacteria can produce when the flora is unbalanced (see notes above on their individual characteristics).

• Chronic muscular pain, such as fibromyalgia, has been shown to be directly associated, in many cases, with a history of bowel dysbiosis and/or candidiasis – both of which are linked to a weakened state of the normal bowel flora (see Ch. 2).

Probiotic nutritional guidelines
(Elmer 1996)

Foods and substances which improve the health of the friendly bacteria (or which encourage their ability to colonise – attach to the lining of the gut – and thrive so that they can provide the many benefits they offer us in return for accommodation) are called bifidogenic foods.

• The friendly bacteria respond badly to sustained stress because of the biochemical changes this produces in the intestines in terms of hormonal changes and alterations in the production of digestive acids and enzymes.

• Complex carbohydrates such as fresh vegetables, pulses (the bean family including lentils, soya beans, etc.), nuts, seeds, whole grains (wheat, rice, oats, etc.) are all bifidogenic – they are welcomed by the friendly bacteria because the offer just the sort of nourishment they need. Refined carbohydrates (sugars, white flour products), however, are harmful to them.

• Particular vegetables which have been shown to help bifidobacteria function because they contain fructo-oligosacharides include carrot, potato and maize extracts.

• Fermented milk products are the perfect bifidogenic food for the lactobacilli and the bifidobacteria – kefir, sour milk, cottage cheese, yogurt, etc. – but they must not contain the antibiotic residues which are present in much commercial dairy food. This calls for extra expense and effort if possible in tracking down sources which guarantee that the herds the dairy products come from are 'organic' or 'free range' or 'chemical free'. Goat and sheep's milk products are usually (but not always) chemical free.

• Fermented soya products (tofu and miso for example) are almost as bifidogenic as dairy foods.

• Low fat meats and fish are good foods for the friendly bacteria, but high fat content in food creates problems for them. Meat and fish which is 'factory farmed' is likely to have antibiotic residues so look for organic or free range poultry and meat and non-farmed fish.

• Removing the fat from milk and replacing it with a vegetable source of oil, such as is found in flax seed oil, enhances bifidobacteria function (i.e. makes it bifidogenic).

• Lactulose – a combination of fruit sugar and galactose – is created by heating milk, and this too is bifidogenic. Lactulose is used when liver function is poor to help bifidobacteria to reduce the load on the liver.

Summary

Reduce stress and eat a diet which emphasises low fat, low sugar, high complex carbohydrate, useful levels of cultured and fermented dairy and other products such as yogurt and tofu, and which avoids toxic and antibiotic residues.

And to really boost friendly bacteria function, consider supplementing with the main probiotic organisms, *L. acidophilus*, the bifidobacteria and *L. bulgaricus*.

Protocol for probiotic replenishment

Whenever purchasing a probiotic product ensure the following:

- The product should ideally contain only one organism, not a cocktail. However, if more than one organism is present in a capsule or container, ensure that the label contains a statement as to minimum numbers of each organism, not just their names.
- The names of the organisms in the container are clearly stated, and that labels which carry vague terms such as 'lactobacilli' or 'lactic acid producing bacteria' are not purchased. The named, beneficial probiotic organism(s) must be clearly listed by both their genus and species, for example *Bifidobacterium* (genus) *bifidum* (species) – and not just 'bifidobacteria'.
- There is a statement as to the guaranteed number of organisms per gram or other measurement (e.g. teaspoon).
- This number is guaranteed to be the case *at the time of opening* and not just at the time of manufacture of the product ('guaranteed shelf-life').
- This number should be of 'viable colony-forming units'.
- Never buy a probiotic which is in tablet form as the process of making tablets severely damages the bacteria's potential for colonisation.
- The organism is a 'human strain'.
- The container is (ideally) made of dark glass.
- The product is a powder or a powder in a capsule and never a liquid or tablet formulation.
- The product also contains some of the supernatant (the culture in which the organism was grown) as this provides nutrition for the organism.
- The product requires refrigeration after opening.
- There is an expiry date and that the product is within that time limit.

- That products designed for those who are dairy sensitive state clearly what culture medium has been used in the production.

General rules for storing and taking probiotic supplements

- Probiotic supplements maintain their potency for much longer periods when not exposed to heat or moisture.
- Keep all probiotic supplements refrigerated for long-term storage.
- For therapeutic dosages, avoid liquids and gelatin capsules, which have a high moisture content, as this causes the probiotics to lose their potency rapidly.
- Before taking the supplement, mix probiotic products in unchlorinated, tepid water to maintain optimum viability of the cells.
- Gradually build up to therapeutic dosage levels to prevent rapid, sometimes uncomfortable, changes in intestinal ecology.
- For best results, *L. acidophilus* and *B. bifidum* should be taken on an empty stomach, 30–45 minutes before meals.
- *L. bulgaricus* should be taken with or immediately following meals.

CAUTION: People with milk intolerance may not be able to use milk-based products. If the condition is a simple lactose intolerance, most people will do very well on a milk-based *L. acidophilus* supplement. The production of lactase as a byproduct of *L. acidophilus* metabolism has been shown to be effective in the management of lactose intolerance (see notes on individual bacteria above). With more sensitive patients who are actually allergic to dairy products the use of a milk-free *L. acidophilus* supplement for a month or two may improve a patient's lactose intolerance enough to tolerate a milk-based supplement.

Protocols for adults

During and following antibiotic therapy

- 1/2 to 1 teaspoon of *L. acidophilus*, three times per day, before meals.

- It is recommended that *B. bifidum* also be taken, 1/2 to 1 teaspoon, three times per day, before meals, for optimum results.
- If possible, take probiotic supplements at a different time of the day than antibiotics.
- Continue supplementation at therapeutic levels for 1 month after discontinuation of antibiotics.

In cases of acute intestinal distress

- 1 teaspoon of both *L. acidophilus* and *B. bifidum* every hour until symptoms cease.

In cases of chronic constipation

- 2 teaspoons *L. bulgaricus*, two to three times per day, with meals, for several weeks.
- Follow with maintenance dosages of *L. acidophilus* and *B. bifidum*.

In cases of infection or to improve white cell counts

- 2 teaspoons of *L. bulgaricus*, three to four times per day, with meals.
- After 2 weeks, add 1/2 teaspoon of both *L. acidophilus* and *B. bifidum*, three times per day, before meals.

In cases of candidiasis

Oral administration

- 1 teaspoon of both *L. acidophilus* and *B. bifidum*, three times per day, before meals.
- It is recommended that 2–3 teaspoons of *L. bulgaricus*, three times per day, with meals, be added to the protocol for several weeks.
- If severe *Candida* die-off symptoms occur, reduce dosage and then gradually increase again.

LOCAL APPLICATION

- Fill two large size 00 or four small size 0 gelatin capsules (obtainable from pharmacies) with *L. acidophilus* and insert vaginally or rectally before bedtime, for 10 days.
- Or, mix 1 rounded teaspoon of *L. acidophilus* with 2 tablespoons of plain regular yoghurt (not low- or non-fat). Insert vaginally or rectally before bedtime, for 10 days.

CAUTION: Do not fill capsules ahead of time as high moisture content may destroy the viability of the acidophilus (the empty two-piece gelatin capsules are available at most health food stores and pharmacies.)

Douche

- Mix 1 teaspoon of *L. acidophilus* in warm water. Stir briskly and let stand for at least 5 minutes. Stir again. Use as a douche each morning for 10 days.

Maintenance dosages

- 1 teaspoon *L. acidophilus* and 1/4 teaspoon *B. bifidum*, once daily, on an empty stomach.
- Lacto-vegetarians, athletes, and those of black or Oriental ancestry may have a need for more *Bifidobacterium* than *L. acidophilus* due to their high intake of complex carbohydrates or ancestral dietary patterns. For such individuals, 3/4 teaspoon *B. bifidum* and 1/2 teaspoon *L. acidophilus*, once daily is suggested.

In Chapter 12 a number of the key associated conditions of fibromyalgia syndrome are evaluated in relation to a variety of treatment strategies ranging from detoxification to hydrotherapy and breathing retraining. Chapter 13 discusses bodywork options.

REFERENCES

Abraham G E, Flechas J D 1992 Hypothesis: management of fibromyalgia: rationale for the use of magnesium and malic acid. Journal of Nutritional Medicine 3: 49–59

Baldry P 1993 Acupuncture, trigger points and musculoskeletal pain. Churchill Livingstone, Edinburgh

Benedetto P Di, Iona L G, Zidarich V 1993 Clinical evaluation of S-adenosyl-L-methionine versus transcutaneous electrical nerve stimulation in primary fibromyalgia. Current Therapeutic Research 53(2): 222

Bengtsson A et al 1988 Regional sympathetic blockade in primary fibromyalgia. Pain 33: 161–167

Bennett R et al 1996 Group treatment of FMS – a 6 month outpatient program. Journal of Rheumatology 23(3): 521–528

Block S 1993 Fibromyalgia and the rheumatisms. Controversies in Clinical Rheumatology 19(1): 61–78

Blunt K, Moez H, Rajivani D, Guerriero R 1997 Effectiveness of chiropractic management of fibromyalgia patients: pilot study. Journal of Manipulative and Physiological Therapeutics 20(6): 389–399

Burckhardt C et al 1994 Randomized controlled clinical trial of education and physical training for women with fibromyalgia. Journal of Rheumatology 21(4): 714–720

Campbell S et al 1985 A double blind study of cyclobenzaprine in patients with primary fibromyalgia. Arthritis and Rheumatism 28: S40

Carette S, Bell M 1994 Comparison of amitriptyline, cyclobenzarapine and placebo in FMS. Arthritis and Rheumatism 37(1): 32–40

Carette S et al 1986 Evaluation of amitripyline in primary fibrositis. Arthritis and Rheumatism 29: 655–659

Caruso I, Puttini P S, Cazzola M, Azzolini V 1990 Double-blind study of 5-hydroxytryptophan versus placebo in the treatment of primary fibromyalgia syndrome. Journal of International Medical Research 18(3): 201–209

Clark S et al 1985 Double blind crossover trial of prednisone in treatment of fibrositis. Journal of Rheumatology 12(5): 980–983

Cracchiolo C 1997 Frequently asked questions about yeast infections. fibrom-1 Internet

DeLuze C et al 1992 Electroacupuncture in fibromyalgia. British Medical Journal 21: 1249–1252

Donovan P 1986 Bowel toxaemia, permeability and disease. In: Pizzorno, Murray (eds) Textbook of natural medicine. JBCNM, Seattle

Dubos R, Schaedler R 1962 Some biological effects of the digestive flora. American Journal of Medical Sciences (September): 265–271

Eisinger J 1987 Cocarboxylase et fibromyalgies, un rendezvous manqué. Lyon Méditerranée Méd 23: 11526

Eisinger J, Ayavou T 1990 Transketolase stimulation in fibromyalgia. Journal of American College of Nutrition 9(1): 56–57

Eisinger J et al 1988 Données actuelles sur les fibromyalgies: traitement des fibromyalgies primitives par la cocarboxylase. Lyon Méditerranée Méd 24: 11585–11586

Eisinger J et al 1988 Données actuelles sur les fibromyalgies: magnésium et transaminases. Lyon Méditerranée Méd

Eisinger J, Zakarian H, Plantamura A et al 1992a Studies of transketolase in chronic pain. Journal of Advanced Medicine 5(2): 105–113

Eisinger J, Arroyo P, Calendini C et al 1992b Anomalies biologiques au cours des fibromyalgies: III. Explorations endocriniennes. Lyon Méditerranée Méd 28: 858–860

Eisinger J, Bagneres D, Arroyo P et al 1994 Effects of magnesium, high energy phosphates, piracetam and thiamin on erythrocyte transketolase. Magnesium Research 7(1): 59–61

Elmer G 1996 Biotherapeutic agents. Journal of the American Medical Association 275(11): 870–876

Felson D, Goldenberg D 1986 The natural history of fibromyalgia. Arthritis and Rheumatism 29: 1522–1526

Ferraccioli G et al 1989 EMG-biofeedback in fibromyalgia syndrome. Journal of Rheumatology 16: 1013–1014

Fibromylagia Network 1996 Report. Fibromyalgia Network, January: 5

Fisher P et al 1989 Effect of homoeopathic treatment of fibrositis (primary fibromyalgia). British Medical Journal 32: 365–366

Friend B, Shahani K 1984 Nutritional and therapeutic aspects of lactobacilli. Journal of Applied Nutrition 36: 125–153

Gatterman M et al 1990 Muscle and myofascial pain syndromes. In: Gatterman M (ed) Chiropractic management of spine related disorders. Williams and Wilkins, Baltimore

Gemmell H et al 1991 Homoeopathic Rhus *Toxicodendron* in treatment of fibromyalgia. Chiropractic Journal of Australia 21(1): 2–6

Gilliland S, Speck M 1977 Antagonistic action of *L. acidophilus* towards intestinal and food borne pathogens. Journal of Food Protection 40: 820–823

Gilliland S et al 1985 Assimilation of cholesterol by *L. acidophilus*. Applied and Environmental Microbiology (February): 377–381

Goldenberg D 1993 Fibromyalgia: treatment programs. Journal of Musculoskeletal Pain 1(3/4): 71–81

Goldenberg D, Felson D, Dinerman H 1986 Randomized, controlled trial of amitripyline anproxine in treatment of patients with fibromyalgia. Arthritis and Rheumatism 29: 1371–1377

Goldenberg D, Kaplan K, Nadan M 1991 Impact of cognitive–behavioural therapy on fibromyalgia. Arthritis and Rheumatism 34(S9): S190

Grassetto M, Varotto A 1994 Primary fibromyalgia is responsiveto S-adenosyl-L-methionine. Current Therapeutic Research 55(7): 797–806

Grutte F et al 1980 Human gastrointestinal microflora. J A Barth, Leipzig

Haanen H et al 1991 Hypnotherapy in treatment of refractory fibromyalgia. Journal of Rheumatology 18: 72–75

Horger I, Moro V, Van Schaik W 1988 Zirkulierende Immunkomplexe bei Polyarthritispatienten. Natur-und Ganzheits-Medizin 1: 177–22 [in German]

Irving R 1981 Pain and the protective reflex generators. Journal of Manipulative and Physiological Therapeutics 4: 69–71

Jacobsen S, Danneskiold-Samsoe B, Andersen R B 1991 Oral S-adenosylmethionine in primary fibromyalgia. Double-blind clinical evaluation. Scandinavian Journal of Rheumatology 20(4): 294–302

James S et al 1985 Effekter av selenvitamin E-behandling till kvinnor medlång variga arbetsrelaterade nack-och skuldersmärtor. En dubbelblindstudie. Läkaresällskapets Riksstämma [in Swedish]

Jameson S et al 1985 Pain relief and selenium balance in patients with connective tissue disease and osteoarthrosis: a double-blind selenium tocopherol supplementation study. Nutr Res 1(Supplement): 391–397

Jiminez C et al 1993 Treatment of FMS with OMT and self-learned techniques. Report in Journal of American Osteopathic Association 93(8): 870

Kirkaldy-Willis W et al 1984 Lumbar spondylosis and stenosis correlation of pathological anatomy with high resolution computed tomographic scanning. In: Donovan Post Medical Journal. Computed tomography of the spine. Williams and Wilkins, Baltimore

Korr I 1975 Proprioceptors and somatic dysfunction. Journal of the American Osteopathic Association 74: 638–650

Lewit K 1985 The muscular and articular factor in movement restriction. Manual Medicine 1: 83–85

McCain G 1986 Role of physical fitness training in fibrositis/fibromyalgia syndrome. American Journal of Medicine (S3A): 73–77

McCain G, Bell D, Mai F et al 1988 Controlled study of supervised cardiovascular fitness training program. Arthritis and Rheumatism 31: 1135–1141

Martin et al 1996 An exercise program in treatment of fibromyalgia. Journal of Rheumatology 23(6): 1050–1053

Prescott E, Nørrgård J, Rotbøl Pedersen L, Danneskiold-Samsøe B 1992 Fibromyalgia and magnesia. Letter. Scandinavian Journal of Rheumatology 21(4): 206

Puttini P S, Caruso I 1992 Primary fibromyalgia syndrome and 5-hydroxy-L-tryptophan: a 90-day open study. J Internal Medicine Research 20(2): 182–189

Rasic L Lj 1990 Chart of microorganisms used as probiotics. In: Chaitow L, Trenev N Probiotics. Thorsons, London pp 198–208

Robinson M F et al 1981 Effect of daily supplements of selenium on patients with muscular complaints in Otago and Canterbury. New Zealand Medical Journal 93: 289–292

Romano T J, Stiller J W 1994 Magnesium deficiency in fibromyalgia syndrome. Journal of Nutritional Medicine 4: 165–167

Rubin B et al 1990 Treatment options in fibromyalgia syndrome. Report in Journal of American Osteopathic Association 90(9): 844–845

Russell I J et al 1995 Treatment of fibromyalgia syndrome with Super Malic: a randomized, doubleblind, placebo controlled, crossover pilot study. Journal of Rheumatology 22: 953–958

SAMe 1997 Part 4. Treatment for arthritis. Life Extension (September): 7–10

Sandford Kiser R et al 1983 Acupuncture relief of chronic pain syndrome correlates with increased plasma metenkephalin concentrations. Lancet ii: 1394–1396

Savage D 1987 Factors influencing biocontrol of bacterial pathogens in the intestines. Food Technology (July): 82–87

Shambaugh P 1987 Changes in electrical activity in muscles resulting from chiropractic adjustment. Journal of Manipulative and Physiological Therapeutics 10: 300–304

Simon G, Gorbach S 1981 Intestinal flora in health and disease. In: Johnson L (ed) Physiology of the Gastrointestinal Tract. Raven Press, New York, pp 1361–1380

Sneath P 1986 Bergey's manual of systematic bacteriology. Williams and Wilkins, Baltimore, vol 2

Speck M 1975 Interactions among lactobacilli and man. Journal of Dairy Sciences 59: 338–343

Stalanyl D, Copeland M 1996 Fibromyalgia and Chronic Fatigue Syndrome Survival Manual. New Harbinger Publications, Oakland, California

Stoltz A 1993 Effects of OMT on the tender points of FMS. Report in Journal of American Osteopathic Association 93(8): 866

Sunshine W, Field T, Quintino O et al 1996 Fibromyalgia benefits from massage therapy and TENS. Journal of Clinical Rheumatology 2: 18–22

Tavoni A, Vitali C, Bombardieri S, Pasero G 1987 The evaluation of S-adenosylmethionine in primary fibromyalgia. A double-blind crossover study. American Journal of Medicine 83(SA): 107–110

Uffelmann K, Vogler W, Fruth C 1990 Der Einsatz hydrolytischer Enzyme beim extraartikularen Rheumatismus. Allgemain Medizin 19: 151–153 [in German]

van Rij A M et al 1979 Selenium deficiency in total parenteral nutrition. American Journal of Clinical Nutrition 32: 2076–2085

Vernon H 1986 Spinal manipulation and beta-endorphins. Journal of Manipulative and Physiological Therapeutics 9: 115–123

Werbach M 1998 Nutritional influences on illness. CD-ROM, Third Line Press, Tarzana, California

Wolfe F 1986 Clinical syndrome of fibromyalgia syndrome. American Journal of Medicine (S3A): 12

Wolfe F 1986 Clinical syndrome of fibrositis. American Journal of Medicine 81(S3A): 7–14

Yunus M B, Dailey J, Aldag J, Masi A, Jobe F 1992 Plasma tryptophan and other amino acids in primary fibromyalgia: a controlled study. Journal of Rheumatology 19(1): 90–94

12

Fibromyalgia: treating associated conditions

The methods briefly outlined in previous chapters represent some of the approaches for which evidence exists of benefit in treating FMS. This chapter concentrates on fibromyalgia's associated conditions and the usefulness in treating them of a variety of the complementary methods discussed previously, as well as a number of additional approaches, ranging from hydrotherapy to exclusion and detoxification diets, along with breathing retraining and relaxation methods. Many of these methods are of proven value while others have a good clinical track record without having research evidence to back up their usefulness. You are asked to evaluate the evidence presented and cited, and to make up your own mind as to what is most useful for you from among this collection of therapeutic possibilities, basing your decisions on your own belief systems and training.

The conditions and symptoms often associated with FMS include:

- Allergy and chemical sensitivity (and hypoglycaemia)
- 'Brain' symptoms
- Candidiasis (yeast overgrowth)
- Depression
- Fatigue
- Infection: viral and bacterial
- Inflammation/pain
- Irritable bowel syndrome
- Gulf War syndrome
- Premenstrual tension syndrome
- Pelvic pain and myofascial pain syndrome
- Raynaud's syndrome
- Sleep (and growth hormone) problems
- Toxicity.

ALLERGY AND CHEMICAL SENSITIVITY/TOXICITY
(Werbach 1990, Balch 1990, Davies 1987, Chaitow 1994; see also Figs 3.1, 3.2 and 11.1, and Table 3.1)

People with allergies are more likely to develop FMS and people with FMS are more likely than not to have allergies. A study in Seattle compared three groups of patients referred to a university-based clinic who already had a diagnosis of chronic fatigue syndrome (CFS), or fibromyalgia syndrome (FMS), or multiple chemical sensitivities (MCS). What emerged was a picture of three conditions which were frequently difficult to distinguish from each other. Fully 70% of the patients with an FMS diagnosis and 30% of those with MCS met all the criteria for chronic fatigue syndrome.The researchers' conclusion was that it was difficult to clearly distinguish patients with CFS, FMS and MCS. Symptoms typical of each disorder are common in the other two conditions (Buchwald 1994).

Recent Turkish research (Tuncer 1997) evaluated the frequency of major symptoms in a group of over 30 patients with a diagnosis of 'primary fibromyalgia' compared with people without FMS, and found that those with fibromyalgia had far more evidence of allergy than the people they were compared with.

Dr Anne Macintyre, medical adviser to ME [CFS] Action, an active patient support group for patients with chronic fatigue conditions in the UK, supports an 'immune dysfunction' model as the underlying mechanism for CFS/FMS: 'The immune dysfunction may be associated with increased sensitivities to chemicals and/or foods, which can cause further symptoms such as joint pain, asthma, IBS and headache' (Macintyre 1993).

According to the Fibromyalgia Network (October 1993, p. 12), the most commonly identified foods which cause problems for many people with FMS and CFS (ME) are wheat and dairy products, sugar, caffeine, Nutra-Sweet®, alcohol and chocolate. Elimination and rotation diets are explained in this chapter.

The chemical sensitivity link

Chemical sensitivities/allergies are also common in people with FMS and it is thought by many experts that a percentage of people with FMS/CFS(ME) have probably been affected by toxic contamination as a major cause of their conditions, and that this has not always happened in industrial settings. In order to assess the involvement of allergic symptoms in CFS patients, a 2-month double blinded placebo controlled study, involving 30 patients, was carried out of the efficacy of antihistamine medication (Seldane) (Steinberg 1996). This was found not to be effective in treating the major symptoms of the condition but alleviated coexisting allergic problems which were noted in 70% of CFS patients.

Yeasts and parasites as a 'cause' of allergy

Infestation of the bowels by yeast or parasites can result in damage to the delicate lining of the intestinal tract as well as reduced health and efficiency of the bowel flora (see Ch. 3). This can lead to substances (food breakdown products, toxins, etc.) being absorbed from the gut into the bloodstream, triggering allergic symptoms (often including fatigue and muscle pain) (Crooke 1983, Truss 1982). In this way, the allergy and irritable bowel conditions can be seen as two links in a chain of events in which fatigue (a common side-effect of allergy) and muscle pain can also occur (see Fig. 11.1).

Exclusion and rotation diets

Food allergy can be dealt with by eliminating the allergen(s) through specific exclusion or hypoallergenic diets. The identification of foods to which we are allergic or intolerant can be difficult. In some cases it is obvious, and we therefore avoid the food; in other cases we may need to undertake long and difficult detective work in order to identify culprits. The notes in Boxes 12.1, 12.2, and 12.3, on exclusion and rotation and oligoantigenic diet, can be adapted for patients to use.

Box 12.1   Notes for exclusion diets

Make notes of the answers to the following questions:

1.   List any foods or drinks that you know disagree with you, or which produce allergic reactions (skin blotches, palpitations, feelings of exhaustion, agitation, or other symptoms).
     NOTES   ....

2.   List any food or beverage that you eat or drink at least once a day
     NOTES   ....

3.   List any foods or drink that if you were unable to obtain, would make you feel really deprived.
     NOTES   ....

4.   List any food that you sometimes have a definite craving for.
     NOTES   ....

5.   What sort of food or drink is it that you use for snacks? List these.
     NOTES   ....

6.   Are there foods which you have begun to eat (or drink) more frequently/more of recently?
     NOTES   ....

7.   Read the following list of foods and highlight in one colour any that you eat at least every day, and in another colour those that you eat three or more times a week: Bread (and other wheat products); milk; potato; tomato; fish; cane sugar or its products; breakfast food; sausages or preserved meat; cheese; coffee; rice; pork; peanuts; corn or its products; margarine; beetroot or beet sugar; tea; yoghurt; soya products; beef; chicken; alcoholic drinks; cake; biscuits; oranges or other citrus fruits; eggs; chocolate; lamb; artificial sweeteners; soft drinks; pasta.
     When it comes to testing by 'exclusion' the foods which appear most often on your list (in questions 1 to 6 and the ones highlighted in the first colour as being eaten daily) are the ones to test first – one by one.

•   Decide which foods on your list are the ones you eat most often (say bread) and test wheat and other grains by excluding these from your diet for at least 3 weeks (wheat, barley, rye, oats and millet).

•   You may not feel any benefit from this exclusion (if wheat or other grains have been causing allergic reactions) for at least a week, and you may even feel worse for that first week (caused by withdrawal symptoms).

•   If after a week your symptoms (fatigue, palpitations, skin reactions, breathing difficulty, muscle or joint ache, feelings of agitation – or whatever) are improving, you should maintain the exclusion for several weeks before reintroducing the excluded foods – to challenge your body – to see whether symptoms return. If they do return after you have eaten the foods and you feel as you did before the exclusion period, you will have shown that your body is better, for the time being at least, without the food you have identified.

•   Remove this from your diet (in this case grains – or wheat if that is the only grain you tested) for at least 6 months before testing it again. By then you may have become desensitised to it and be able to tolerate it again.

•   If nothing was proved by the wheat/grain exclusion, similar elimination periods on a diet free of dairy produce, or fish, or citrus, or soya products, etc. can also be attempted – using your questionnaire results to guide you – always choosing the next most frequently listed food (or food family).

This method is often effective. Dairy products, for example, are among the commonest allergens in asthma and hay fever problems. A range of gluten-free and dairy-free foods are now available from health stores which makes such elimination far easier.

Rotation diet

There are other ways of reducing the stress of irritant foods, and one of these involves the use of a rotation diet (Box 12.2).

Another way of 'unmasking' allergy provoking foods is the 'oligoantigenic diet' developed at

Great Ormond Street Hospital for Sick Children (below and Box 12.3).

Oligoantigenic diet

The oligoantigenic diet (Box 12.3) was developed at Great Ormond Street Hospital for Sick

---

Box 12.2 The rotation diet

In the rotation diet, foods from any particular family of suspect foods (identified by the questionnaire) are eaten only once in 5 days or so. This system is effective, especially if a detailed 'food and symptom' diary is kept, in which all deviations from your normal state of health are noted down, as are all foods eaten.

- Symptoms such as feelings of unusual fatigue, or irritability, or difficulty in concentrating, or muscular pains or actual breathing difficulties should be listed and given a daily score out of (say) 10, where 0 = no problems and 10 = the worst it has ever been. Make sure to score each symptom each day to see how it varies, and to link this to when suspect foods are eaten (sometimes reaction to foods takes up to 12 hours to be noticed).

- If such a score sheet is kept and note is made of suspect foods, a link may be uncovered.

- By comparing the two lists (suspect foods and symptoms) it is often possible to note a pattern connecting particular foods and symptoms, at which time the exclusion diet (Box 12.1) can be started.

Children, London, and at Addenbrookes Hospital, Cambridge, as a means of identifying foods which might be causing or aggravating the conditions of young patients.

By avoiding foods which may be provoking symptoms for not less than 5 days, all traces of any of the food will have cleared the system and any symptoms caused by these should have vanished. Symptoms which remain are either caused by something else altogether (infection for example, or hormonal imbalance or emotions) or by other foods or substances. On reintroduction of foods in a carefully controlled sequence (the 'challenge'), symptoms which reappear are shown to derive from a reaction to particular foods which are then eliminated from the diet for at least 6 months.

There is some evidence to support the idea that those foods which have become a major part of human diet since stone-age times, mainly grains (particularly wheat) of all sorts, and dairy produce, are the most likely to provoke reactions. All modern processed foods involving any chemicals, colourings, flavourings, etc., are also suspect.

The oligoantigenic diet is usually followed for 3 weeks while a careful check is kept on symp-

toms (pain, stiffness, mobility etc.). If symptoms improve or vanish, then one or more of the foods being avoided may be to blame. Identification and subsequent avoidance of the culprit food(s) depends upon the symptom returning upon the reintroduction (challenge) of the food. The eating pattern listed in Box 12.3 is a modified version of the hospital pattern.

Box 12.3 Oligoantigenic diet

- To try a modified oligoantigenic exclusion diet, evaluate the effect of following a pattern of eating in which the foods as listed below are excluded for 3 weeks.

Fish
Allowed: white fish, oily fish
Forbidden: All smoked fish

Vegetables
None are forbidden but people with bowel problems are asked to avoid beans, lentils, Brussels sprouts and cabbage

Fruit
Allowed: bananas, passion fruit, peeled pears, pomegranates, paw-paw, mango
Forbidden: all fruits except the six allowed ones

Cereals
Allowed: rice, sago, millet, buckwheat, quinoa
Forbidden: wheat, oats, rye, barley, corn

Oils
Allowed: sunflower, safflower, linseed, olive
Forbidden: corn, soya, 'vegetable', nut (especially peanut)

Dairy
Allowed: none
Forbidden: cow's milk and all its products including yoghurt, butter, most margarine, all goat, sheep and soya milk products, eggs

Drinks
Allowed: herbal teas such as camomile and peppermint
Forbidden: tea, coffee, fruit squashes, citrus drinks, apple juice, alcohol, tapwater, carbonated drinks

Miscellaneous
Allowed: sea salt
Forbidden: all yeast products, chocolate, preservatives, all food additives, herbs, spices, honey, *sugar of any sort*

- If benefits are felt after this exclusion, a gradual introduction of *one food at a time*, leaving at least 4 days between each reintroduction, will allow you to identify those foods which should be left out altogether – if symptoms reappear when they are reintroduced.

Box 12.3 (Contd.)   Oligoantigenic diet

- If a reaction occurs (symptoms return having eased or vanished during the 3-week exclusion trial), the offending food is eliminated for at least 6 months and a 5-day period of no further experimentation is followed (to clear the body of all traces of the offending food), after which testing (challenge) can start again, one food at a time, involving anything you have previously been eating which was eliminated by the oligoantigenic diet.

CAUTION: When a food to which you are strongly allergic and which you have been consuming regularly is stopped, you may experience 'withdrawal' symptoms for a week or so, including flu–like symptoms and marked mood–swings, anxiety, restlessness, etc. This will pass after a few days. This can be a strong indication that whatever you have eliminated from the diet is responsible for a 'masked' allergy, which may be producing many of your symptoms.

CAUTIONS: No one with a history of eating disorder should be encouraged to follow exclusion diets unless they have a great deal of support and supervision.

If bowel malabsorption problems exist, resulting perhaps from yeast or parasite activity, then the bowel condition needs to be addressed, concurrently or before the allergy is tackled (see IBS and Candida below).

Sometimes allergy occurs when incomplete digestion of food takes place due to inadequate hydrochloric acid levels or poor digestive enzyme production, and expert nutritional and herbal methods can help in normalising these imbalances.

Chemical sensitivities

Supplementation with antioxidant nutrients such as:

- vitamin C (1–3 g daily)
- vitamin E (400 IU daily)
- selenium (200 µg daily)
- zinc (15–30 mg daily)

can all be useful in helping to increase the tolerance of the body for chemicals as well as for neutralising many of their harmful oxidation effects. Vitamin C acts as mild antihistamine (Pizzorno 1996).

CAUTION: The text below highlights the connection between anxiety, hyperventilation, hypoglycaemia and allergy.

ANXIETY/HYPERVENTILATION/ HYPOGLYCAEMIA (see also Fig. 3.3)

In Chapter 3 there was a discussion of the possible direct connection between the symptoms of hyperventilation and those of CFS/FMS. A summary of the major influences follows, as well as a listing of additional connections between breathing dysfunction and allergy, and also low blood-sugar tendencies.

Summary

Hypoxia ('reduced oxygen tension') which results from hyperventilation has the following effects (Timmons 1994):

1. The first and most direct response to hyperventilation is cerebral vascular constriction – reducing oxygen availability by about 50%.
2. Of all body tissues, the cerebral cortex is the most vulnerable to hypoxia.
3. This depresses cortical activity causing dizziness, vasomotor instability, blurring of consciousness ('foggy brain') and vision.
4. Loss of cortical inhibition results in crying and emotional lability.

Neural repercussions

1. Loss of CO_2 ions from neurons during moderate hyperventilation stimulates neuronal activity, producing muscular tension and spasm, speeding spinal reflexes as well as producing heightened perception (pain, photophobia, hyperacusis).
2. When hypocapnia is more severe, it depresses activity until the nerve cell becomes inert.

Tetany

1. Tetany is secondary to alkalosis. Muscles which maintain 'attack–defense' mode –

hunched shoulders, jutting head, clenched teeth, scowling – are those most likely to be affected.
2. Painful nodules develop and are easily felt in nape of neck, anterior chest and shoulder girdle.
3. Temporal headache centred on painful nodules in the parietal region are common.
4. Also present in some but not all are painful legs.
5. 'The whole body expresses tension and patients cannot relax in any position'.
6. Sympathetic dominance is evident by virtue of dilated pupils, dry mouth, sweaty palms, gut and digestive dysfunction, abdominal bloating, tachycardia.
7. Allergies and food intolerances are common due to increased circulating histamines (see also allergy notes above).
8. Hyperventilation increases circulating histamines making allergic reactions more violent and possibly more likely.

Nasal connection with breathing dysfunction

A high proportion of people with CFS/FMS suffer from rhinitis – possibly allergic in origin. Barelli (1994) states that reflex effects and referred phenomena exist between nose and heart, lungs and diaphragm. Unilateral nasal obstruction/narrowing can decrease movement of the diaphragm on that side.

Nasal reflexes influence cardiac and peripheral circulation – these being among the most powerful reflexes observed in experimental settings.

• On lying down on one side, the lower nostril normally narrows and becomes congested, the lumen closes during sleep, breathing becomes unilateral, movement of the head and turning of body are inaugurated.
• With poorly functioning nasal function (blocked due to allergic rhinitis for example), the head remains in one position, and symptoms such as backache, numbness, cramp, circulatory deficit become more likely. When normal nasal function is disturbed a poor sleep pattern is more likely.

Low blood glucose and hyperventilation (Lum 1994)

1. The symptoms of hypocapnia resemble hypoglycaemia.
2. The brain is fuelled by glucose as well as by oxygen, therefore feelings of faintness, cold sweats, weakness, disturbed consciousness are common to both hyperventilation and hypoglycaemia.
3. Coincident hypoxia and hyperventilation increase such symptoms, which are reduced when blood sugar and oxygenation (paO_2) are both high.
4. During overbreathing both EEG and cortical functions deteriorate as glucose values fall below 100 mg%.
5. 3 minutes of hyperventilation has minimal effects when the blood sugar is in the range of 85–90mg%, but with blood sugar at 70–75% gross disturbances can be noted. Note: these values of blood sugar are well within normal ranges of fasting blood sugar.
6. Hypoglycaemic effects are greater when clustered late morning and late afternoon when blood sugar is likely to be lowest.
7. Hypoglycaemic symptoms are greater in the autumn (fall) – even if glucose levels are in the normal range.
8. High carbohydrate diets are not considered desirable in cases of hypoglycaemia as these lead to increased blood sugar levels followed by sharp falls to fasting levels or below.
9. Proteins (little and often) produce moderate and prolonged glucose rise. This is particularly important relative to panic attacks and any type of seizure.

Dr Jonathan Brostoff (Brostoff 1992) states that some experts are dismissive of the concept of food intolerance and believe that a large number of people so diagnosed are actually hyperventilators. He considers the picture to be more complex: 'Hyperventilation is relatively uncommon and can masquerade as food sensitivity'. Others maintain that anxiety brought on by the food reaction produces breathing changes and the two disorders can aggravate each other.

Some experts believe mild hyperventilation is a symptom of food reactions which vanishes if the intolerance is dealt with (by elimination or desensitisation). Brostoff says that if symptoms vanish when air is rebreathed (paper bag treatment) the cause lies in the breathing, but if not it may lie in food intolerance.

Action on hyperventilation/hypoglycaemia/allergy involvement in CFS/FMS

- Understand the processes involved
- Avoid coffee and other stimulants which raise blood sugar and stimulate sympathetic nervous system
- Eat little and often – especially protein
- Avoid sugar rich foods; start detoxification
- Eliminate likely culprit foods to assess effects (see allergy notes earlier this chapter)
- Practice relaxation and breathing retraining exercises (see below)
- Identify vulnerable periods (premenstrual, stress, etc.)
- Have regular constructive therapeutic, as well as relaxation, bodywork
- Use natural relaxing and sleep-enhancing herbs
- Employ appropriate nutritional supplements such as glucose tolerance factor (GTF) (chromium)
- A combination of relaxed muscles, full breathing, mental calm and nutritional excellence offer protection from the worst effects of stress as well as reducing sympathetic over-arousal.

This scenario is not meant to suggest that FMS is always caused by a shallow overbreathing tendency, but it can certainly be seen to link with many of the common symptoms and to need attention (such as appropriate bodywork methods and breathing retraining) in order to minimise the waste of energy and the mechanical stress to the muscles and joints of the neck, shoulder and chest region in particular. The main author has seldom, if ever, failed to find at least some degree of breathing dysfunction in people with CFS(ME) or FMS (or its previous incarnation of 'fibrositis'). Sometimes it is a major element and sometimes only a part of the picture, but it is almost always involved.

Anti-arousal breathing technique

To start to retrain breathing and help reduce the tendency it produces towards hyperventilation/anxiety the following exercise should be performed regularly:

1. Sit in a chair which has arms and rest your arms on the chair.
2. As you practise deep breathing, make sure your elbows are firmly pressed downwards towards the floor, against the arms of the chair during inhalation (or interlink hands on lap, palms upwards, with fingertip pads pressing into dorsum of hand on inhalation, releasing on exhalation). As you breathe (to the timing described in the next exercise) try to observe whether or not – without making any particular effort to make it happen – your abdomen moves forward at the start of inhalation and flattens on exhalation. (While pressing down with the elbows it is impossible to use the neck/shoulder muscles – you are obliged to use correct breathing muscles.)

Pranayama breathing (Cappo & Holmes 1984, Readhead 1984)

There are many exercises to help improve breathing but there is just one which has been shown in research studies to effectively reduce arousal and anxiety levels. This is an exercise based on traditional yogic breathing. The pattern is as follows:

1. Having placed yourself in a comfortable (ideally seated/reclining) position, exhale FULLY through your partially open mouth, lips just barely separated. This out breath should be slowly performed. Imagine if you will that a candle flame is just about 6 inches from your mouth and exhale in such a way as to not blow this out. As you exhale count silently to yourself to establish the length of the out breath. An effective method for counting 1 second at a time is to say (silently) 'one hundred, two hundred, three hundred, etc.' Each count lasts about 1 second.
2. When you have exhaled fully, without causing any sense of strain to yourself in any way, allow the inhalation through the nose which follows to be full, free and uncontrolled. The

complete exhalation which preceded the inhalation will have created a 'coiled spring' which you do not have to control in order to inhale. Once again, count to yourself to establish how long your in breath lasts.

3. Without pausing to hold the breath exhale FULLY, again as before through the mouth (again you count to yourself at the same speed).

4. Continue to repeat the inhalation and the exhalation for between 20 and 30 cycles.

5. The objective is that in time you should achieve an inhalation phase which lasts 2–3 seconds while the exhalation phase lasts 6–8 seconds – without any strain at all.

6. Most importantly, the exhalation should be slow and continuous (it is no use breathing the air out in 2 seconds and then simply waiting until the count reaches 6, 7 or 8 before inhaling again).

7. By the time you have completed 15 or so cycles, any sense of anxiety which you previously felt should be much reduced and awareness of pain should also have lessened.

8. Repeat this exercise for a few minutes every hour if you are anxious or whenever stress seems to be increasing. At the very least it should be practised on waking, and before bedtime, and if at all possible before meals.

⚠️ CAUTION: Note that there are no contraindications to this breathing exercise. However, individuals with a tendency to anxiety and panic attacks may need to be very carefully tutored in the method to avoid over-concentration on the mechanics of the process, possibly leading to increased anxiety and even panic.

Relaxation methods compared in fibromyalgia

Italian researchers compared the benefits of autogenic training (AT) and progressive muscular relaxation (PMR – also called Erickson's technique) for patients with FMS (Rucco et al 1995). They found that both groups benefited in terms of pain relief *if they carried out the exercise regularly*, but that because PMR is easier and quicker to learn, patients are more likely to perform this regularly compared with AT. Those learning AT

complained of 'too many intrusive thoughts' which is precisely what AT is designed to eventually quieten – that is the 'training' part of the exercise.

Relaxation technique 1: autogenic training
(Jevning 1992, Schultz 1959)

The following modified form of AT is an excellent way of achieving some degree of control over muscle tone and/or circulation, and therefore over pain.

Every day, ideally twice a day, for 10 minutes at a time, do the following:

1. Lie on the floor or bed in a comfortable position, small cushion under the head, knees bent if that makes the back feel easier, eyes closed. Do the yoga breathing exercise described above for 5 cycles (1 cycle equals an inhalation and an exhalation) then let breathing resume its normal rhythm.

2. When you feel calm and still, focus attention on your right hand/arm and silently say to yourself 'my right arm (or hand) feels heavy'.

Try to see/sense the arm relaxed and heavy, its weight sinking into the surface it is resting on. Feel its weight. Over a period of about a minute repeat the affirmation as to its heaviness several times and try to stay focused on its weight and heaviness.

You will almost certainly lose focus as your attention wanders from time to time. This is part of the training in the exercise – to stay focused – so don't feel angry, just go back to the arm and its heaviness.

You may or may not be able to sense the heaviness – it doesn't matter too much at first. If you do, stay with it and enjoy the sense of release – of letting go – that comes with it.

3. Next, focus on your left hand/arm and do exactly the same thing for about a minute.

4. Move to the left leg and then the right leg, for about a minute each, with the same messages and focused attention.

5. Go back to your right hand/arm and this time affirm a message which tells you that you sense a greater degree of warmth there. 'My hand is feeling warm (or hot).'

6. After a minute or so go to the left hand/arm, the left leg and then finally the right leg, each time with the 'warming' message and focused attention. If warmth is sensed stay with it for a while and feel it spread. Enjoy it.

7. Finally focus on your forehead and affirm that it feels cool and refreshed. Stay with this cool and calm thought for a minute before completing the exercise.

By repeating the whole exercise at least once a day (10–15 minutes is all it will take) you will gradually find you can stay focused on each region and sensation. 'Heaviness' represents what you feel when muscles relax and 'warmth' is what you feel when your circulation to an area is increased, while 'coolness' is the opposite, a reduction in circulation for a short while – usually followed by an increase due to the overall relaxation of the muscles. Measurable changes occur in circulation and temperature in the regions being focused on during these training sessions and the benefits of this technique to people with Raynaud's phenomenon and to anyone with pain problems is proven by years of research. Success requires persistence – daily use for at least 6 weeks – before benefits are noticed, notably a sense of relaxation and better sleep.

CAUTION: There are no contraindications to autogenic training as described in this modified form. Any focus on breathing or heart function during autogenic training should be under supervision of a trained expert.

Relaxation technique 2: progressive muscular relaxation

- Wearing loose clothing, lie with arms and legs outstretched.
- Clench one fist. Hold for 10 seconds.
- Release your fist, relax for 10–20 seconds and then repeat exactly as before.
- Do the same with the other hand (twice).
- Draw the toes of one foot towards knee. Hold for 10 seconds. Relax. Repeat and then do same with the other foot.
- Perform the same sequence in 5 other sites

(one side of your body and then the other, making 10 more muscles) such as:
- back of the lower legs: point and tense your toes downwards and then relax
- upper leg: pull your kneecap towards your hip and then relax
- buttocks: squeeze together and then relax
- back of shoulders: draw the shoulder blades together and then relax
- abdominal area: pull in or push out the abdomen strongly and then relax
- arms and shoulders: draw the upper arm into your shoulder and then relax
- neck area: push neck down towards the floor and then relax
- face: tighten and contract muscles around eyes and mouth or frown strongly and then relax

After one week combine muscle groups:
- hand/arm on both sides: tense and then relaxed together
- face and neck: tense and relax all the muscles at the same time
- chest, shoulders and back: tense and relax all the muscles at the same time
- pelvic area: tense and relax all the muscles at the same time
- legs and feet: tense and relax all the muscles at the same time.

After another week abandon the 'tightening up' part of the exercise – simply lie and focus on different regions, noting whether they are tense. Instruct them to relax if they are.
Do the exercise daily.

CAUTION: There are no contraindications to these relaxation exercises.

Hydrotherapy for anxiety/stress reduction (Chaitow 1993, Buchman 1979, Thrash & Home 1981)

Neutral bath for inducing deep relaxation /sleep enhancement. A neutral bath in which the body temperature is the same as that of the water produces a relaxing influence on the nervous system (this was the main method of calming violent and disturbed patients in mental asylums before tranquillisers appeared).

Indications In all cases of anxiety, feelings of 'being stressed' and for relieving chronic pain and/or insomnia. Ideal for reducing excessive fluid retention by means of hydrostatic pressure.

Materials required A bathtub, water and a bath thermometer.

Method Run a bath as full as possible and with the water as close to 97°F (36.1°C) as possible, and certainly not exceeding that level. The bath has its effect by being as close to body temperature as possible. Immersion in water at this neutral temperature has a profoundly relaxing, sedating effect and a calming influence on nervous system activity.

Get into the bath so that, if possible, water covers the shoulders. Support the head on a towel or sponge. The thermometer should be in the bath and the temperature should not be allowed to drop below 92°F/33.3°C. It can be topped up periodically but must not exceed the 97°F/36.1°C limit. The duration of the bath should be anything from 30 minutes to 4 hours – the longer the better as far as relaxation effects are concerned. After the bath, pat dry quickly and get into bed for at least 1 hour.

CAUTION: Neutral baths are suitable for most people but contraindicated in skin conditions which react badly to water or if there is serious cardiac disease.

Aromatherapy for sleep enhancement/stress reduction

The oils described below have proven herbal properties – *none are meant to be consumed*. When being added to a bath, the oils are used neat in the running water which disperses and mixes them. If used for massage they should be combined with a neutral carrier oil.

Basil On its own this can be used (10–20 drops in a bath) to treat weakness, fatigue (including mental tiredness/fogginess) headaches, nausea, feelings of tension or faintness and depression.

Chamomile It can be used on its own (10–20 drops in a bath) to treat sleep and digestive disturbances, skin conditions, neuralgia, and inflammation. Combined with *sage* for menopausal problems (10 drops of each in bath).

Cypress. It can be used alone (10–20 drops in a bath) to treat rheumatic and muscular conditions, coughs, flu and nervous tension. Combined with *lavender* (10–20 drops of each in warm water) it can be used for menopausal problems or for general nervous system treatment.

Lavender with cypress (as above) For menopausal or 'nervous system' problems and with *vetiver* for anxiety (10 drops of each).

Neroli Used alone (10–20 drops in a bath) to treat depression, insomnia and nervous tension, digestive upsets and lack of sexual interest. Together with *basil* (10 drops of each) in bath in cases of anxiety, tension or depression.

CAUTION: The only contraindications to any of these essential oils would be an intolerance to them indicated by prior allergic reaction. Intolerance to lavender is extremely rare.

Constitutional hydrotherapy (CH): home application

Effects CH has a non-specific 'balancing' effect, inducing relaxation, reducing chronic pain, enhancing immune function and promoting healing. This method cannot be self-applied, help is needed.

Materials

- Somewhere to lie down
- A full-sized sheet folded in two, or two single sheets
- Two blankets (wool if possible)
- Three bath towels (when folded in two each should be able to reach side to side and from shoulders to hips)
- One hand towel (each should as a single layer be the same size as the large towel folded in two)
- Hot and cold water.

Method

1. Patient undresses and lies supine between sheets and under blanket.

2. Place two hot folded bath towels (four layers) onto patient's trunk, shoulders to hips, side to side.

3. Cover with sheet and blanket and leave for 5 minutes.

4. Return with a single layer (small) hot towel and a single layer cold towel.

5. Place 'new' hot towel onto top of four 'old' hot towels and 'flip' so that hot towel is on skin and remove old towels. Immediately place cold towel onto new hot towel and flip again so that cold is on the skin, remove single hot towel.

6. Cover patient with sheet and leave for 10 minutes or until the cold towel is warmed.

7. Remove previously cold, now warm, towel and turn patient onto stomach.

8. Repeat steps 2 to 6 to the back of the patient.

Suggestions and notes:

1. If using a bed take precautions not to get this wet.

2. 'Hot' water in this context is a temperature high enough to prevent you leaving your hand in it for more than 5 seconds.

3. The coldest water from a running tap is adequate for the 'cold' towel. On hot days, adding ice to the water in which this towel is rung out is acceptable if the temperature contrast is acceptable to the patient.

4. If the patient feels cold after the cold towel is placed, use back massage, foot or hand massage (through the blanket and towel) and/or use visualisation – ask the patient to think of a sunny beach for example.

5. Most importantly, by varying the differential between hot and cold, making it a small difference for someone whose immune function and overall degree of vulnerability is poor, for example, and using a large contrast, very hot and very cold, for someone whose constitution is robust, allows for the application of the method to anyone at all.

6. Apply daily or twice daily

CAUTION: There are no contraindications to constitutional hydrotherapy since the degree of temperature contrast in its application can be modified to take account of any degree of sensitivity, frailty, etc.

BRAIN SYMPTOMS/'FOGGY BRAIN SYNDROME' (Journal for Action for ME 1994, Fibromyalgia Network 1993–94)

Memory lapses, inability to concentrate, dyslexic episodes, inability to recall simple words, are all part of many people's fibromyalgia (and of most people's chronic fatigue) and modern technology has now identified what may be happening in the brain with these conditions.

Among the abnormalities so-far found in the brains of many patients with FMS and CFS(ME) are reduced blood flow and energy production in key sites of the brain. While any such changes might themselves merely be symptoms of the syndrome, it is thought by many researchers that the most important imbalance in these conditions probably lies in the brain and central nervous system itself. New technologies for visualising the brain in a non-invasive manner (SPECT, BEAM, PET) show that there are few, if any, differences in the scans of patients with CFS(ME) and FMS.

Scan evidence (Komaroff 1996)

- 80% of 144 CFS patients displayed small areas of 'high signals' compared with 20% of controls on MRI scans
- SPECT scans showed significant reduction in brain blood flow in CFS patients compared with healthy controls – similar to changes seen in AIDS patients
- Over 50% of CFS patients displayed abnormal vestibular function tests – which may result from balance control centres in the brain
- Tilt-table testing of CFS patients reveals that autonomic function is dysfunctional.

See also Dr Jay Goldstein's work in this area, as described in Box 7.3.

Treatment possibilities

- Autogenic training combined with the anti-arousal breathing techniques as described above are two excellent methods for starting to improve circulation to and through the brain.

- Thermoregulatory hydrotherapy (see below) will further improve circulatory function.
- Bodywork options include attention to the vital area of the suboccipital triangles, as described in Chapter 3. Refer back to research into the influence on traumatised muscles in this area and FMS (see notes on whiplash injury in Ch. 3).
- Allergy, toxicity, candidiasis or viral problems can cause or aggravate the brain-related typical symptoms. Appropriate treatment protocols are outlined elsewhere in these notes.
- A herbal approach involving the taking of standardised extracts of the plant *Ginkgo biloba* is suggested for a 6 month trial since this has been shown in medical studies (using between 120 and 240 mg daily) to improve memory and reduce the symptoms of inadequate circulation to the brain (Foster 1991). This herb has no side-effects or contraindications. It is now one of the most prescribed medications in Germany and Scandinavia for cerebral dysfunction, specifically indicated for dizziness, memory loss, tinnitus, headaches, emotional instability combined with anxiety. It is also used for treating peripheral circulation (involved in cold hands and feet).
- Additional circulatory support is available by taking not less than 90 mg daily of the nutrient coenzyme Q_{10}. This takes up to a month to be effective in enhancing oxygen transportation and easing fatigue (Kamikawa 1985, Biomedical and clinical aspects of CoQ10 1980, Wanfraechem 1981)

⚠️ CAUTION: The same cautions suggested earlier should be applied to these specialised nutrients and herbs, most notably, stick to suggested dosages and make only one change at a time and evaluate for reactions before making any additional change in prescribed substances or treatment.

Thermoregulatory hydrotherapy (TRH)

Method 1 (Ernst 1990). In 1990, at Hanover Medical School in Germany, volunteer students were asked to take either warm morning showers or cold morning showers, and their levels and intensity of infection (colds mainly) over the following 6 months were monitored.

Those taking cold showers were asked to gradually increase the degree of coldness so that by the end of the first 3 weeks they were taking a 2–3 minute shower with the water as cold as possible (if any of them developed a cold during the 6 month trial they were told to stop for its duration and for 1 week afterwards). By the end of the 6 month trial those students taking cold showers had had half the number of colds compared with the group taking warm showers, and the colds they did have lasted half as long – they were less acute, their immune systems cleared them up faster.

This trial gives clear evidence that regular cold showers offer an increase in resistance to infection as well as enhanced efficiency of immune function should infection occur. The London research (below) takes this much further and is of specific interest in cases of CFS/FMS.

Method 2 (Pizzorno & Murray 1989, Chaitow 1994, Boyle 1991). The results of important hydrotherapy research in London involving 100 volunteers were published in *The European*, on 22 and 29 April 1993. The Thrombosis Research Institute (who conducted the research) claims that the use of this form of self-treatment proves without question the dramatic value of carefully graduated cold baths, regularly taken (6 months daily use for optimal results). The institute, under its director, Dr Vijay Kakkar, have now gathered 5000 volunteers, many of them suffering from CFS(ME), for the next stage of this research into the benefits of what has been called thermoregulatory hydrotherapy (TRH). The results of the first study showed that when applied correctly the effect of TRH was:

- A boost to sex hormone production which helps regulate both potency in men and fertility in women.
- Renewed energy. Many sufferers from chronic fatigue syndrome (ME) were found to improve dramatically. In one case, a person confined to bed 18 hours a day in a state of exhaustion acquired 'a new lease of life'. The person is quoted in *The European* as stating: 'From the first day I have regularly undertaken the hydrotherapy. With each day the feeling of well-being

increases to such an extent that I can hardly wait for the next morning.'

• Improved circulation in people with cold extremities. Circulation is found to improve rapidly with TRH along with levels of specific enzymes which help circulation.

• Reduced chances of heart attack and stroke because of improved blood clotting function.

• Increased levels of white blood cells.

• Reduced levels of unpleasant menopausal symptoms.

• Some of the volunteers found that their nails became harder and their hair growth improved.

Method

There are four stages to TRH and it is essential to 'train' the body towards the beneficial response by going through these stages.

Equipment needed

A bath, a bath thermometer, a watch and a bath mat.

The bathroom needs to be at a reasonably comfortable temperature – not too cold and not very hot. The temperature of the water should eventually be as it comes from the tap – cold – however, it is possible to train towards the cold bath by first having a tepid bath for a few weeks, and gradually making the water colder so that it goes below body heat, until having a really cold bath is no longer a shock. The timing described below can also be modified so that at first the whole process takes just a few minutes as the various stages of immersion are passed through, with a slow increase in the timing of each stage as well as a reduction in temperature.

CAUTION: When cold water treatments are prescribed for people with FMS/CFS, the degree of stimulus used (how cold the water is, and how long a time is spent immersed) needs to be modified so that a very SLOW increment in contrast is achieved, gradually training and 'hardening' the body to what is potentially a stress factor.

The original TRH programme ran for 80 days and the degree of coldness and the length of time in the water was only gradually increased. It makes sense in cases of extreme sensitivity to cold to make this an even slower process, taking 6 months if necessary to reach the degree of cold achieved in 80 days in the initial studies. To plunge someone who is extremely fragile in their ability to handle stress of any sort into cold water straight from the tap would be foolhardy, whereas taking a shower or bath in 'neutral' (body heat) water for a week before extremely gradually starting the process of, day by day, getting the water cooler and cooler, perhaps over a period of many months before tap-cold water is used, is both sensible and effective.

Stage 1: Stand in the bath in cold water (the range recommended is between 12.7°C and 18.3°C (N.B. 10°C = 50°F while 15°C = 59°F) (but take account of the note above as to how cold the water should be in relation to the degree of fragility/robustness) for about 1 minute, increasing to 5 minutes when fully used to the process, perhaps after some weeks, as the internal thermostat (in the hypothalamus) responds.

Have a non-slip mat in place and avoid standing still but 'walk' up and down the bath or march on the spot.

Stage 2: The internal thermostat is now primed. Sit in cold water for another 1–5 minutes (5 when fully used to the process, perhaps after some weeks) – up to the waist ideally – so that the pooled blood in the lower half of the body is cooled, further influencing the hypothalamus.

Stage 3: This is the most important part of the programme in which it is necessary to immerse the entire body up to the neck and back of the head in cold water. Gently and slowly move the arms and legs to ensure that the slightly warmer water touching the skin is not static, so that the cooling effect continues. This stage ultimately lasts between 10 and 20 minutes but could be for as little as 2 minutes at first, with the degree of coldness being adjustable according to sensitivity.

Stage 4: This is for 'rewarming'. Get out of the bath, towel dry and move around for a few minutes. As warming takes place, a pleasant glowing sensation will usually be felt in the chest, feet and between the shoulder blades.

The whole sequence, *modified at first by reducing time and temperature*, needs to be done daily if the training or hardening effect is to be achieved, with some people finding that several cold baths daily improves their function and energy.

⚠ CAUTION: Despite possibly having value in such conditions, this cold water bath method (TRH) is not recommended as a self-help measure for people with well-established heart disease, high blood pressure or other chronic diseases which require regular prescription medication, unless a suitably qualified physician has been consulted as to safety and supervision.

CANDIDA (YEAST) CONNECTIONS
(Chaitow 1991, Fibromyalgia Network Newsletters 1990–94; see also Fig. 11.1)

Dr Carol Jessop (see Ch. 2) reported that nearly 90% of her patients with FMS (men and women) had yeast infections and that the vast majority had records of recurrent antibiotic use (for sinus, acne, prostate, urinary tract and chest infections in the main); 70% of the women with CFS/FMS had been on the contraceptive pill for 3 years or more; and 63% reported a sugar craving.

The use of antibiotics and steroid medication (including the contraceptive pill) can lead to the spread in the intestinal tract and the body generally of yeasts which are normally controlled by 'friendly' bacteria which are damaged by this medication. (Refer to the notes on probiotics in Ch. 11 for more information on this.)

The main yeast engaged in such activity is *Candida albicans,* best known for causing thrush. Candida is dangerous because of its ability to turn from a simple yeast into an aggressive mycelial fungus which puts down 'rootlets' (rhizomes) into the mucous membrane of the intestinal tract, so permitting undesirable toxins to move from the gut into the bloodstream, with the strong possibility of allergic and toxic reactions taking place (Truss 1982). Among the many symptoms which have been catalogued in people affected in this way are a range of digestive symptoms (bloating, swings from diarrhoea to constipation and back), urinary tract infections, menstrual disturbances, fatigue, muscle aches, emotional disturbances, 'foggy brain' symptoms and skin problems (Crooke 1983). The frequency

with which such symptoms are suffered by people with FMS is enormous. Laboratory tests are commonly inaccurate although one of the most useful involves a sugar loading test which assesses blood alcohol levels before and after the sugar intake (yeast – and some bacteria – can turn sugar into alcohol rapidly in the intestines).

Three month anti-candida strategy
(Chaitow 1991)

- Antifungal medication (or herbs), as advised by a qualified practitioner.
- To encourage repopulation of intestinal flora: between meals (three times daily) a high quality acidophilus and bifidobacteria (powder or capsule form – see Ch. 11) – either a capsule of each, or between a quarter and a whole teaspoon of powdered versions of each, should be taken.
- General nutritional support is useful: a well formulated, yeast-free, hypoallergenic, multivitamin/multimineral to provide at least the recommended daily allowance for the major nutrients is suggested.

Dietary suggestions for candida

- Eat three small main meals daily as well as two snack meals where possible (no sugar-rich food).
- Include in the diet as much ginger, cinnamon and garlic (as well as other aromatic herbs such as oregano) as possible, as these are all antifungal and most also aid digestive processes.
- Avoid all refined sugars and for the first few weeks avoid very sweet fruit as well (melon, sweet grapes).
- Eat vegetables – cooked or raw – pulses (bean family), fish, poultry (avoid skin), whole grains, seeds, nuts (fresh) and after the first few weeks, fruit.
- To assist with bowel function take at least a tablespoonful of linseed, swallowed unchewed with water to provide a soft fibre.
- Avoid aged cheeses, dried fruits (because of their fungal and mould content) and any

food obviously derived from or containing yeast (in case of sensitisation).

- Avoid caffeine-containing drinks and foods (coffee, tea, chocolate, cola) as these produce a sugar release which encourages yeast activity.
- Avoid alcohol.
- If possible avoid all yeast-based foods, including bread and anything that has contained yeast in its manufacture or which might contain mould.

CAUTIONS: The patient may feel off colour for the first week of such a programme as yeast 'die-off' (Herxheimer's reaction) takes place. This will pass on its own; however, anyone with a severe and longstanding yeast problem might consider supplementing with high doses of probiotics for a week or so before starting the anti-candida programme to reduce the intensity of the 'die-off' reaction. Increased thrush activity may be noticed after starting the diet, this will usually calm down after a few days.

Local treatment

- Mix 1 rounded teaspoon of *L. acidophilus* with 2 tablespoons of plain regular yoghourt (not low or non–fat). Insert vaginally or rectally before bedtime as needed.

Douche

- Mix 1 teaspoon of *L. acidophilus* in warm water. Stir briskly and let stand for at least 5 minutes. Stir again. Use as a douche each morning for 10 days.
- Use diluted tea tree oil (15% solution) directly onto irritated areas or pure tea tree oil, 10 drops in warm bath.

CAUTION: Treatment of yeast overgrowth can result in the patient feeling intensely unwell, especially at the outset when yeast 'die-off' occurs (Herxheimer's reaction). The process of recovery from yeast overgrowth (candidiasis) can be slow (seldom less than 3 months and usually 6 months or more of strict adherence to the

diet and nutrient/herbal protocol) and many setbacks are commonly experienced, especially when the patient attempts to return to a normal eating pattern. Patients need to be given a great deal of support and the process can be almost as draining for the practitioner as for the patient.

DEPRESSION

Signs of depression are often noted in people with CFS(ME) and FMS. This, however, is not surprising, since there can be few more depressing situations than being constantly tired, lethargic and in pain, with matters made worse when there is a lack of understanding on the part of doctors. The diagnosis of depression as the 'cause' of the condition is now discredited, since most depression related to FMS is a direct reaction to the condition (loss of health) and is not a clinical depression which has no obvious external cause. The fact that antidepressant medication helps to restore some degree of sleep normality and therefore minimises the symptoms of FMS should not be taken to indicate that depression causes FMS – it does not (see Ch. 4).

Treatment choices

- Low dosage antidepressant medication under medical direction.
- St John's wort (*Hypericum perforatum*) has an excellent record of helping 'long-term, low-grade depression and for mild to moderate major depression' with a number of double-blind placebo controlled trials. Pizzorno reports that studies comparing St John's wort to regular medication (imipramine) produced comparable results, and that there have been '28 controlled studies involving 1500 depressed patients with consistently positive results in mild-to-moderate depression' (Pizzorno 1996). The recommended dosage is 300 mg three times daily. Side-effects are very rare (Muldner et al 1984)

Nutritional tactics

These might include :

1. Cut out/down sugar/caffeine. Approximately half of a depressed group of 23 demonstrated significant and sustained mood deterioration following caffeine or refined sucrose challenge (with cellulose and aspartame as placebo) (Kreitsch et al 1988). In another experimental double blind study, seven out of 16 patients complaining of depression and fatigue improved on a 2 week sucrose- and caffeine-free diet and had a return of symptoms when challenged with caffeine and refined sucrose for 6 days (with cellulose and aspartame as placebo) (Christensen 1988).

2. Folic acid supplementation (200 μg daily) may be useful, especially in patients whose depression is secondary to easy fatiguability (experimental double-blind study) (Coppen 1986).

3. Nutritional interventions which help to balance serotonin levels (see notes on 5–hydroxy–l–tryptophan, p. 155). If the pain and fatigue elements can be modified, depression usually improves.

FATIGUE

In Chapter 5 the fatigue link with FMS was examined and the caution offered that doing too much too soon is a major cause of setbacks for patients with this chronic condition.

Treatment choices

- Use of constitutional hydrotherapy, relaxation methods, appropriate bodywork, a structured and balanced diet which considers both toxicity and allergy factors as well as specific medical or herbal/homoeopathic/acupuncture interventions, where appropriate, form the 'team' approach for restoration of energy and well-being. This will be individual to each person.
- Particular emphasis on the restoration of normal breathing function is also suggested (see this chapter, above).
- Low thyroid function (hypothyroidism – see Ch. 10) as well as adrenal dysfunction ('adrenal exhaustion') can also produce or contribute to chronic fatigue.

- Allergy and fatigue: in one study of what was called 'the allergic tension–fatigue syndrome' it was found that 75% of 50 patients (diagnosed as having FMS) with 'tension/fatigue' had a history of nasal, ocular, respiratory or skin allergy, and that over half the patients treated by elimination diets (see earlier in this chapter) had excellent results, while a further 16 of the 50 had good results (Cleveland et al 1992).
- Deficiencies and fatigue: Professor Melvyn Werbach of UCLA has shown that nutritional deficiencies of potassium, magnesium, iron, folic acid, pantothenic acid (vitamin B_5), pyridoxine (B_6), B_{12}, vitamin C, zinc, aspartic acid, the amino acids carnitine, glutamine, inosine and coenzyme Q10 have *all* been shown, in various studies, to link with fatigue, and that supplementation, as appropriate, based on individual requirements, can be helpful (Werbach 1991).
- Low blood sugar and fatigue: if there is a tendency towards hypoglycaemia (characterised by mood swings, sugar and stimulant craving, a feeling of being spaced out and anxious if meals are missed, as well as fatigue) then the author has found that it is useful to suggest:
  — Taking twice daily, between meals, 4–5 g of full spectrum amino acid complex, in powder or capsule form, in order to help stabilise blood sugar fluctuations and to decrease sugar craving episodes
  — Six small meals should be eaten daily, avoiding sugar and stimulants (caffeine and alcohol in particular) while concentrating on obtaining adequate protein
  — To facilitate a more balanced sugar management glucose tolerance factor (GTF), incorporating the vital nutrient chromium, should be taken (100–200 μg daily).

Clinical observation: In one study of FMS about one-half of the patients seen were found to have reactive hypoglycaemia (St Amand 1996).

INFECTION: VIRAL AND BACTERIAL

In Ch. 3 the possibility of a viral connection with CFS/FMS was explored. Low grade or recurrent viral or bacterial infections can be treated using herbal products without the risks of side-effects of antibiotics and with no risk of resistance being encouraged. In this way antibiotics can be reserved for use in life-threatening situations. Focus on enhancing immune function through sound nutrition, reduced stress levels and reduction in environmental stressors (pollutants, etc.) would seem to offer a singularly little explored approach to containment of viral and bacterial activity.

Herbal methods using echinacea, hydrastis and berberine plus a host of other antiviral and antibacterial products emerging from traditional Chinese and Western medicine can be safely used, ideally under expert supervision. If antibiotics are required these should of course be used, but with due regard to:

- their specificity and precise dosage being established
- the use of probiotics to replenish damaged bowel flora subsequently (see probiotic notes below and Ch. 11) (Mose 1983).

Allium sativum (garlic)

This is a powerful antibacterial, antiviral, antiparasitic and antifungal agent with recent evidence of anti-HIV potential (Pizzorno & Murray 1989). It is also effective against worms and protozoa including organisms resistant to standard antibiotics (Adetumbi et al 1983, Vahora et al 1973, Hu Nan Medical College 1980). Garlic has been used for thousands of years as a food and a medicine, and is currently attracting enormous research interest because of its safety and efficacy. The active ingredient of garlic (which has the antibiotic effects) is allicin; this also carries the most obvious indication of its use – the smell. Fortunately methods have been found to develop garlic with all its potency intact and without the odour.

Astragalus membranaceus

Long used to enhance immune function in Chinese medicine (increased phagocytosis, enhanced T–cell transformation, increased numbers of macrophages, increased IgA and IgG levels, induced formation of interferon, enhanced blastogenesis in white blood cells of normal and cancer patients) (Sun et al 1983a, 1983b).

Dionaea muscipula (Venus fly trap plant) (carnivora)

Immune stimulator and modulator (increases number and activity of T-cells, increases phagocytosis of macrophages). Used intravenously, intramuscularly by inhalation and orally (Walker 1991, 1992a, 1992b).

Echinacea angustifolia (and E. purpurea)

This is an amazingly useful and safe herb which has powerful immune enhancing properties including macrophage activation, as well as inhibiting viral, fungal and bacterial activity. The effect of echinacea seems to be directly on the thymus gland, which is a vital component of immune defence. Research has shown extracts of the root of echinacea to include substances such as inulin which activates the production of a wide range of immune chemicals. Echinacea has been a traditional Native American herbal substance for centuries, and has now been widely researched and used throughout the world.

It can be taken in capsule form or as a liquid (as an alcohol extract). Many experts believe this (liquid) form to be superior in that it is absorbed and used by the body more efficiently. Liquid extract of echinacea, taken by healthy individuals (30 drops three times a day for 5 days) boosts the presence of leukocytes by about 40% (Stimpel et al 1984, Wacker et al 1978). A dose of three or four 500 mg capsules at least twice daily is usually suggested during an infection. Combination capsules and liquids are now available in which echinacea and other herbs are combined for a potent effect against infection and to enhance immune function.

Ginseng (or Eleutherococcus: 'Siberian ginseng')

These are adaptogens which enhance resistance to all forms of stress and which have tonic effects on the thymus gland which is vital for production of T cells (Brekhmann 1980, Takada 1981).

Glycyrrhiza glabra *(liquorice)*

This is an immune system enhancer (Abe et al 1982). Improves macrophage activity, improves production of interferon. Liquorice extract also has broad spectrum antimicrobial effects (Mischer et al 1980). In addition, it is an antioxidant, protecting tissues from free radical damage, especially the liver (Kiso et al 1984). Glycyrrhizin is also an anti-inflammatory agent and protects against allergy and its effects, most notably related to skin conditions (Juroyanagi et al 1966, Onuchi 1981). It protects the thymus from shrinking when steroids such as cortisone are used as well as enhancing the anti-inflammatory effects of cortisone (Kumazi et al 1967).

As far as immune support is concerned this remarkable herb acts against numerous undesirable pathogenic bacteria (*Staphylococcus aureus*, for example, and *Candida albicans*) but for many naturopathic and herbal practitioners this is the herb of first choice in dealing with viral infections (3 x 500 mg capsules four times daily during infection) (Abe et al 1982, Pompei et al 1979, Ito et al 1988).

Hydrastis canadensis *(golden seal)*

Immune enhancer, macrophage activator, increases natural killer cells activity, enhances gastrointestinal function (especially diarrhoea) antibacterial, antifungal, anti-*Candida albicans*. For many naturopathic and herbal practitioners this is the first choice herb for use in treating bacterial infection (4 x 500mg capsules four times daily during infection) (Sharma et al 1978, Choudray et al 1972, Sack et al 1982).

Hypericum perforatum *(St John's wort)*

Apart from its usefulness in treating mild to moderate depression (see notes above), this is commonly used for its antibacterial and antiviral qualities and for its specific anti–retroviral effects. In doses of around 1500 mg daily (in divided doses) it enhances the function of the immune system – apparently by improving circulation to the spleen – with macrophage activity being increased (Meruelo et al 1988, Someya 1985, Barbagallo et al 1987).

Usnea barbata

The extract of this European 'plant' (a lichen – so it is not really a plant, more of a cross between a fungus and an algae) has powerful antibiotic effects, on some of the nastiest bacterial agents, including *Staphylococcus* spp. and *Mycobacterium tuberculosis*. It is taken as a liquid extract, starting (to ensure tolerance) with three to four drops in water twice a day and building up to around 10 drops three times a day during an active infection. It can also be used for sore throats as a gargle (one drop in sufficient water with which to gargle), and for a douche for vaginal infections. Ideally it should be used under expert guidance as it can irritate the stomach and bowels if used excessively. Some experts claim that it is a more powerful antibacterial agent than penicillin, but far safer (Wagner & Prokcsh 1983).

CAUTION: All herbal compounds and many individual herbs are toxic if used in excessive amounts. Many produce mild digestive side-effects (Chen & Chen 1992). Advice from an expert is always prudent if consideration is being given to embarking on use of herbal products.

INFLAMMATION/PAIN

Fibrositis/FMS does not usually involve active inflammation; however, many of the associated muscle, soft tissue and joint problems involving pain certainly do. The dietary strategies outlined below are effective and safe and can be incorporated into a normal eating pattern without difficulty.

There are two major anti-inflammatory nutritional methods which are useful in most pain situations: the dietary approach and the enzyme approach, and both or either can be used if appropriate. Inflammation is a natural and mostly useful response by the body to irritation, injury and infection. To drastically alter or reduce inflammation may be counterproductive and therefore a mistake, as has been shown in the treatment of arthritis using non-steroidal anti-inflammatory drugs over the past 30 years or so – untreated patients and joints have been shown over these years to be better off than those treated.

Nutritional anti-inflammatory treatment approaches

1. Reduce animal fats. A major part of pain/inflammation processes involves particular prostaglandins and leukotrienes. These are themselves to a great extent dependent upon the presence of arachidonic acid which humans manufacture mainly from animal fats. Reducing animal fat intake cuts down access to the enzymes which help to produce arachidonic acid and therefore lowers the levels of the inflammatory substances released in tissues which contribute so greatly to pain (Donowitz 1985, Ford-Hutchinson 1985).

— The first priority in an anti-inflammatory dietary approach is to cut down or eliminate dairy fat.
— Fat free or low fat milk, yoghurt and cheese should be eaten in preference to full fat varieties, and butter avoided altogether.
— Meat fat should be completely avoided, and since much fat in meat is invisible, meat itself can be left out of the diet for a time (or permanently).
— Poultry skin should be avoided.
— Hidden fats in products such as biscuits and other manufactured foods should be looked for on packages and avoided.

2. Eating fish or taking fish oil helps (Moncada et al 1986). Fish which come from cold water areas contain high levels of eicosapentenoic acid (EPA) which reduces levels of arachidonic acid in tissues and therefore helps to create fewer inflammatory precursors. Fish oil has these anti-inflammatory effects without interfering with those prostaglandins which protect the stomach lining and maintain the correct level of blood clotting. This is important because drugs which do just what fish oil can do commonly cause new problems by interfering with prostaglandin function.

Research has shown the use of EPA in rheumatic and arthritic conditions to offer relief from swelling, stiffness and pain, although benefits do not usually become evident until 3 months of supplementation, reaching their most effective level after about 6 months.

Advice for patients:
— Eat fish such as herring, sardine, salmon and mackerel at least twice weekly – more if desired.
— Take EPA capsules (5–10 daily) regularly when inflammation is at its worst until relief appears and then a maintenance dose of 6 daily.

3. Anti-inflammatory (proteolytic) enzymes. It has been found that proteolytic enzymes derived from plants have a gentle but substantial anti-inflammatory influence. These include bromelaine which comes from the pineapple plant (stem not fruit) and papain from the papaya plant. It is necessary to ensure around 2–3 g of one or other are taken (bromelaine is more effective) spread through the day away from meal times (or all they will do is help digest protein) as part of an anti-inflammatory, pain relieving strategy (Taussig 1988, Chichoke 1981).

IRRITABLE BOWEL SYNDROME (IBS)
(see also Fig. 11.1)

This condition has been shown in research to affect at least three quarters of FMS patients – fewer in some studies than others but always a significant number (see Dr Jessop's figures Ch. 2). The symptoms of IBS range from alternating diarrhoea and constipation to abdominal gas/bloating, nausea, just diarrhoea or just constipation.

An Irish study examined people who had been diagnosed as having IBS and found that 65% of these could also be diagnosed as having

FMS, so it is clear that the two conditions are closely associated.

Treatment

- Stress reduction is usually useful. Allergic elements need to be considered and dealt with (see allergy, p. 168). The commonest sensitivities are to grains (wheat especially), corn, yeasts, food colourings, coffee, citrus and dairy products. 'Safe' dietary intake usually consists of lamb, fresh white fish, cabbage, peas, carrots, rye based biscuits/crispbreads (no wheat), rice cakes, milk–free margarine, weak black tea.
- Candidiasis (see above) is a common cause as are parasites (commonest is *Giardia lamblia*). (See also probiotic notes in Ch. 11.)
- Hydrochloric acid deficiencies (and therefore possibly zinc) are common in IBS as are deficiencies of digestive enzymes. Expert advice is required to help normalise such problems but the supplementation of probiotic substances (acidophilus, bifidobacteria and *L. bulgaricus* – all dairy free if possible) is a safe and effective method for starting to normalise bowel health. The detoxification programme outlined below, plus the stress reduction methods (above) are all recommended.
- Fat seems to be a major stimulant of gastro-colonic response and its dietary intake should be controlled (Wright et al 1980, Kellow et al 1988).
- Diets high in refined carbohydrate have been implicated in many studies in aetiology of IBS, encouraging intense smooth-muscle spasm (Grimes 1976, Kruis et al 1987).
- Review articles indicate a subset of IBS patients with strong history of atopy and immunologically linked food allergy, possibly via increased bowel permeability. Elimination diets improve symptoms in these patients. Experimental studies confirm this. Foods most implicated were dairy produce and grains (Petitpierre et al 1985).
- Enteric coated peppermint oil capsules have been shown in experimental double-blind crossover trials to reduce abdominal symptoms.

⚠️ CAUTION: Enteric coated capsules are essential for this effect to prevent too rapid release.

Dosage is 1–2 enteric coated capsules (0.2 ml/cap) three times daily between meals (Dew et al 1984, Rees et al 1995).

GULF WAR SYNDROME
(see also allergy/chemical sensitivity above)

Many thousands of veterans of the Gulf War are now reporting a long list of symptoms: unexplained joint and muscle pain, fatigue, difficulty sleeping, memory/concentration problems, headaches, chest pain, breathing problems, gastrointestinal problems, skin rashes, allergies to foods and odours . . . and so on. Experts state that in many instances what is being complained of is the same as FMS.

Most participants in the Gulf War received numerous immunisation procedures against usual diseases as well as against anthrax and botulinus toxin (in anticipation of biological warfare) while also taking anti-nerve gas pills (pyridostigmine bromide). Vehicles were sprayed with chemical agent resistant coatings and areas surrounding the military operations were sprayed with pesticides. There were also numerous oil well fires and atmospheric pollution, diesel exhausts, solvents vaporised by intense heat, poor hygiene (despite the best efforts) and extremes of stress.

In investigating the condition, experts note that there is a direct link between what is inhaled and the brain since there is no protective shield for the brain at this level of acquiring chemicals into the body. Limbic dysfunction due to chemical overload (multiple chemical sensitivities, or MCS) is therefore one explanation for the symptoms described above. In a review article in the July 1994 issue of Fibromyalgia Network these possibilities are discussed, as is the alternative diagnosis of post traumatic stress disorder (PTSD).

Treatment has apparently been attempted at some VA centres which involves a very pure environment (air purifiers used throughout), stress reduction programmes, endurance and exercise classes along with detoxification through rotation and elimination diets. So far results are not available but this approach at least seems to be dealing with some aspects of the toxic overload imposed on the some 30 000 individuals who have reported symptoms of Gulf War syndrome (many thousands are probably still in military service and statistics on these are not available). The possible immune system damage caused by the cocktail of immunisations received would seem to be far more difficult to evaluate or correct (see detoxification notes below).

PELVIC PAIN (Fibromyalgia Network 1996)

In Brazil, 80 people with disabling pelvic pain were evaluated. MPS was diagnosed in all 80. Treatment using heat, stretching, massage and injection of trigger points resulted in significant improvement in pain levels in 60% of patients. Triggers are common in this region, especially in muscles on the pelvic floor. Yunus (1997) reports that pelvic pain is common in FMS, and that research has shown:

- Pain thresholds in dysmenorrhoeic women were lower than controls at all body sites
- The pelvic region had lower pain thresholds than other body areas in all women tested
- During premenstruation all women in the study were more sensitive in the pelvic area
- At the same time that dysmenorrhoeic women experienced their greatest levels of pain they were hypersensitive to pain elsewhere (limbs, etc.) – something not noted in women in the control group.

(See notes on facilitation and trigger points for a greater understanding of these phenomena (Box 6.1 and Ch. 1).)

Premenstrual syndrome and chronic pelvic pain

Of Dr Carol Jessop's patients, 90% had symptoms of premenstrual tension. Most of them had these symptoms well before their FMS/CFS symptoms started. Nearly 65% had endometriosis symptoms as well (see Ch. 2).

Many of the symptoms associated with premenstrual syndrome (fatigue, bloating, muscular pains, sleep disturbance, headaches, anxiety, swelling in extremities, depression, confusion, emotional lability, etc.) are common to CFS(ME) and FMS. The fact that these symptoms are periodic and not constant shows the distinction from the more chronic conditions of FMS/CFS(ME) and also allows us to glimpse certain possible contributing elements in the maze of potential causes involved in CFS(ME) and FMS.

Dr G. Abraham (Abraham 1981, 1982) has clinically treated and classified premenstrual symptoms into the following categories:

'A' (for 'anxiety' – involving nervous tension, mood swings, irritability, anxiety, insomnia).

This relates to elevated oestrogen and low progesterone and usually a tendency to a high sugar and dairy food diet.

- Nutritional treatment requires taking between 200 and 800 mg of vitamin B_6 daily . . .

CAUTION: [high dosage under expert guidance only] . . . to reduce blood oestrogen levels and increase progesterone.

- Also useful is the taking of omega-6 fatty acids (either as borage oil, flaxseed oil, evening primrose oil) in doses of 1–2 g daily.
- All caffeine and sugar intake should be reduced or eliminated for at least 3 days prior to onset of premenstrual symptoms, and dairy products (and calcium) cut back.

'C' (for 'craving' – involving headache, cravings for sweets, increased appetite, pounding heart, dizziness or fainting, fatigue).

This form of PMT is associated with poor carbohydrate tolerance, low blood magnesium levels and possible prostaglandin imbalances.

- Nutritional treatment requires taking magnesium in supplemental form: at least 500 mg daily (usually combined calcium 1 g, and magnesium 0.5 g is suggested).
- Also useful is the taking of omega-6 fatty acids (either as borage oil, flaxseed oil, evening primrose oil) in doses of 1–2 g daily.
- All caffeine and sugar intake should be reduced or eliminated for at least 3 days prior to onset of premenstrual symptoms. Salt

intake should be reduced to no more than 3 g daily for the 3 days prior to symptom onset.

'D' (for 'depression' – involving depression, forgetfulness, tearfulness, confusion).

This form of PMT relates to high levels of progesterone during the mid-luteal phase and sometimes elevated adrenal androgens (in hairy people). Sometimes lead toxicity seems to be involved in this type of PMT.

- Expert advice is required once the individual's hormonal pattern has been established but caffeine should be reduced or eliminated.
- Vitamin E (300 to 600 IU daily for at least 2 months to assess effect).
- Omega-6 fatty acids (either as borage oil, flaxseed oil, evening primrose oil) in doses of 1–2 g daily.

'H' (for 'hyperhydration' – involving weight gain above 3 lb, swelling of extremities, breast tenderness, abdominal bloating).

This form of PMS is associated with fluid retention and may relate to elevated levels of aldosterone.

- This can be reduced by vitamin B_6 supplementation (500 mg daily under supervision by a health care professional).
- Also (under supervision only) the taking of between 200 000 and 300 000 IU daily of vitamin A has been shown to help this form of PMT if taken from day 15 of cycle until symptom onset.
- Found useful in clinical trials has been omega-6 fatty acids (either as borage oil, flaxseed oil, evening primrose oil) in doses of 1–2 g daily.
- Vitamin E can usually help reduce breast symptoms (300 to 600 IU daily) but *in some studies the symptoms were worse* when PMT-H patients supplemented with Vitamin E.
- Salt intake must be kept low – 3 g daily at most.

 CAUTION: Vitamin A can be toxic in high doses and is contraindicated in pregnancy; vitamin B_6 should not be taken in doses higher than 400 mg daily unless under supervision.

RAYNAUD'S PHENOMENON

This is also known as cold-induced vasospasm, and has been observed in up to 40% of FMS patients in some studies. Bennett (1996) reports that in FMS/CFS patients the syndrome does not always manifest in the classical manner of altered hand colour. There may be a great deal of pain but no colour changes may be observed. He believes that the mechanism for the production of these symptoms in CFS/FMS patients may relate to autonomic nervous system changes.

Treatment

- There are specific biochemical changes involved in this condition, which has been helped by various forms of medication as well as by bodywork techniques, acupuncture and deep relaxation induced by biofeedback or autogenic training techniques, in which the person learns to partially influence the flow of blood to the hands or feet (see autogenic training exercise above).
- There are often links to food allergy and certain nutrient supplements and herbs have been shown to help this problem (CoQ10, ginkgo, vitamins E and C and bioflavonoids).
- Numbness and tingling of the hands/feet may have a mechanical aetiology, involving a restriction in circulation or nerve supply due to tense muscles or joint restriction which can affect the thoracic outlet. Bodywork methods can usually help such problems (Cantu & Grodin 1992).

SLEEP (AND GROWTH HORMONE) PROBLEMS (see Fig. 4.2)

Sleep laboratories have found that nearly half of all people with fibromyalgia have disturbed (by intrusive alpha wave periods) delta stages, and tend to wake up feeling as tired as – or more tired than – they did when they went to bed. A large percentage of the remainder of FMS patients suffer from other forms of sleep disturbance (see below). Prescription antidepressant medication which has successfully reduced many of the symptoms of fibromyalgia includes various drugs which, while they increase the amount of sleep have not been shown to alter the disturbed and limited delta stages by more than a small amount.

The growth hormone connection

Delta stage sleep involves growth hormone being released by the pituitary gland as well as immune system repair functions being more active. Growth hormone, 80% of which is produced during delta stage sleep, has a direct effect on the quality of repair and regeneration of muscles; when deficient because of sleep disturbance this can account, at least in part, for the muscular symptoms of FMS. There is evidence that growth hormone production can be encouraged by specific dietary strategies.

How muscles are affected by sleep disturbance

Dr H. Moldofsky conducted a study in which six volunteers had their stage four sleep disrupted for three nights in a row. They all developed fatigue, widespread aching muscles and specific tenderness on palpation of the appropriate sites used to diagnose fibromyalgia. Interestingly, when the same sleep disruption pattern was used on volunteer long-distance runners there was no fatigue and no pain. Carefully constructed 'training' can be an effective method in recovery from fibromyalgia (Moldofsky 1993).

Some studies show that 'normal' insomnia does not involve the same degree of disturbance of delta stage sleep (by alpha waves) as we see in FMS. When normal sleep is disturbed by insomnia there is also often a greater degree of 'arousal' or increased neurological excitability than is evident in FMS patients. In other words, it is a different form of sleep disturbance, and because delta wave sleep is not upset, growth hormone production remains normal, and muscular dysfunction does not occur when 'normal' insomnia occurs (Lue 1994).

Other sleep anomalies in FMS patients include sleep apnoea (about 25% of FMS patients), nocturnal myoclonus (about 16% of FMS patients) and bruxism (affecting between 10 and 15% of FMS patients) (Maryon 1991):

- Moldofsky (1993) reports that all substances containing caffeine (coffee, tea, chocolate, cola) are contraindicated for people with sleep apnoea as are alcohol and tricyclic (antidepressant) medication.
- Nutritional treatment of myoclonus includes supplementation with vitamin E (400 mg daily) and folic acid (200 µg daily) as well as avoidance of caffeine (Werbach 1993).
- Bruxism is best treated by a dentist/orthodontist who may provide special plates to be worn at night to protect the teeth from damage due to the grinding.

A return to a better sleep pattern is clearly a key, some say the major key, to normalising or helping people with fibromyalgia, but the same treatment is not required for all forms of sleep abnormality.

Supplementation for sleep and growth hormone production (Weindruch & Walford 1988, Chaitow 1992, Kenton 1988)

1. 5-l-HTP (5-hydroxy-l-tryptophan), a tryptophan-like substance derived from an African bean, is now available and clinical experience suggests it is useful in sleep enhancement (Puttini & Caruso 1992).

2. The plant proteins in chlorella and other blue-green algae are ideal sources and a drink containing this (available most health stores) in the evening will provide tryptophan, as will a full spectrum amino acid powder (or capsules) available from health stores.

3. Calcium and magnesium (in a ratio of 2:1) is another useful relaxing nutrient and a gram of calcium/half a gram of magnesium (tablet, capsule, powder or liquid) taken at night helps the relaxation process.

4. Herbs such as valerian, passiflora, hops, chamomile in various combinations are helpful as teas, capsules, etc.

TOXICITY (AND DETOXIFICATION STRATEGIES) (Wing 1983, Burton 1987, Keys 1950, Hoefel 1928, Imamura et al 1958, Kroker 1983, Kjeldsen-Kragh et al 1991, Chaitow 1990, Chaitow 1991, Kernt et al 1982)

Toxicity can be usefully reduced by following a pattern of regular 'detoxification days' (see Box 12.4). Other methods which can help in this task are hydrotherapy methods, skin brushing, sauna baths, aerobic exercise, specific herbal liver treatments, and bodywork to assist in lymphatic drainage.

It is known from research that everyone on the planet has deposits of DDT, petrochemicals, pesticides, lead, cadmium and dioxin in their bodies, as well as measurable serum levels of chlorinated hydrocarbons. As a rule, these are significantly higher in people with CFS (Dunstan et al 1995).

Self-help

A number of methods for safe detoxification exist. These include repetitive short fasting periods which allow the liver in particular to recover from toxic stress. Of particular importance in fibromyalgia is the fact that, on short fasts, growth hormone production is stimulated (see citations contained in Weindruch & Walford 1988).

Detoxification and dietary programmes

If someone is robust and vital a more vigorous detoxification programme will be appropriate than if they are unwell and somewhat fragile in health. The detoxification programme in Box 12. 4 is safe for *almost* everyone.

CAUTION: If someone is a recovering drug user, or an alcoholic, or has an eating disorder, or is a diabetic, then these methods *should not be applied* without professional advice. If there is a candida or bowel problem then self-help and/or professional guidance to help normalise this should be used before starting on the detoxification methods outlined in this chapter.

Bland's detoxification approach (Bland 1995)

Other forms of detoxification are being researched. For example, noted nutritional expert Dr Jeffrey Bland has formulated a meal-replacement product (Ultra-Clear) which is based on rice protein and which is also rich in detoxifying nutrients. By combining avoidance of allergenic foods and using products such as this, a modified fast/detoxification programme can be carried out while continuing with normal activities. Research has shown this to be very helpful for many people with FMS/CFS. A study of Bland's detoxification methods involved 106 patients at different clinics, with either CFS or FMS (plus IBS). The programme called for avoidance of known food allergens, encouragement of intestinal repair, stimulation of liver detoxification and a modified fast using the rice protein powder. Over a 10 week period there was a greater than 50% reduction in symptoms as well as laboratory evidence of improved liver and digestive function.

Joseph Pizzorno ND, one of America's leading naturopathic physicians and founder president of Bastyr University, Seattle, encourages liver detoxification in such cases by means of increased eating of brassica family foods (cabbage, etc.), the use of specific nutrients such as N–acetyl–cysteine and glutathione, as well as taking the herb *Silybum marianum* (milk thistle) 12 mg three times daily. He also encourages adrenal gland function (supplementing with vitamins C and B_5). He states: 'The strong correlation between chronic fatigue syndrome, fibromyalgia and multiple chemical sensitivities suggests that all may respond to hepatic (liver) detoxification, food allergy control and a gut restoration diet' (Pizzorno 1996).

Box 12.4   Detoxification programme

Over almost every weekend for a few months (and thereafter once a month at least) choose between:

Method 1
Short water-only fast (24–36 hours) conducted over a weekend (starting Friday evening and ending Saturday evening or Sunday morning; or just all day Saturday, so that work schedules are not interfered with), making sure that not less than 4 and not more than 8 pints of water are consumed during the day. After fasting for 24–36 hours, break the fast with stewed pears or apples (no sweetening) or with a light vegetable soup, or with plain, low-fat, unsweetened yoghurt.

On the Sunday have a raw food day (fruit/salad only, well chewed, plus water ad lib), or, if the individual has a sensitive digestion, lightly cooked (steamed, stir-fried) vegetables, baked potato and stewed fruit (no sugar) plus yoghurt could be chosen.

Method 2
A full weekend monodiet (Friday night to Sunday evening on a single food as described below):

- Up to 3 lb daily of any of a single (organic, unsprayed if possible) fruit choice such as grapes, apples, pears (best choice if an allergy history exists) or papaya (ideal if digestive problems exist), OR

- Organic (unsprayed) brown rice or buckwheat, or millet or potatoes (skin and all), boiled and eaten whenever desired (up to 1 lb dry weight of any of the grains, which can be made palatable by the addition of a little lemon juice and olive oil, or 3 lb of potatoes daily).

If fruit only is chosen it can be raw or lightly cooked without sweetening.

Whichever type of weekend detoxification is chosen, rest and warmth are essential with no engagements/dates – this is a time to allow energy to focus on the repairing and cleansing processes of detoxification.

Method 3
Milder midweek detoxification days, in between these weekend detoxification intensives:

Breakfast:
- Fresh fruit (raw or lightly cooked – no sweetening) and live yoghurt, OR

- Home made muesli (seeds and nuts and grains) and live yoghurt, OR

- Cooked grains and yoghurt (buckwheat, millet, linseed, barley, rice, etc.).

Drink:
Herbal tea (linden blossom, chamomile, mint, sage, lemon verbena) or lemon and hot water drink.

Lunch/evening meal:
- One of these could be a raw salad with jacket potato or brown rice and either bean curd (tofu) or low fat cheese or nuts/seeds, OR

- If raw food is a problem, a stir fried vegetable/tofu meal or steamed vegetables eaten with potato or rice together with low fat cheese or nuts and seeds.

- The other main meal should be a choice between fish, chicken, game or vegetarian savoury (pulse/grain combination) and vegetables lightly steamed, baked or stir fried.

Desserts:
Lightly stewed fruit – add apple or lemon juice (not sugar) or live natural yoghurt.

Food should be seasoned with garlic and herbs, avoiding salt as much as possible.

At least 2 litres of liquid should be consumed daily between meals.

What to expect during detoxification
In the early days (for the first few weekends of short-term fasting or monodiet) a headache and furred tongue are likely. These side-effects of detoxification will slowly become less obvious as detoxification progresses weekend by weekend.

Nothing should be taken to stop the headache.

As the weeks pass, skin should become clearer (it may get a bit spotty for a while), eyes clearer, brain sharper, digestion more efficient, energy levels should start to rise. When the tongue no longer becomes furred with the weekend detoxification, and headaches no longer appear, the detoxification days can be spread apart – three a month and then two a month and then maintenance of once a month.

When a definite change is noticed, and there is far less reaction to the weekend fasts, the in-between, milder detoxification pattern can also be relaxed a bit.

Detoxification enhancement
1. Skin brushing: frictioning skin before bathing or showering enhances skin function/elimination
2. The Salt glow: a skin friction using wet coarse (sea) salt or Epsom salts before a bath or shower is particularly beneficial for people who have difficulty sweating or who have poor circulation to their hands and/or feet; it is also useful for people prone to rheumatic aches and pains and so is ideal for people with fibromyalgia
3. Sauna – if not too enervating
4. Lymphatic drainage massage, and general massage.

CAUTION: If someone is a recovering drug user, or an alcoholic, or has an eating disorder, or is a diabetic, then these methods *should not be applied* without professional advice. If there is a candida or bowel problem then self-help and/or professional guidance to help normalise this should be used before starting on the detoxification methods outlined in this chapter.

REFERENCES

Abe N, Ebina T, Ishida N 1982 Interferon induction by glycyrrhizen in mice. Microbiology and Immunology 26(6): 535–539

Abraham G, Lubran H 1981 Serum and red cell magnesium levels in patients with PMT. American Journal of Clinical Nutrition 34(11): 2364–2366

Abraham G 1982 Premenstrual blues. Free booklet. Call: Optimox Corporation 800–223–1601

Adetumbi, Lau B 1983 Allium sativum: a natural antibiotic. Medical Hypothesis 12: 227–237

Balch J 1990 Prescription for nutritional healing. Avery, New York

Barbagallo C et al 1987 Antimicrobial activity of three Hypericum species. Fitoteripia 58(3): 175–177

Barelli P 1994 Nasopulmonary physiology. In: Timmons B Behavioural and psychological approaches to breathing disorders. Plenum Press, New York

Bennett R 1996 Report in Fibromyalgia Network, April, p 8

Biomedical and clinical aspects of CoQ10. 1980 Elsevier Science, Amsterdam, vol 2

Bland J 1995 A medical food-supplemented detoxification program in the management of chronic health problems. Alternative Therapies 1: 62–71

Boyle W 1991 Lectures in naturopathic hydrotherapy. Buckeye Press, East Palestine OH

Brekhmann E 1980 Man and biologically active substances. Pergamon Press, London

Brostoff J 1992 Complete guide to food allergy. Bloomsbury, London

Buchman D D 1979 The complete book of water therapy. Dutton, New York

Buchwald D 1994 Comparison of patients with CFS, FMS and MCS. Archives of Internal Medicine 154(18): 2049–2053

Burton A 1987 Therapeutic fasting. In: Pizzorno J, Murray M (eds) Textbook of natural medicine. Bastyr University, Seattle

Cantu R, Grodin A 1992 Myofascial manipulation. Aspen Publications, Gaithersberg, Maryland, ch 5

Cappo B, Holmes D 1984 Utility of prolonged respiratory exhalation for reducing physiological and psychological arousal in non-threatening and threatening situations. Journal of Psychosomatic Research 28: 265–273

Chaitow L 1991 Candida Albicans. Healing Arts Press, Rochester, Vermont

Chaitow L 1992 Natural life extension. Thorsons, Wellingborough, UK

Chaitow L 1993 Water therapy. Harper, San Francisco

Chaitow L (med ed) 1994 Alternative medicine. Future Medicine, San Francisco

Chaitow L, Trenev N 1990 Probiotics. Thorsons, London

Chen Z-L, Chen M–F 1992 Foundations of Chinese herb prescribing. Oriental Healing Arts Institute, Long Beach, California

Choudray V, Sabir M, Bhide V 1972 Berberine in giardiasis. Indian Pediatrics 9: 143–146

Christensen L 1988 Psychological distress and diet – effects of sucrose and caffeine. Journal of Applied Nutrition 40(1): 44–50

Cichoke A 1981 The use of proteolytic enzymes with soft tissue athletic injuries. American Chiropractor (October): 32

Cleveland C et al 1992 Chronic rhinitis and underrecognised association with fibromyalgia. Allergy Proceedings 13(5): 263–267

Coppen A 1986 Folic acid enhances lithium prophylaxis. Journal of Affective Disorders 10: 9–13

Crooke W 1983 The yeast connection. Professional Books, Jackson, Tennessee

Davies S 1987 Nutritional medicine. Pan, London

Dew M, Evans B, Rhodes J 1984 Peppermint oil for IBS – a multicentre trial. British Journal of Clinical Practice 38: 394–398

Donowitz M 1985 Arachidonic acid metabolites and their role in inflammatory bowel disease. Gastroenterology 88: 580–587

Dunstan R et al 1995 Preliminary investigation of chlorinated hydrocarbons and CFS. Medical Journal of Australia 163(September 18): 294–297

Ernst E 1990 Hydrotherapy research. Physiotherapy 76(4): 207–210

Fibromyalgia Network Newsletters 1990–94 (October 1990–January 1992, (Compendium No. 2), January 1993, May 1993, (Compendium, January 1994), July 1994

Fibromyalgia Network 1993–94 May 1993, Compendium, July 1993, January 1994

Fibromyalgia Network. 1996 Report. 32: 6–7

Ford-Hutchinson A 1985 Leukotrienes their formation and role as inflammatory mediators. Federal Proceedings 44:25–29

Foster S 1991 Ginko. Botanical series 304. American Botanical Council, Austin, Texas

Grimes D 1976 Refined carbohydrate, smooth muscle spasm and disease of the colon. Lancet 1: 395–397 (Review article)

Hoefel G 1928 Effects of fasting on metabolism. American Journal of Diseases in Children 28: 16–24

Hu Nan Medical College 1980 Garlic in cryptococcal meningitis. Chinese Medical Journal 93: 123–126

Imamura M et al 1958 Trial of fasting on immunological reactions. Lancet pp 760–763

Ito M et al 1988 Mechanism of inhibitory effect of glycyrrhizin on replication of HIV. Antiviral Research 10: 289–298

Jevning R 1992 The physiology of meditation – a wakeful hypometabolic integrated response. Neuroscience and Biobehavioural Reviews 16: 415–424

Journal for Action for ME 1994 No.15, Spring (Box 1302, Wells BA52WE, UK)

Journal of the Royal Society of Medicine 1981 Hyperventilation and the anxiety state. Editorial. Journal of the Royal Society of Medicine 74(January): 1–4

Juroyanagi T et al 1966 Effect of prednisone and glycyrrhizin on passive transfer of experimental allergic encephalomyitis. Allergy 15: 670–675

Kamikawa T et al 1985 Effects of CoQ10 on exercise tolerance in chronic stable angina pectoris. American Journal of Cardiology 56: 247

Kellow J F et al 1988 Dysmotility of the small intestine in irritable bowel syndrome. Gut 29(9): 1236–1243

Kenton L 1988 Ageless ageing. Century Arrow, London

Kernt P et al 1982 Fasting – pathophysiology and complications. Western Journal of Medicine 137: 379–399

Keys A 1950 Biology of human starvation. University of Minnesota Press, vols 1 and 2, Minneapolis

Kiso Y et al 1984 Mechanism of antihepatotoxic activity of glycyrrhizin. Planta Medica 50(4): 298–302

Kjeldsen-Kragh J et al 1991 Controlled trial of fasting and one year vegetarian diet in rheumatoid arthritis. Lancet pp 899–904

Kleijnen J 1992 Ginko biloba. Lancet 340: 8828; Nov 1992 1136–1139

Komaroff K 1996 CFS – is it real? Fibromyalgia Network 33: 4–5

Kreitsch K et al 1988 Prevalence, presenting symptoms and psychological characteristics of individuals experiencing a diet-related mood disturbance. Behavioural Therapy 19: 593–604

Kroker G 1983 Fasting and rheumatoid arthritis. Clinical Ecology 2(3): 137–144

Kruis W et al 1987 Influence of diets high and low in refined sugar on stool qualities, gastrointestinal transit time and faecal bile acid secretion. Gastroenterology 92: 395–397

Kumazai A, Nanaboshi M, Asanuma Y et al 1967 Effects of glycyrrhizin on thymolytic and immunosuppressive action of cortisone. Endocrinology Japan 14(1): 39–42

Lue F 1994 Sleep and fibromyalgia. Journal of Musculoskeletal Pain 2(3): 89–100

Lum L 1994 Hyperventilation syndromes. In: Timmons B Behavioural and psychological approaches to breathing disorders. Plenum Press, New York

Macintyre A 1993 The immune dysfunction hypothesis. Journal of Action for ME 14: 24–25

Maryon F 1991 Fibrositis (fibromyalgia syndrome) and the dental clinician. Journal of Craniomandibular Practice 9(1): 64–70

Meruelo D et al 1988 Therapeutic agents with dramatic retroviral activity. Proceedings of National Academy of Sciences 85: 5230–5234

Mischer L et al 1980 Antimicrobial agents from higher plants. Journal of Natural Products 43(2): 259–269

Moldofsky H 1993 Fibromyalgia, sleep disorder and chronic fatigue syndrome. CIBA Symposium 173, pp 262–279

Moncada S et al 1986 Leucocytes and tissue injury: the use of eicosapentenoic acid in the control of white cell activation. Wiener Klinische Wochenschrift 98(4): 104–106

Mose J 1983 Effects of echinacin on phagocytosis of NK cells. Medical Welt 34: 1463–1467

Muldner Von H et al 1984 Antidepressivewirkung eines auf den wirkstoffkomplex hypericin standardisierten hypericum-extraktes. Arzneimittel-forschung 34: 918

Onuchi K 1981 Glycyrrhizin inhibits prostaglandin E2 production. Prostaglandins in Medicine 7(5): 457–463

Petitpierre M et al 1985 IBS and hypersensitivity to food. Annals of Allergy 54: 538–540

Pizzorno J 1996 Total wellness. Prima Publishing, Rocklin, California

Pizzorno J, Murray M (eds) 1989 Textbook of natural medicine. Hydrotherapy section. Bastyr University, Seattle

Pompei R, Pani R, Flore O et al 1979 Glycyrrhizic acid inhibits virus growth and inactivates virus particles. Nature 281: 689–690

Puttini P S, Caruso I 1992 Primary fibromyalgia syndrome and 5-hydroxy-L-tryptophan: a90-day open study. Journal of Inernal Medicine Research 20(2): 182–189

Readhead C 1984 Enhanced adaptive behavioural response through breathing retraining. Lancet (22 September): 665–668

Rees W et al 1995 Capsules of enteric coated peppermint oil significantly reduce abdominal symptoms. British Medical Journal 2(6194): 835–836

Rucco V et al 1995 Autogenic training versus Erickson's analogical technique in treatment of fibromyalgia syndrome. Rev. European Sci. Med. Farmacol 17(1): 41–50

Sack R, Froelich J 1982 Berberine inhibits intestinal secretory response of *Vibrio cholerae, E. coli* enterotoxins. Infection and Immunity 35(2): 471–475

St Amand R P 1996 Exploring the fibromyalgia connection. The Vulvar Pain Newsletter, Fall,1: 4–6

Schaffler V 1985 Double blind study of the hypoxia protective effect of standardised Ginko biloba. Arzneimittel-forschung 35: 1283–1286

Schultz J 1959 Autogenic training – psychophysiological approach to psychotherapy. Grune and Stratton, New York

Sharma R et al 1978 Berberine tannate in acute diarrhoea. Indian Pediatric Journal 7: 496–502

Someya H 1985 Effect of a constituent of hypericum on infection and multiplication of Epstein-Barr virus. Journal of Tokyo Medical College 43(5): 815–826

Steinberg P 1996 Double blind placebo controlled study of efficacy of oral terfenadine in treatment of CFS. Journal of Allergy and Clinical Immunology 97(1): 119–126

Stimpel M et al 1984 Macrophage activation and induction of cytotoxicity by purified polysaccharide fractions from Echinacea purpurea. Infection and Immunity 46: 845–849

Sun Y et al 1983a Preliminary observation on the effects of Chinese herbs. Journal of Biological Response Modifiers 2: 227–237

Sun Y et al 1983b Immune restoration and/or augmentation of local versus host reaction by traditional Chinese herbs. Cancer 52(1): 70–73

Takada A et al 1981 Restoration of radiation injury by Ginseng. Journal of Radiation 22: 323–325

Taussig S 1988 Bromelain and its clinical application – update. Journal of Ethnopharmacology 22: 191–203

Thrash A, Home C 1981 Remedies. New Life Books, Groveland CA

Timmons B 1994 Behavioural and psychological approaches to breathing disorders. Plenum Press, New York

Truss C O 1982 The missing diagnosis. The Missing Diagnosis Inc, Birmingham, Alabama

Tuncer T 1997 Primary fibromyalgia and allergy. Clinical Rheumatology 16(1): 9–12

Vahora S et al 1973 Medicinal use of Indian vegetables. Planta Medica 23: 381–393

Vanfraechem J H P 1981 CoQ10 and physical performance. In: Biomedical and Clinical Aspects of CoQ10 3: 235–41

Vorberg G 1985 Ginko extract – a long term study of chronic cerebral insufficiency. Clinical Trials Journal 22: 149–157

Wacker A et al 1978 Virus inhibition by Echinacea purpurea. Planta Medica 33: 89–102

Wagner H, Prokcsh A 1983 Immunostimulating drugs from fungi and higher plants. In: Progress in medicinal and economic plant research. Academic Press, London, vol 1

Walker M 1991 Carnivora therapy. Raum & Zeit 4(2)

Walker M 1992a Carnivora therapy in cancer and AIDS. Explore 3(5): 10–15

Walker M 1992b Carnivora and AIDS. Townsend Letter for Doctors May 1992

Weindruch R, Walford R 1988 Retardation of aging and disease by dietary restriction. Charles Thomas, Springfield, Illinois

Werbach M 1990 Nutritional influences on illness. Third Line Press, Los Angeles

Werbach M 1991 Nutritional influences on illness. Third Line Press, Tarzana, California

Wing E 1983 Fasting enhanced immune effector mechanism. American Journal of Medicine 75: 91–96

Wright S et al 1980 Effect of dietary components on the gastrocolonic response. American Journal of Physiology 238(3): G228–232

Yunus M 1997 FMS: Clinical Features and Spectrum. The Fibromyalgia Syndrome. Haworth Press, Binghampton, NY

13

Bodywork approaches to fibromyalgia

Although muscular pain is the defining component of fibromyalgia, the consensus is that FMS is not primarily a musculoskeletal problem, but one which emerges as a result of neurohumoral imbalances caused by any of a combination of inherited and acquired factors. The solution, as far as it exists, therefore lies in restoring neurohumoral balance utilising biochemical, educational and psychosocial tools, as well as biomechanical tools to ease musculoskeletal discomfort, pain and restriction.

Despite most of the theorising as to causal agents ending up with biochemical and psychosocial 'causes', there are in fact some very specific musculoskeletal features involved in FMS; these are sometimes aetiological, sometimes symptomatic of the condition, and not unusually both. Amongst these biomechanical features – in no particular order of importance – are the following:

• The evidence regarding whiplash injury and the changes this involves in the suboccipital region offer compelling impetus to focus attention to this area (see Ch. 3).
• The evidence that in many instances a history exists of hypermobility suggests that compensation patterns will have evolved and that these deserve attention.
• The powerful relationship between the symptoms of over-breathing (hyperventilation tendency) and those of FMS, and the almost universal presence of breathing dysfunction in this patient population, calls for a major focus on restoration of both structural and functional integrity of respiratory function (see Ch. 3).

- The overwhelming evidence of the involvement of myofascial trigger point activity as a part (perhaps the major part in some instances) of the pain experienced by the patient with FMS points to this being an area of primary interest for pain relief (see Ch. 6).
- The degree of emotional distress which accompanies FMS, whether as part of the cause or as a result of the condition, will always have associated with it patterns of myofascial compensation and adaptation.

PATTERNS OF DYSFUNCTION

In order to address identified dysfunctional patterns in the musculoskeletal system, a variety of treatment approaches exist, and some of these will be described in detail. Before investigating these, however, it is necessary to briefly summarise what can happen to the human body in musculoskeletal terms, as it adapts to the 'normal' stresses of life.

As we follow this journey towards dysfunction (which most of us make) it will be clear that particular patterns emerge, and that these can be used diagnostically and prognostically, in either a 'normal' or a fibromyalgia setting. This also helps to identify the areas where therapeutic interventions are most likely to be helpful.

In brief, the progression is one which involves all or some of following elements (more closely detailed below):

- Inborn anomalies (short leg, hypermobility, fascial distortion, etc.)
- Acquired habits of misuse (posture, breathing imbalance, etc.)
- Overuse factors (repetitive movement patterns in sport, work, general activities, etc.)
- Trauma
- Emotional patterns which have musculoskeletal influences (chronic anger, fear, anxiety, depression, etc.)
- Additional stressors (toxicity, deficiency, infection, allergy, hormonal imbalance, etc.)
- Frank musculoskeletal disease (osteoarthritis)
- Reflexive activity (myofascial trigger points or areas of segmental facilitation).

A model which bases itself on the work of Hans Selye is useful in establishing the patterns of dysfunction which can emerge from the sort of of inputs listed above.

GAS and LAS

Selye (1956) called stress the non-specific element in disease production. He described the relationship between the general adaptation syndrome (GAS), i.e.:

- alarm reaction
- resistance (adaptation) phase, followed by
- exhaustion phase (when adaptation finally fails),

which affects the organism as a whole, and the local adaptation syndrome (LAS), which affects a specific stressed area of the body, and demonstrated that stress results in a pattern of adaptation individual to each organism. He also showed that when an individual is acutely alarmed, stressed or aroused, homeostatic (self-normalising) mechanisms are activated.

This is the alarm reaction of Selye's general adaptation syndrome and local adaptation syndrome. If the alarm status is prolonged, or if repetitive defensive adaptation processes commence, long-term chronic changes arise. The results of the repeated postural and traumatic insults of a lifetime combined with tensions of emotional and psychological origin will often present a confusing pattern of tense, contracted, bunched, fatigued and ultimately fibrous tissue (Chaitow 1989). Researchers have shown that the type of stress involved can be entirely biomechanical in nature (Wall & Melzack 1989) (e.g. a single injury or repetitive postural strain) or purely psychic in nature (Latey 1983) (e.g. chronically repressed anger). More often than not though, a combination of emotional and physical stresses will so alter neuromusculoskeletal structures as to create a series of identifiable physical changes which will themselves generate further stress such as pain, joint restriction, general discomfort and fatigue.

Predictable chain-reactions of compensating changes will evolve in the soft tissues in most instances of this sort of chronic adaptation to bio-mechanical and psychogenic stress (Lewit 1992). Such adaptation will be seen almost always to be at the expense of optimal function as well as also being an ongoing source of further physiological embarrassment.

Soft tissue: stress response sequence

When the musculoskeletal system is 'stressed' a sequence occurs which can be summarised as:

1. 'Something' (listed above) occurs which leads to increased muscular tone.

2. Increased tone, if anything but short-term, leads to a retention of metabolic wastes.

3. Increased tone simultaneously leads to a degree of localised oxygen lack (relative to the efforts being demanded of the tissues) – resulting in ischaemia.

4. Increased tone might also lead to a degree of oedema.

5. These factors (retention of wastes/ischaemia/oedema) result in discomfort/pain.

6. Discomfort/pain leads to increased or maintained hypertonicity.

7. Inflammation – or at least chronic irritation – may be a result.

At this stage the patient will experience intermittent stiffness, discomfort and possibly some pain. Relaxation methods and simple stretching may be all that is needed to ease the soft tissue changes, along with re-education. If this is not achieved and the pattern continues as above:

8. Neurological reporting stations in hypertonic tissues will bombard the CNS with information regarding their status, leading to a degree of sensitisation of neural structures and the evolution of facilitation – hyper-reactivity.

9. Macrophages are activated, as is increased vascularity and fibroblastic activity.

10. Connective tissue production increases with cross linkage leading to shortened fascia.

11. Since all fascia/connective tissue is continuous throughout the body, any distortions which develop in one region can potentially create distortions elsewhere, so negatively influencing structures which are supported or attached to the fascia, including nerves, muscles, lymph structures and blood vessels.

12. Changes occur in the elastic (muscle) tissues, leading to chronic hypertonicity and ultimately to fibrotic changes.

13. Hypertonicity in a muscle will produce inhibition of its antagonist muscles.

14. Chain reactions evolve in which some muscles (postural – Type I) shorten while others (phasic – Type II) weaken (these muscle types are described and listed below).

15. Because of sustained increased muscle tension, ischaemia in tendinous structures occurs, as it does in localised areas of muscles. Periosteal pain areas develop.

16. Malcoordination of movement occurs with antagonist muscle groups being hypertonic (e.g. erector spinae) or weak (e.g. weak rectus abdominis group) (Fig. 13.1).

At this stage therapeutic interventions may need to be more aggressive, attempting to restore shortened structures to their normal length; enhancing strength in inhibited (by hypertonic antagonists) muscles; re-educating patterns of

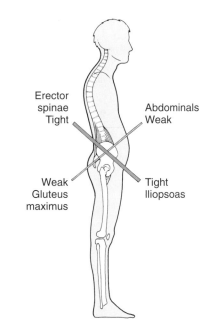

Erector spinae Tight

Abdominals Weak

Weak Gluteus maximus

Tight Iliopsoas

Figure 13.1 The lower crossed syndrome, as described by Janda (1982).

use, etc. If this is not achieved and the pattern described above continues:

17. Joint restrictions and/or imbalances as well as fascial shortenings develop.

18. Localised areas of hyper-reactivity of neural structures occur (facilitated areas) in paraspinal regions or within the myofascia – i.e. trigger points.

19. Energy wastage due to unnecessarily maintained hypertonicity leads to fatigue.

20. Widespread functional changes develop as particular muscle groups modify – for example affecting respiratory function – with repercussions on the total economy of the body. (Fig. 13.2)

21. Heightened arousal results, with an inability to relax adequately and consequent increased hypertonicity.

22. Functional patterns of use of a biologically unsustainable nature emerge, involving chronic musculoskeletal problems and pain.

At this stage, restoration of normal function requires therapeutic input which addresses the multiple changes which have occurred, as well as the need for a re-education of the individual as to how to use their body, to breathe, carry and use themselves in less stressful ways. The chronic adaptive changes which develop lead to the likelihood of future acute exacerbations as the increasingly chronic, less supple structures attempt to cope with new stress factors resulting from the normal demands of modern living (Janda 1982, 1983, Travell & Simon 1983, 1991, Basmajian 1974, Lewit 1992, Korr 1978, Dvorak & Dvorak 1984).

As a result of the processes described above – which affect each and every one of us to some degree – acute and painful problems overlaid on chronic soft tissue changes become the norm.

Source of pain

Where pain exists in tense musculature, Barlow suggests that in the absence of other pathology such pain results from:

• The muscle itself through some noxious metabolic product (e.g. Factor P – see Fig. 3.5, Ch. 3) (Lewis 1942) or an interference in blood circulation due to spasm, resulting in relative ischaemia.

• The muscular insertion into the periosteum, involving a lifting of the periosteal tissue following marked, sustained or repetitive muscular tension (Lewit 1992).

• The joint, which can become restricted and over-approximated. In advanced cases, osteoarthritic changes can result from the repeated microtrauma of ongoing muscular imbalances. Over-approximation of joint surfaces due to soft tissue shortening can also lead to uneven wear and tear, as for example when the tensor fascia lata structure shortens and crowds both the hip and lateral knee joint structures.

• Neural irritation, which can be produced spinally or along the course of the nerve as a result of chronic muscular contractions. These can involve disc and general spinal mechanical faults (Korr 1976).

Variations in pain threshold which have to do with perception (Melzack 1983) or interpretation in FMS (see Fig. 4.4, Ch. 4) will make all these factors more or less significant and obvious.

Baldry (1993) describes the progression of normal muscle to one in painful chronic distress as commonly involving initial or repetitive trauma (strain or excessive use) resulting in the

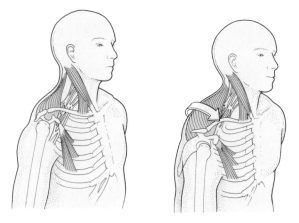

Figure 13.2 A progressive pattern of postural and biomechanical dysfunction develops resulting in, and aggravated by, inappropriate breathing function.

release of chemical substances such as bradykinin, prostaglandins, histamine, serotonin and potassium ions. Sensitisation of A–δ and C (Group IV) sensory nerve fibres may follow with involvement of the limbic system and the frontal lobe (see Ch. 6).

Trigger points (see Figs. 6.4 and 6.5) which evolve from such a progression themselves become the source of new problems, locally as well as at distant sites, as their sarcoplasmic reticulum is damaged and free calcium ions are released, leading to the formation of localised taut bands of tissue (involving the actin–myosin contractile mechanisms in the muscle sarcomeres). If free calcium and energy-producing ATP are present, this becomes a self-perpetuating feature compounded by the relative (to surrounding tissues) ischaemia which has been identified in such chronically contracted tissues (Simons 1987).

Where pain has been produced by repetitive habits, postural and otherwise, with emotional and psychological overtones, the task of therapeutic intervention is complex since hypertonicity can often only be partially released or relaxed without resolving the underlying pattern of use (posture, overuse, etc.).

Different responses in postural and phasic muscles
(Woo et al 1987, Engel et al 1986)

Muscles have a mixture of fibre types although in most there is a predominance of one sort or another. There are those which contract slowly ('slow twitch fibres') which are classified as Type I. These have very low stores of energy-supplying glycogen but carry high concentrations of myoglobulin and mitochondria. These fibres fatigue slowly and are mainly involved in postural and stabilising tasks.

There are also several phasic/active Type II fibre forms, notably:

• Type IIa fibres which ('fast twitch') which contract more speedily than Type I and are moderately resistant to fatigue with relatively high concentrations of mitochondria and myoglobulin.
• Type IIb fibres ('fast twitch/glycolytic fibres')

which are less fatigue-resistant and depend more on glycolytic sources of energy, with low levels of mitochondria and myoglobulin.
• Type IIm ('super fast fibre'), found mainly in the jaw muscles, which depend upon a unique myosin structure which, along with a high glycogen content, differentiates it from the other Type II fibres (Rowlerson 1981).

Long-term stress involving Type I muscles (postural) leads to them shortening, whereas Type II muscles (phasic) undergoing similar stress will weaken without shortening over their whole length (they may, however, develop shortened areas within the muscle). It is important to emphasise that shortness and tightness of a postural muscle does not imply strength. Such muscles may test as strong or weak. However, a weak phasic muscle will not shorten overall and will always test as weak.

Evidence exists as to the potential for adaptability of muscles, so that committed muscle fibres can be transformed from slow-twitch to fast-twitch and vice versa depending upon the patterns of use to which they are put (Lin 1994). An example of this potential involves the scalene muscles, which Lewit (1985) confirms can be classified as either postural or phasic. If the largely phasic (dedicated to movement) scalene muscles have postural functions thrust upon them (as in an asthmatic condition or in chronic hyperventilation) in which they will attempt to maintain the upper ribs in elevation so as to enhance lung capacity, their fibre type will alter and they will shorten – becoming postural muscles.

Postural muscles

Postural muscles which shorten in response to dysfunction include:

• Trapezius (upper), sternocleidomastoid, levator scapulae and upper aspects of pectoralis major, in the upper trunk, and the flexors of the arms
• Quadratus lumborum, erector spinae, oblique abdominals and iliopsoas, in the lower trunk

- Tensor fascia lata, rectus femoris, biceps femoris, adductors (longus, brevis and magnus), piriformis, hamstrings, semitendinosus, in the pelvic and lower extremity region.

Phasic muscles

Phasic muscles which weaken in response to dysfunction (i.e. are inhibited) include:

- The paravertebral muscles (not erector spinae) and scaleni (which can become postural through stress), the extensors of the upper extremity, the abdominal aspects of pectoralis major; middle and inferior aspects of trapezius; the rhomboids, serratus anterior, rectus abdominus; the internal and external obliques, gluteals, the peroneal muscles and the extensors of the arms.

Indications of soft tissue adaptation

A fully functional muscle or joint will be pain free and have a normal firing sequence, range, motion and end feel, while a dysfunctional one will not. Evidence of dysfunction is found by assessing for altered range, modified quality during motion and a changed 'end feel'. Commonly, the firing sequence of dysfunctional muscles alters (as associated structures undertake its tasks) offering further evidence of dysfunction.

The checklist in Box 13.1 can be used to follow (and record results of) the simple sequence of postural muscle assessment, some of which are described in detail below.

Palpatory diagnosis (Baldry 1993, DiGiovanna 1991, Beal 1983, Travell & Simons 1986, 1993)

One of the most successful methods of palpatory diagnosis is to run the pads of a finger (or several fingers) extremely lightly over the area being checked, assessing for changes in the skin and thereby the tissues below it. After localising any changes in this way, deeper periaxial structures can be evaluated by means of the application of

greater pressure, although in cases involving FMS pressure should always be minimised.

There are a number of specific changes to be sought in light palpatory examination; this applies to both acute and chronic dysfunction:

1. Skin changes (Lewit 1992)

Over an area of acute or chronic dysfunction, skin will feel tense and will be relatively difficult

---

Box 13.1   Postural muscle assessment sequence

NAME _____

01. Gastrocnemius	E L R
02. Soleus	E L R
03. Medial hamstrings	E L R
04. Short adductors	E L R
05. Rectus femoris	E L R
06. Psoas	E L R
07. Hamstrings: a. upper fibres	E L R
b. lower fibres	E L R
08. Tensor fascia lata	E L R
09. Piriformis	E L R
10. Quadratus lumborum	E L R
11. Pectoralis major	E L R
12. Latissimus dorsi	E L R
13. Upper trapezius	E L R
14. Scalenes	E L R
15. Sternocleidomastoid	E L R
16. Levator scapulae	E L R
17. Infraspinatus	E L R
18. Subscapularis	E L R
19. Supraspinatus	E L R
20. Flexors of the arm	E L R

21. Spinal flattening:
    a. seated legs straight LL LDJ LT MT UT
    b. seated legs flexed LL LDJ LT MT UT
    c. cervical spine extensors short? Yes   No

KEY: E = Equal (circle both if both are short)
L & R are circled if left or right are short
Spinal abbreviations indicate low lumbar, lumbodorsal junction, low thoracic, mid-thoracic and upper thoracic areas (of flatness and therefore reduced ability to flex – short erector spinae)

to move or glide over the underlying structures, i.e. there will be greater adherence between the skin and the underlying fascia (Fig. 13.3).

The skin overlying reflexively active areas such as trigger points (or active acupuncture points) tends to produce a sensation of 'drag' as it is very lightly stroked ('feather-light'), due to increased hydrosis resulting from increased sympathetic activity (Fig. 13.4).

There is also an apparent undulation sensation, a rising and falling, palpable on an extremely light stroke (as above), described illustratively as 'hills and valleys'.

The skin will lose a degree of its fully elastic quality, so that on light stretching (easing an area of skin to its easy resistance barrier by placing two fingers touching and separating and taking the underlying skin with them) it will test as less elastic than neighbouring skin (Fig. 13.5).

2. Induration

A slight increase in diagnostic pressure will ascertain whether or not the superficial musculature has an increased indurated feeling (Fig. 13.6).

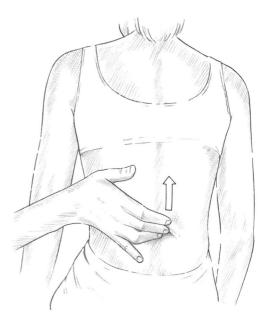

Figure 13.4   Assessing variations in skin friction (drag, resistance).

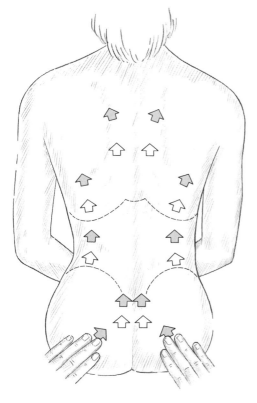

Figure 13.3   Testing tissue mobility by bilaterally 'pushing' skin with fingertip.

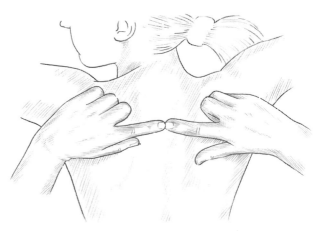

Figure 13.5   Fingers touch each other directly over skin to be tested – very light skin contact assesses degree of skin elasticity – compared with neighbouring skin area.

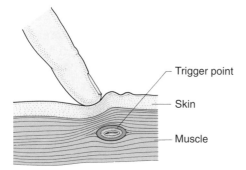

Figure 13.6 Trigger points are areas of local facilitation which can be housed in any soft tissue structure, most usually muscle and/or fascia. Palpation from the skin or at depth may be required to localise these.

When chronic dysfunction exists, the superficial musculature will demonstrate a tension and immobility indicating fibrotic changes within and below these structures. These changes are further discussed in the text dealing with the application of basic spinal and abdominal NMT in its assessment mode (p. 209).

3. Temperature changes

In acute dysfunction a localised increase in temperature may be evident.

A 'scan' of the tissues being investigated, keeping the hand approximately 1 inch from the skin surface, is used by some practitioners (manual thermal diagnosis) as a means of establishing areas which apparently differ from each other in temperature. Using sophisticated equipment, French osteopath Jean-Pierre Barrell has established that areas which scan (non-touching) as 'hot' are only truly warmer/hotter than surrounding areas in 75% of instances. It seems that scanning for hot and cold areas results in the perception of greater heat being noted whenever a major difference occurs in one area compared to a neighbouring one. This means that scanning over a 'normal' then a cold area will often (usually) result in a perception that greater heat is being sensed. This does not nullify the usefulness of such approaches in attempting to identify dysfunctional tissues without being invasive, but does mean that what seems 'hot' may actually be 'cold' (ischaemic?) (Barrell 1996).

In chronic lesion conditions there may, because of relative ischaemia, be a reduced temperature of the tissues which may indicate that fibrotic changes have occurred.

4. Tenderness

Tenderness of palpated tissues requires investigation:

- Is the tissue inflamed?
- Is the local area reflexively active?
- What is the nature and cause of the sensitivity?
- Is it worse when passively moved?

5. Oedema

An impression of swelling, fullness and congestion can often be obtained in the overlying tissues in acute dysfunction. In chronic dysfunction this is usually absent, possibly having been replaced by fibrotic changes.

Questions we need to answer via palpation:

- What am I feeling?
- What significance does it have in relation to the patient's condition/symptoms?
- How does this relate to any other areas of dysfunction I have noted?
- Is this a local problem or part of a larger pattern of dysfunction?
- What does what I am feeling mean?

Deeper palpation

In deep palpation the pressure of the palpating fingers or thumb needs to increase sufficiently to make contact with deeper structures such as the periaxial (paravertebral) musculature without provoking a defensive response. Amongst the changes which might be noted may be immobility, tenderness, oedema, deep muscle tension, fibrotic and interosseous changes. Apart from the fibrotic changes, which are indicative of chronic dysfunctions, all these changes can be found in either acute or chronic problems. All trigger points, tender points, connective tissue zones, etc. are characterised by the presence of hyperalgesic skin zones (HSZ) in the overlying tissues, allowing for easy identification of reflex activity by means of changes (discussed above) in skin elasticity and adherence (Lewit 1992).

Palpation exercise (suggested time 20 minutes)

Select a local area and identify local soft tissue distress, especially trigger points, utilising the following approaches, charting what is found:

1. Off-body scan for temperature variations (remembering that cold may suggest ischaemia, hot may indicate irritation/inflammation). Using the palm or back of the hand, approximately 1 inch from the surface, move steadily across the tissues, ensuring that the scan starts 'off' the body so that a norm can be established of no radiant heat reaching the hand. Movement should be steady – too slow and the chance for discrimination is lost, and too fast precludes anything meaningful being assessed.

2. Evaluate skin adherence to underlying fascia using light but firm 'pushing'. Place three fingerpads of each hand bilaterally alongside the spine, an inch or two away from it, and apply a very light pressure so that the skin on the fascia is taken superiorly to its elastic barrier. Sequentially test the entire thoracic area in this way. Asymmetry is being evaluated. Any skin-on-fascia glide which seems resistant, compared with the opposite side, or in which both glides seem restricted, suggests the tissues below it deserve further investigation. Do such areas correspond with information gained from other assessments such as scanning?

3. Evaluate for reflexively active areas (triggers, etc.) by means of very light single digit palpation seeking the phenomenon of 'drag' and/or 'hills and valleys'. By using no pressure at all, simply touch of skin-on-skin, and moving gently along a line to be evaluated, try to sense either a slight degree of hesitation, 'roughness', 'drag' – which suggests greater hydrosis in the tissues directly below the sensation or, as the light stroke is being made, sense a rise and fall, and pay attention to tissues below the 'hills'. Which method is more sensitive? When identified in

this way light compression of the underlying tissues should reveal the presence of an active trigger point (Fig. 13.6).

4. Next use the method of assessing skin elasticity and compare the accuracy of this with the methods previously attempted (above). Assess variations in local skin elasticity (Lewit's 'skin stretch') by placing two digits (both index fingers usually) so that they touch, and simply separate the fingers, taking the skin with them to the elastic barrier. Repeat this in a steady sequential series so that one stretch is compared with the previous one, not too slowly or the differential is lost and not too fast or it is irritating. Any area where the stretch is reduced compared to the previous stretch is likely to be directly over an active trigger point. Lewit claims that loss of elastic quality indicates a hyperalgesic zone and probable deeper dysfunction (e.g. trigger point) or pathology (Lewit 1992).

Non-nvasive therapeutic possibilities emerging from this exercise

A number of important therapeutic possibilities of particular value in FMS emerge from this assessment exercise:

1. Having found an area where the skin seems less elastic than that previously assessed, experiment by holding the skin at its elastic barrier (unforced) for 10–15 seconds.

What happens? The skin should slowly release, stretch and lengthen. This is a miniature example of myofascial release, and can be effectively used on very sensitive areas/patients to begin the process of deactivating myofascial trigger points.

Having established that holding skin at its barrier (unforced) changes its length/elasticity, test this phenomenon on larger areas of tissue (e.g. paraspinal muscle mass).

2. Introduce a 'C' or 'S' bend – ease a muscle (or part of it) into a 'bent' position and hold the tissue at its elastic barrier without force for 15–20 seconds and note how it gradually lengthens without force.

3. Place two or three finger pads – no pressure just the weight of the fingers – onto the skin

surface over an area where the skin did not seem to glide as freely on underlying fascia as did surrounding skin. Test for the preferred directions of glide of the skin on the fascia. Take it superiorly and then inferiorly (Fig. 13.7).

Which was 'easier'? Which was the direction of tissue preference?

Ease the skin towards that direction and then test a different plane of movement – lateral and medial. Having established which way the skin travels most easily between these two directions, hold it there. You have now 'stacked' one position of ease onto another. Now, while holding the tissues in their combined ease position, test a third possibility. Does the tissue 'rotate' clockwise or anticlockwise more easily? Whichever it is, take it in that direction and hold for not less than 20 seconds. Release the held tissues and go back to the start and reevaluate.

Has anything changed? Almost certainly one or more of the directions which were previously restricted ('bound') will now test as being more normal, with a more symmetrical facility of gliding available of skin on fascia. You have positionally released the tissues, to an extent. A repeat of the whole exercise would give additional freedom of movement to these superficial tissues, with an influence on underlying structures as well. The mechanisms involved will be explained when we examine positional release phenomena later in this chapter. This is a superbly gentle approach to tissue normalisation and is ideal for FMS.

4. If instead of seeking the combined position of ease, as in the previous example, you had taken the tissues to their 'combined position of bind' (restriction) you would have identified a barrier which could be eased either by simply leaning against it (just as in the examples of holding skin at its elastic barrier or the 'C' and 'S' bends described above) or by introducing an isometric contraction for 5–7 seconds, following which the barrier would almost always retreat and the tissues would be more symmetrically relaxed.

Try this by identifying the tight directions as you glide the skin on fascia first in one plane, then while holding the tissues towards the restricted direction, another plane and finally a third plane. In this way you would move in precisely the opposite directions to those you would choose if you were performing the exercise above. Having found this 'bound' or 'restricted' barrier, ask the patient with a minimum of force to contract the tissues you are holding for 5–7 seconds. On releasing, retest and compare the release you have achieved using muscle energy technique (MET) in this way with that you achieved using directions of ease.

Whether you take tissues to a barrier and wait, or take them away from a barrier into an ease position and wait, or take them to the barrier and use isometric activity to induce a release, you will achieve a reduction in hypertonicity, enhancement of local circulation and some degree of neural resetting of resting muscle length. These possibilities will be referred to later in the treatment protocol segment of this chapter.

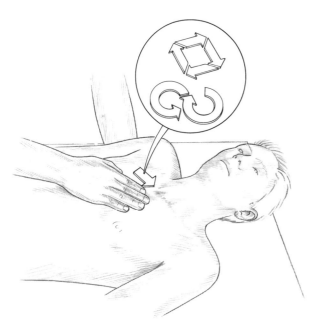

Figure 13.7 Release of traumatised fascial structures. In this figure, the operator's left hand lies between the patient's scapulae while the right hand lies on the sternum. The hands independently assess the 'tissue preference patterns' (Dickey 1989). These positions of ease are held in order to allow distorted fascial patterns to modify or normalise.

Patterns of dysfunction: 'crossed syndromes'

When a chain reaction evolves in which some muscles shorten and others weaken, predictable patterns involving imbalances develop: Czech researcher Vladimir Janda MD (1982) describes the so-called 'upper' and 'lower crossed' syndromes, as follows:

Upper crossed syndrome (Fig. 13.8)

This involves the following basic imbalance:

Pectoralis major and minor
Upper trapezius
Levator scapulae
Sternomastoid
} all tighten and shorten

while

Lower and middle trapezius
Serratus anterior and rhomboids
} all weaken

As these changes take place they alter the relative positions of the head, neck and shoulders as follows:

- The occiput and C1/2 will hyperextend, with the head being pushed forward.
- The lower cervical to fourth thoracic vertebrae will be posturally stressed as a result.
- Rotation and abduction of the scapulae occurs.
- An altered direction of the axis of the glenoid fossa will develop, resulting in the humerus needing to be stabilised by additional levator scapula and upper trapezius activity, with additional activity from supraspinatus as well.

The result of these changes is greater cervical segment strain plus referred pain to the chest, shoulders and arms. Pain mimicking angina may be noted plus a decline in respiratory efficiency.

The solution according to Janda (1982) is to be able to identify the shortened structures and to release (stretch and relax) them, followed by re-education towards more appropriate function.

Lower crossed syndrome (Fig. 13.1)

This involves the following basic imbalance:

Hip flexors
Iliopsoas, rectus femoris
TFL, short adductors
Erector spinae group of the trunk
} all tighten and shorten

while

Abdominal and gluteal muscles   all weaken

The result of this chain reaction is to tilt the pelvis forward on the frontal plane, flexing the hip joints and producing lumbar lordosis and stress in L5–S1 with pain and irritation (see Fig. 13.1).

A further stress commonly appears in the sagittal plane in which:

Quadratus lumborum   tightens
while
Gluteus maximus and medius   weakens

When this 'lateral corset' becomes unstable the pelvis is held in increased elevation, accentuated when walking, resulting in L5–S1 stress in the sagittal plane. One result is low back pain. The combined stresses described produce instability at the lumbodorsal junction, an unstable transition point at best. Also commonly involved are the piriformis muscles which in 20% of individuals are penetrated by the sciatic nerve so that piriformis syndrome can produce direct sciatic pressure and pain. Arterial involvement of piriformis shortness produces ischaemia of the lower extremity, and through a relative fixation of the sacrum, sacroiliac dysfunction and pain in the hip.

The solution for an all too common pattern such as this is to identify the shortened structures and to release them, ideally using variations on the theme of MET, followed by re-education of posture and use.

Hypertonicity: implications

In palpation/evaluation hypertonicity is a common finding. What does it actually represent? According to experts we need to consider a

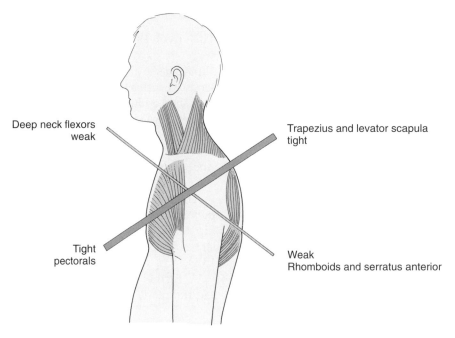

Deep neck flexors
weak

Trapezius and levator scapula
tight

Tight
pectorals

Weak
Rhomboids and serratus anterior

Figure 13.8 The upper crossed syndrome, as described by Janda (1982).

number of possibilities. Janda notes that the word 'spasm' is commonly used without attention to various functional causes of hypertonicity and he has divided this phenomenon into five variants (Janda 1989a):

1. Hypertonicity of limbic system origin which may be accompanied by evidence of stress, and be associated with, for example, tension-type headaches.

2. Hypertonicity of a segmental origin, involving interneuron influence. The muscle is likely to be spontaneously painful, and will probably be painful to stretch and will certainly have weak (inhibited) antagonists.

3. Hypertonicity due to uncoordinated muscle contraction resulting from myofascial trigger point activity. The muscle will be painful spontaneously if triggers are active. There may only be increased tone in part of the muscle which will be hyper-irritable while neighbouring areas of the same muscle may be inhibited.

4. Hypertonicity resulting from direct pain irritation, such as might occur in torticollis.

This muscle would be painful at rest, not only when palpated, and would demonstrate electromyographic evidence of increased activity even at rest. This could be described as reflex spasm due to nociceptive (pain receptor) influence.

5. Overuse hypertonicity results in muscles becoming increasingly irritable, with reduced range of motion, tightness and painful only on palpation.

Thus, increased tone of functional origin can result from pain sources, from trigger point activity, from higher centres or CNS influences and from overuse.

Liebenson (1990) suggests that each type of hypertonicity requires different therapeutic approaches, ranging from adjustment (joint manipulation) through use of soft tissue and rehabilitation and facilitation approaches. The many different MET variations described offer the opportunity to influence all stages of dysfunction – the acute, the chronic and everything in between.

Inappropriate breathing

Garland (1994) has described the somatic changes which follow from a pattern of upper chest breathing (which at its extreme becomes hyperventilation); these are summarised in Chapter 3. As we consider soft tissue dysfunction in this chapter, in particular its relationship with overuse and misuse, the outline given by Garland should be borne in mind (see also Fig. 3.3). The direct influence on the upper fixator muscles of the shoulders (accessory breathing muscles) and their influence on the cervical and cranial structures are of particular relevance to people with FMS.

Garland points to the likelihood of counselling (for associated anxiety or depression for example) and breathing retraining being far more likely to be successfully initiated if the structural component(s) are dealt with in such a way as to minimise the effects of the somatic changes described.

ASSESSMENT AND TREATMENT

Functional assessment

The following simple observation and palpation tests allow for a rapid gathering of information with a minimum of effort for the patient. They are based on the work of Dr Vladimir Janda (Janda 1983) and interpretations of these by Dr Craig Liebenson (Liebenson 1996).

Prone hip extension test (Fig. 13.9)

The patient lies prone and the operator stands at waist level with hands placed so that the cephalad one spans the lower erector spinae on both sides and the caudad hand rests with the thenar eminence on gluteus maximus and the fingertips on the hamstrings. The patient is asked to raise the leg into extension of the hip.

The normal activation sequence is gluteus maximus and hamstrings, followed by erector spinae (contralateral then ipsilateral). If the hamstrings and/or the erectors adopt the role of gluteus, as indicated by their firing first, they are working inappropriately, are therefore 'stressed' and will by implication have shortened (see discussion of postural and phasic muscles earlier in this chapter)

Trunk flexion test (Figs. 13.10A, 13.10B)

Patient lies supine, no pillow for the head, with arms folded across chest high on body. The oper-

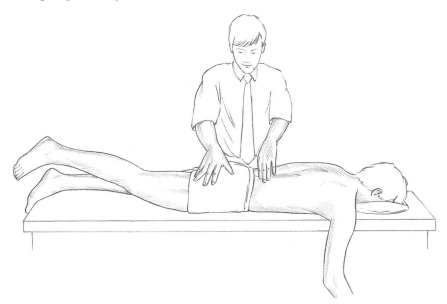

Figure 13.9 Hip extension test. The normal activation sequence is gluteus maximus and hamstrings, followed by erector spinae (contralateral then ipsilateral).

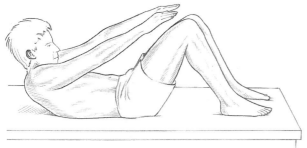

Figure 13.10 Trunk flexion test.
Figure 13.10A Normal – ability to raise trunk until scapulae are off table without feet lifting off or low back arching.

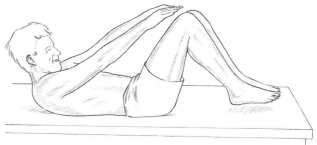

Figure 13.10B Abnormal – when feet rise up or low back arches before scapulae are raised from the table.

ator observes (no hands on) as the patient is asked to slowly raise the head, the shoulder and the shoulderblades from the table.

Normal. Ability to raise trunk until scapulae are off table without feet lifting off the table or low back arching.

Abnormal. When the feet rise up or low back arches before scapulae are raised from the table, indicating psoas overactivity and weak abdominals (lower crossed syndrome, see above).

Hip abduction test (Figs. 13.11A, 13.11B)

Patient lies on the side with lower leg flexed to provide support and the upper leg straight, in line with trunk. The operator stands in front of the patient at the level of the feet and observes (no hands on) as the patient is asked to abduct the leg slowly.

Normal. Hip abduction to 45°.

Abnormal. If hip flexion occurs (indicating TFL shortness), and/or leg externally rotates (indicating piriformis shortening) and/or 'hiking' of the hip occurs at the outset of the movement (indicating quadratus overactivity, and therefore, by implication, shortness).

The test can be repeated with the operator standing behind the patient at waist level, with a finger pad on the lateral margin of quadratus lumborum. As the leg is abducted, if quadratus fires strongly and first (before gluteus medius) this indicates overactivity and probable shortness of quadratus lumborum (this would show visually as a 'hip-hike' as mentioned in the first part of the test).

Scapulohumeral rhythm test (Figs. 13.12A, 13.12B)

This is an important assessment which can give information as to the status of some of the most important upper fixators of the shoulder.

The patient is seated with arm at the side, elbow flexed and facing forwards. The operator stands behind and observes as the patient is asked to raise the elbow towards the horizontal.

Normal. Elevation of shoulder after 60° of arm abduction.

Abnormal. If elevation of the shoulder, or obvious 'bunching' occurs between shoulder and neck, or winging of the scapulae occurs within the first 60° of shoulder abduction (indicating levator scapulae and upper trapezius tightness, and lower and middle trapezius, as well as serratus anterior weakness).

This pattern, of weak lower fixators and overworked and probably shortened upper fixators is characteristic of the upper crossed syndrome (see above) and is commonly associated with respiratory dysfunction.

Neck flexion test (Figs. 13.13A, 13.13B)

The patient lies supine without a pillow. Operator kneels to one side at level of the patient's chin and asks the patient to 'lift your head and put your chin on your chest'.

Normal. Ability to hold chin tucked while flexing the head/neck.

Abnormal. If the chin pokes forwards while attempting head flexion (indicating sternocleido-

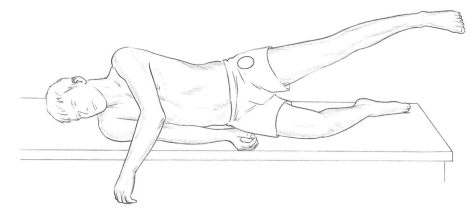

Figure 13.11A Normal – hip abduction to 45°.

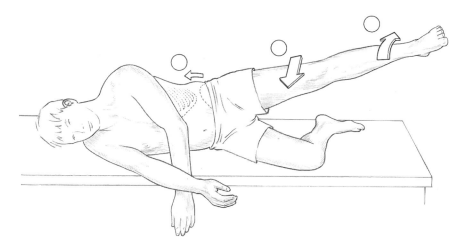

Figure 13.11B Abnormal – if hip flexion, external rotation or 'hiking' occurs, or pelvic rotation takes place during hip abduction.

mastoid and scalenes tightness and weakness of the deep neck flexors – also part of the upper crossed syndrome and characteristic of postural distress, and often of breathing dysfunction).

There are many methods for gathering information by palpation and introduction of specific testing movements and activities. The skin palpation methods listed above and the functional assessments developed by Janda, however, offer very easily applied, non-invasive and non-stressful methods suitable for use in conditions such as FMS. Neuromuscular technique, in its assessment mode (below), offers another choice.

NEUROMUSCULAR TECHNIQUE
(Chaitow 1996a)

In Europe, neuromuscular technique (NMT) refers to a method of assessment and treatment developed in the 1930s by Stanley Lief DC DO, and its evolution since that time. In the USA, the method known as neuromuscular therapy (also NMT) refers to the method first promoted in the 1950s by Raymond Nimmo DC in treating myofascial dysfunction (trigger points) (Nimmo 1969). In recent years the European and American versions of NMT have acquired elements of each others methodologies.

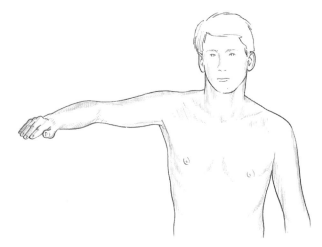

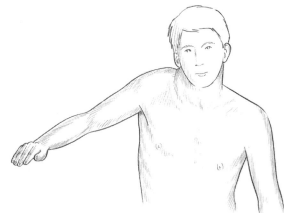

Figure 13.12 Scapulohumeral rhythm test.
Figure 13.12A Normal – elevation of shoulder after 60° of arm abduction.

Figure 13.12B Abnormal – if elevation of the shoulder or winging of the scapulae occurs within the first 60° of shoulder abduction.

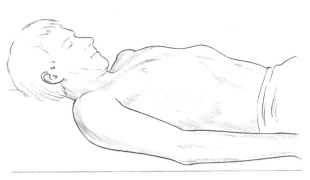

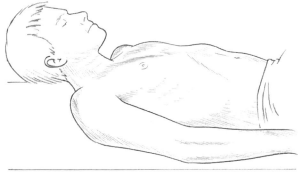

Figure 13.13 Neck flexion test.
Figure 13.13A Normal – ability to hold chin tucked while flexing the head/neck.

Figure 13.13B Abnormal – if the chin pokes forwards while attempting head flexion.

NMT aims to produce modifications in dysfunctional tissue, encouraging a restoration of normality, with a primary focus of deactivating focal points of reflexogenic activity such as myofascial trigger points. An alternative focus of NMT application is towards normalising imbalances in hypertonic and/or fibrotic tissues either as an end in itself or as a precursor to rehabilitation. The technique utilises physiological responses involving neurological mechanoreceptors, golgi tendon organs, muscle spindles and other proprioceptors, in order to achieve the desired responses.

Insofar as they integrate with NMT, other means of influencing such neural reporting stations, including positional release (SCS – strain/counterstrain, see below) and muscle energy methods (MET – such as reciprocal inhibition and postisometric relaxation induction, see below) form a natural set of allied approaches. Traditional massage methods which encourage a reduction in the retention of metabolic wastes and which enhance circulation to dysfunctional tissues are also included in this category of allied approaches.

NMT can usefully be integrated in treatment aimed at postural reintegration, tension release, pain relief, improvement of joint mobility, reflex stimulation/modulation or sedation. There are many variations of the basic technique as developed by Lief, the choice of which will depend upon particular presenting factors or personal preference. Similarities between some aspects of NMT and other manual systems should be anticipated since techniques have been 'borrowed' from other systems where appropriate.

NMT can be applied generally or locally and in a variety of positions (sitting, lying, etc.). The order in which body areas are dealt with is not regarded as critical in general treatment but is of some consequence in postural reintegration. The methods described are in essence those of Stanley Lief and Boris Chaitow (personal communication 1983), both of whom achieved a degree of skill in the application of NMT that is unsurpassed. The inclusion of data on reflex areas and effects, together with basic NMT methods, provides the operator with a useful therapeutic tool, the limitations of which will be largely determined by the degree of intelligence and understanding with which it is employed.

In the description of NMT below only selected regions of particular importance in FMS will be utilised as examples.

NMT thumb technique (Fig. 13.14)

Thumb technique as employed in NMT in either assessment or treatment modes enables a wide variety of therapeutic effects to be produced. The tip of the thumb can deliver varying degrees of pressure via any of four facets, the very tip may be employed, or the medial or lateral aspect of the tip can be used to make contact with angled surfaces. For more general (less localised and less specific) contact, of a diagnostic or therapeutic type, the broad surface of the distal phalange of the thumb is often used. It is usual for a light, non-oily lubricant to be used to facilitate easy, non-dragging, passage of the palpating digit.

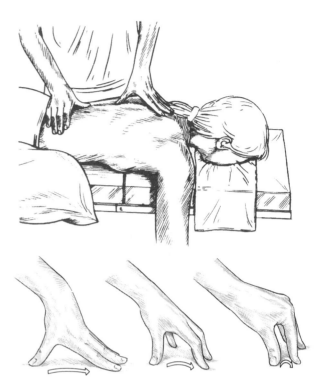

Figure 13.14 NMT thumb technique.

For balance and control the hand should be spread, tips of fingers providing a fulcrum or 'bridge' in which the palm is arched in order to allow free passage of the thumb towards one of the fingertips as the thumb moves in a direction which takes it away from the operator's body. During a single stroke, which covers between 2 and 3 inches (5–8 cm), the fingertips act as a point of balance, while the chief force is imparted to the thumb tip via controlled application of body weight through the long axis of the extended arm.

The thumb therefore never leads the hand but always trails behind the stable fingers, the tips of which rest just beyond the end of the stroke. Unlike many bodywork/massage strokes, the hand and arm remain still as the thumb, applying variable pressure, moves through its pathway of tissue.

The extreme versatility of the thumb enables it to modify the direction of imparted force in accordance with the indications of the tissue being tested/treated. As the thumb glides across and through those tissues it becomes an extension of the operator's brain. In fact, for the clearest assessment of what is being palpated the operator should have the eyes closed in order that every minute change in the tissue can be felt and reacted to. The thumb and hand seldom impart their own muscular force except in dealing with small localised contractures or fibrotic nodules.

In order that pressure/force be transmitted directly to its target, the weight being imparted should travel in as straight a line as possible which is why the arm should not be flexed at the elbow or the wrist by more than a few degrees.

The positioning of the operator's body in relation to the area being treated is also of the utmost importance in order to facilitate economy of effort and comfort. (Fig. 13.15)

The optimum height vis-à-vis the couch and the most effective angle of approach to the body areas being addressed must be considered; the descriptions and illustrations will help to make this clearer.

The degree of pressure imparted will depend upon the nature of the tissue resistance being met during the application of thumb strokes across and through the tissues. The usual degree of pressure is sufficient to 'meet the tissue' precisely, taking out available slack, without any invasive degree of force. When being treated, the patient should not feel strong pain but a general degree of discomfort is usually acceptable as the seldom stationary thumb varies its penetration of dysfunctional tissues. A stroke or glide of 2–3 inches (5–8 cm) will usually take 4–5 seconds, seldom more unless a particularly obstructive indurated area is being dealt with.

If reflex pressure techniques or ischaemic compression are being employed (only with extreme caution in cases of FMS because of sensitivity), a much longer stay on a point will be needed, but in normal diagnostic and therapeutic use the thumb continues to move as it intelligently probes, decongests and generally treats the tissues.

It is not possible to state the exact pressures necessary in NMT application because of the very nature of the objective, which in assessment

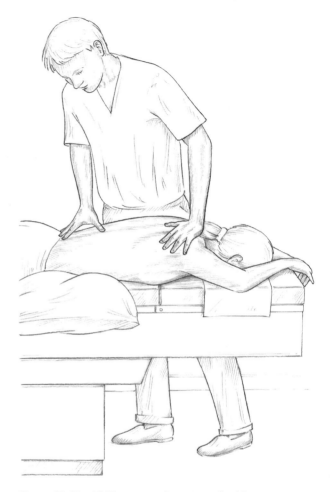

Figure 13.15 NMT – operator's posture should ensure a straight treating arm for ease of transmission of body weight, as well as leg positions which allow for the easy transfer of weight and the centre of gravity. These postures assist in reducing energy expenditure and ease spinal stress.

mode attempts to precisely meet and match the tissue resistance, to vary pressure constantly in response to what is being felt. In effect this means that the firmer and more tense the tissues, the lighter the pressure, since the degree of 'slack' will be minimal. Conversely, the more relaxed and 'soft' the tissues, the greater the penetration possible as slack is taken out.

In subsequent or synchronous (with assessment) treatment of whatever is uncovered during the evaluation stage of NMT application, a greater degree of pressure is used and this will vary depending upon the objective – whether this is to inhibit, to produce localised stretching, to decongest and so on. Obviously on areas with relatively thin muscular covering the applied pressure would be lighter than in tense or thick, well-covered areas such as the buttocks.

Attention should always be paid to the relative sensitivity of different areas and different patients. The thumb should not just mechanically stroke across or through tissue but should become an intelligent extension of the operator's diagnostic sensitivities so that the contact feels to the patient as though it is sequentially assessing every important nook and cranny of the soft tissues. Pain should be transient and no bruising should result if the above advice is followed.

The treating arm and thumb should be relatively straight since a 'hooked' thumb in which all the work is done by the distal phalange will become extremely tired and will not achieve the degree of penetration possible via a fairly rigid thumb.

Hypermobile thumbs

Some operators have hypermobile joints and it is difficult for them to maintain sustained pressure without the thumb giving way and bending back on itself. This is a problem which can only be overcome by attempting to build up the muscular strength of the hand or by using a variation of the above technique (e.g. a knuckle or even the elbow may be used to achieve deep pressure in very tense musculature). Alternatively, the finger stroke as described below can take over from a hypermobile thumb.

NMT finger technique (Fig. 13.16)

In certain localities the thumb's width prevents the degree of tissue penetration suitable for successful assessment and/or treatment and the middle or index finger can usually be suitably employed in such regions. The most usual area for use of finger rather than thumb contact is in the intercostal musculature and in attempting to penetrate beneath the scapula borders in tense fibrotic conditions.

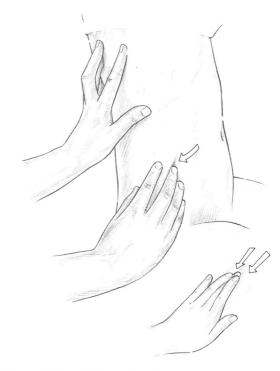

Figure 13.16 NMT finger technique.

The middle or index finger should be slightly flexed and, depending upon the direction of the stroke and density of the tissues, supported by one of its adjacent members.

As the treating finger strokes with a firm contact and usually a minimum of lubricant, a tensile strain is created between its tip and the tissue underlying it. This is stretched and lifted by the passage of the finger which, like the thumb, should continue moving unless or until dense, indurated tissue prevents its easy passage. These strokes can be repeated once or twice as tissue changes dictate.

The ideal angle of pressure to the skin surface is between 40° and 50° (Fig. 13.6).

The fingertip should never lead the stroke but should always follow the wrist, the palmar surface of which should lead as the hand is drawn towards the operator. It is possible to impart a great degree of pull on underlying tissues and the patient's reactions must be taken into account in deciding on the degree of force to be used.

Transient pain or mild discomfort are to be expected but no more than that. All sensitive areas are indicative of some degree of dysfunction, local or reflex, and are thus important and their presence should be recorded. The patient should be told what to expect so that a cooperative unworried attitude evolves.

Unlike the thumb technique, in which force is largely directed away from the operator's body, in finger treatment the motive force is usually towards the operator. The arm position therefore alters and a degree of flexion is necessary to ensure that the pull or drag of the finger across the lightly lubricated tissues is smooth.

Unlike the thumb, which makes a sweep towards the fingertips whilst the rest of the hand remains relatively stationary, the whole hand will move as finger pressure is applied. Certainly some variation in the degree of angle between fingertip and skin is allowable during a stroke and some slight variation in the degree of 'hooking' of the finger is sometimes also necessary. However, the main motive force is applied by pulling the slightly flexed middle or index finger towards the operator with the possibility of some lateral emphasis if needed. The treating finger should always be supported by one of its neighbours.

Application of NMT

It should be clear to the operator that underlying tissues being treated should be visualised and, depending upon the presenting symptoms and the area involved, any of a number of procedures may be undertaken as the hand moves from one site to another.

There may be superficial stroking in the direction of lymphatic flow, or direct pressure along the line of axis of stress fibres, or deeper alternating 'make and break' stretching and pressure or traction on fascial tissue. As variable pressure is being applied, the operator needs to be constantly aware of diagnostic information which is being received via the contact hands and this is what determines the variations in pressure and the direction of force being applied.

Any changes in direction or degree of applied pressure should ideally take place without any sudden release or application of force which could irritate the tissues and produce pain or a defensive contraction.

Lief's basic spinal treatment followed the pattern of which examples will be illustrated and described below. The fact that the same pattern is followed at each treatment does not mean that the treatment is necessarily the same. The pattern gives a framework and a useful starting and ending point, but the degree of emphasis applied to the various areas of dysfunction that manifest themselves is a variable factor based always on what information the palpating hands are picking up. This is what makes each treatment different.

Areas of dysfunction should be recorded on a case card together with all relevant material and diagnostic findings relating to myofascial tissue changes, trigger points and reference zones, areas of sensitivity, restricted motion and so on.

Lief's basic spinal treatment

Lief's basic spinal NMT treatment follows a pattern of placing the patient prone with a medium thickness pillow under the abdomen to prevent undue arching of the lumbodorsal area, forehead ideally resting in a split headpiece or face-hole. The whole spine from occiput to sacrum, including the gluteal area, is lightly oiled or creamed.

A series of different regions are sequentially assessed and/or treated using NMT (and combinations of other methods which integrate into the requirements of the situation demanded by the information gleaned from the assessment). In many instances a full assessment is given without treatment interrupting the flow of the sequence, from neck to mid-thigh, taking approximately 20 minutes and yielding a great deal of information.

Whichever hand is operating at any given time, the other hand can give assistance by means of gently rocking or stretching tissues to complement the efforts of the assessing/treating hand, or it can be useful in distracting tissues which are 'mounding' as the working hand addresses them.

Whenever the operator changes to the other side of the table it is suggested that one hand always maintains light contact with the patient. Indeed it is suggested that once treatment has commenced no breaks in contact be allowed. There is often a noticeable increase in tension in the tissues of the patient if the series of strokes, stretching movements and pressure techniques, etc. which make up NMT is interrupted by even a few seconds, because of a break in contact. Continuity would seem, in itself, to be of therapeutic value, simply as a reassuring and calming feature.

What the treating thumb feels

The movement of the thumb through the tissue should be slow, not uniformly slow but deliberately seeking and feeling for 'contractions' and 'congestions' (to use two words which will be meaningful to any manual therapist). If and when such localised areas are felt, the degree of pressure can be increased and applied in a variable manner.

Variable pressure can relatively painlessly carry the thumb tip across or through restricted tissue, decongesting, stretching and easing. The patient will often report a degree of pain but may say that it 'feels good'. It is a contradiction in terms, but constructive pain is usually felt as a 'nice hurt'.

Practitioner's posture

The treating arm should not be flexed, since the optimum transmission of weight from the operator's shoulder through the arm to the thumb tip is best achieved with a relatively straight arm. This demands that the practitioner ensures table height is suitable. The operator should not be forced to stand on tip-toe to treat patients, nor to adopt an unhealthy bent posture.

The operator's weight should be evenly spread between the separated feet, both of which are forward facing at this stage. In this way the operator, by slightly altering his or her own weight distribution from the front to the back foot and vice versa, can exert an accurate, controlled degree of pressure with minimum arm or hand effort.

Weight transfer: key to economy of effort

The hand itself should not be rigid but in a relaxed state, moulding itself to the contours of the neck or back tissues. To some extent the fingertips stabilise the hand. The thumb's glide is stabilised in this way so that the actual stroke is achieved by the tip of the extended thumb being brought slowly across the palm towards the fingertips. The fingers maintain their position as the thumb performs its diagnostic/therapeutic glide (the illustrations will aid in better understanding of this description). Were all the effort to be on the part of the thumb it would soon tire.

What is working when the thumb applies NMT?

Consider which parts of the operator's body/arm/hand will be involved with the various aspects of the glide/stroke as delivered by the thumb (finger strokes involve completely different mechanics):

- The transverse movement of the thumb is a hand or forearm effort
- The relative straightness or rigidity of the thumb is also a local muscular responsibility
- The vast majority of the energy imparted via the thumb results from transmission of body weight through the straight arm into the thumb
- Any increase in pressure can be speedily achieved by simple weight transfer from back towards front foot and a slight 'lean' onto the thumb from the shoulders
- A lessening of imparted pressure is achieved by reversing this body movement.

Origins and insertions

During NMT treatment special notice should be given to the origins and insertions of the muscles of the area. Wherever these bony landmarks are palpable by the thumb tip they should be treated by the slow, variably applied pressure technique.

All bony surfaces within reach of the probing digit should be searched for undue sensitivity and dysfunction of their attachments, which are amongst the commonest sites of trigger points according to Travell.

NMT application to cervical region using Lief's method (Figs. 13.17A,B).

The area to be treated should be lightly oiled or creamed. The operator should begin by standing half-facing the head of the couch on the left of the patient with his/her hips level with the midthoracic area.

The first contact to the left side of the patient's head is a gliding, light-pressured movement of the medial tip of the right thumb, from the mastoid process along the nuchal line to the external occipital protuberance. This same stroke, or glide, is then repeated with deeper pressure. The operator's left hand rests on the upper thoracic or shoulder area as a stabilising contact.

The treating/assessing hand should be relaxed, moulding itself to the contours of tissues. The fingertips stabilise the hand.

After the first two strokes of the right thumb – one shallow and diagnostic, the second, deeper, imparting therapeutic effort – the next stroke is half a thumb-width caudal to the first. A degree of overlap occurs as these strokes, starting on the belly of the sternocleidomastoid, glide across and through the trapezius, splenius capitus and posterior cervical muscles. A progressive series of strokes is applied in this way until the level of the cervicodorsal junction is reached. Unless serious underlying dysfunction is found it is seldom necessary to repeat the two superimposed strokes at each level of the cervical region. If underlying fibrotic tissue appears unyielding a third or fourth slow, deep glide may be necessary.

For appropriate attention to trigger points found during the assessment, see below (p. 234).

NMT assessment continues

A series of strokes should be applied by the left thumb, upward from the left of the upper dorsal area towards the base of the skull.

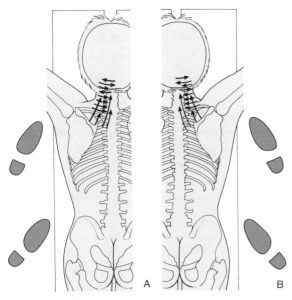

Figure 13.17A,B First two positions of suggested sequence of applications of NMT, to ensure optimal thumb and/or finger contact with primary trigger point sites and with the origins and insertions of most muscles. Note foot positions.

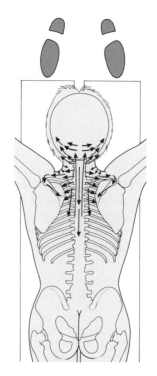

Figure 13.18 Third position of suggested sequence of application of NMT.

The fingers of the left hand rest (and act as a fulcrum) on the front of the shoulder area at the level of the medial aspect of the clavicle. The treating thumb tip should be angled to allow direct pressure to be exerted against the left lateral aspects of the upper dorsal and the lower cervical spinous processes as it glides cephalad.

Subsequent strokes should be in the same direction but slightly more laterally placed. The fingers should then be placed on the patient's head at about the temporooccipital articulation. The left thumb deals in the same way with the mid and upper cervical soft tissues, finishing with a lateral stroke or two across the insertions on the occiput itself.

In this way common sites of a number of possible trigger points will have been evaluated. Following the treatment of the left side of the cervical area, the same procedures are repeated on the right.

The next position (Fig. 13.18)

Once both left and right cervical areas have been treated the operator moves to the head of the table. Resting the tips of the fingers on the lower, lateral aspect of the neck, the thumb tips are placed just lateral to the first dorsal–spinal process.

A degree of downward pressure is applied via the thumbs which are drawn cephalad along the lateral margins of the cervical spinous processes, culminating at the occiput where a bilateral stretch or pull is introduced laterally across the fibres of the muscles inserting into the base of the skull. The upward stroke directs pressure medially towards the spinous process so that the pad of the thumb is pressing downward (towards the

floor) whilst the lateral thumb tip is directed towards the centre, attempting to contact the bony contours of the spine, all the time being drawn slowly cephalad towards the occiput.

The thumbs are then drawn laterally across the fibres of muscular insertion into the skull, in a series of strokes culminating at the occipitoparietal junction. Several strokes are then performed by one thumb or the other running caudad directly over the spinous process from the base of the skull towards the upper dorsal area.

Pressure should be moderate and movement deliberate. From the same position, the left thumb is placed on the right lateral aspect of the first dorsal vertebra and a series of strokes are performed caudad and laterally as well as diagonally towards the scapula.

A series of strokes, shallow and then deep, is applied caudad from D1 to about D4 or 5 and laterally towards the scapula and along and across the upper trapezius fibres and the rhomboids. The left hand treats the right side, and vice versa with the nonoperative hand stabilising the neck or head.

By moving to one side it is possible to apply a series of sensitively searching contacts into the area of the thoracic outlet. Strokes which start in this triangular depression move towards the trapezius fibres and through them towards the upper margins of the scapula.

Several strokes should also be applied directly over the spinous processes, caudad, towards the mid-dorsal area. Triggers sometimes lie on the attachments to the spinous processes or between them. (Figs. 13.19A, 13.19B, 13.20A, 13.20B, 13.21A, 13.21B)

Figure 13.19–13.21. These treatment 'maps' are not described in the text but offer an indication of the comprehensive evaluation pattern followed in NMT as areas of local dysfunction are assessed.

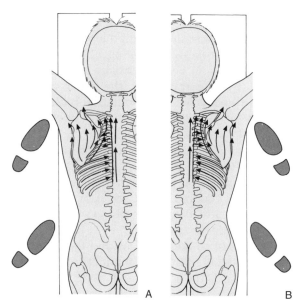

Figure 13.19A, B Fourth (A) and fifth (B) positions of suggested sequence of applications of NMT.

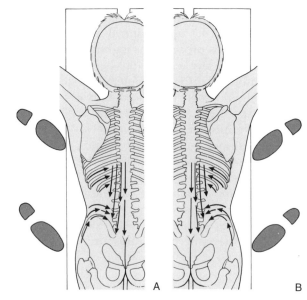

Figure 13.20A, B Sixth position of suggested sequence of applications of NMT.

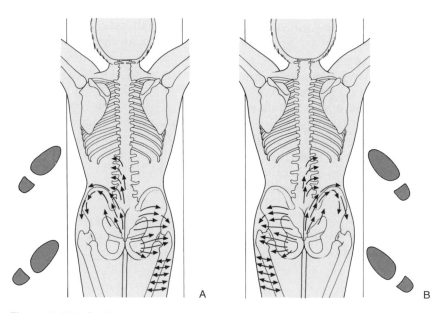

Figure 13.21 A, B Seventh positions of suggested sequence of applications of NMT.

MUSCLE ENERGY TECHNIQUES

Evjenth succinctly summarises when tissues can benefit from MET (Evjenth & Hamberg 1984): 'Every patient with symptoms involving the locomotor system, particularly symptoms of pain and/or constrained movement, should be examined to assess joint and muscle function. If examination shows joint play to be normal, but reveals shortened muscles or muscle spasm, then treatment by stretching [and by implication MET] is indicated' (Evjenth & Hamberg 1984).

Summary of variations (Greenman 1989, DiGiovanna 1991, Travell & Simons 1992, Liebenson 1990, Mitchell 1967, Janda 1989b, Lewit 1986)

There are many variations on the use of muscle energy technique; however, only two will be detailed here as being most appropriate for use in FMS.

1. Isometric contraction: using reciprocal inhibition (Fig. 13.22)

Indications
- Relaxing muscular spasm or contraction or preparing for stretch
- Mobilising restricted joints
- Preparing joint for manipulation.

Contraction starting point
- At barrier for acute problem or for individuals with acute FMS
- Short of restriction barrier, mid-range for chronic problem.

Modus operandi The affected muscle(s) is not employed and therefore this approach is more acceptable in cases where muscular activity produces pain. The antagonists are used in an isometric contraction, obliging shortened muscles (agonists) to relax via reciprocal inhibition. The patient is attempting to push through the barrier of restriction against the operator's precisely-matched counterforce.

Forces Operator's and patient's forces are matched. Initial effort involves approximately 20% of patient's strength; an increase to no more

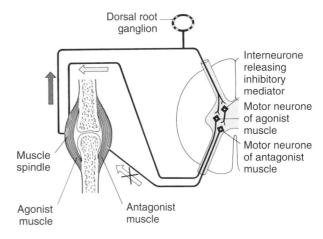

Figure 13.22 Schematic representation of the reciprocal effect of an isometric contraction of a skeletal muscle, resulting in an inhibitory influence on its antagonist.

than 50% on subsequent contractions is appropriate if no pain is felt during the contraction. Increase of the duration of the contraction – up to 20 seconds – is more effective than an increase in force.

Duration of contraction 7–10 seconds initially, increasing to up to 20 seconds in subsequent contractions, if greater effect (recruitment of more fibres) is required.

Action following contraction
- In acute conditions (FMS, recent trauma, etc.) the area (muscle/joint) is taken to its new restriction barrier without stretch, after ensuring complete relaxation.
- In chronic conditions, on an exhalation, the muscle is taken through the barrier (muscle only, never joints) with the patient's assistance. Stretch is held in chronic states for 10–30 seconds.
- Movement to or through the barrier should be performed on an exhalation.

Repetitions 3–5 times or until no further gain in range of motion is possible.

2. Isometric contraction: using postisometric relaxation (Fig. 13.23)

Indications
- Relaxing muscular spasm or contraction or preparing for stretch

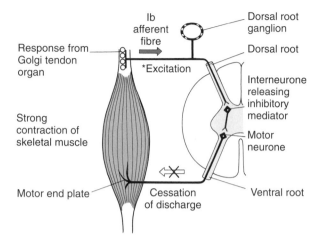

Figure 13.23 Schematic representation of the neurological effects of the loading of the Golgi tendon organs of a skeletal muscle by means of an isometric contraction, which produces a postisometric relaxation effect in that muscle.

- Mobilising restricted joints
- Preparing joint for manipulation.

Contraction starting point
- At the restriction barrier for acute problems
- Short of the restriction barrier, mid-range, for chronic problem.

Modus operandi Affected muscles (agonists) are used in the isometric contraction, therefore the shortened muscles subsequently relax via postisometric relaxation. Operator is attempting to push through the barrier of restriction against the patient's precisely-matched counter effort.

Forces Operator's and patient's forces are matched. Initial effort involves approximately 20% of the patient's strength; an increase to no more than 50% on subsequent contractions is appropriate. Increase of the duration of the contraction – up to 20 seconds – may be more effective (in recruiting more fibres) than an increase in force.

Duration of contraction 7–10 seconds initially, increasing to up to 20 seconds in subsequent contractions, if greater effect (more recruitment) is required.

Action following contraction
- In acute settings (FMS, recent trauma, etc.) the area (muscle/joint) is taken to its new restriction barrier without stretch, after ensuring complete relaxation.

- In chronic settings the muscle is taken through the restriction barrier (muscle only, never joints) with the patient's assistance. Stretch is held in chronic for 10–30 seconds.
- Movement to or through the barrier should be performed on an exhalation.

Repetitions 3–5 times or until no further gain in range of motion is possible.

Important notes on assessments and use of MET

When the term 'restriction barrier' is used in relation to soft tissue structures it is meant to indicate the first signs of resistance (as palpated by sense of 'bind', or sense of effort required to move the area, or by visual or other palpable evidence) not the greatest possible range of movement obtainable.

In all treatment descriptions involving MET it will be assumed that the 'shorthand' reference to 'acute' and 'chronic' will be adequate to alert you to the variations in methodology which these variants call for, especially in terms of the starting position for contractions (acute starts at the barrier, chronic short of the barrier) and the need to take the area to (acute) or through (chronic) the resistance barrier subsequent to the contraction.

CAUTION: In treating fibromyalgia patients with MET the 'acute' mode is always adopted – i.e. no stretching!

Assistance from the patient is valuable as movement is made to or through a barrier, providing the patient can be educated to gentle cooperation and not to use excessive effort.

In most MET treatment guidelines the method described will involve isometric contraction of the agonist(s), the muscle(s) which require stretching. It is assumed that you are now familiar with the possibility of using the antagonists to achieve reciprocal inhibition (RI) before initiating stretch or movement to a new barrier and will use this alternative when appropriate (pain on use of agonist; prior trauma to agonist).

There should be no pain experienced during application of MET although mild discomfort (stretching) is acceptable.

The methods of assessment and treatment of postural muscles, as described, are far from comprehensive or definitive. There are many other assessment approaches, and numerous treatment/stretch approaches using variations on the theme of MET, as evidenced by excellent texts by, among others, Janda, Basmajian, Lewit, Liebenson, Greenman, Grieve, Hartman, Evjenth and Dvorak (see also References list).

Breathing

Breathing cooperation can and should be used as part of the methodology of MET. Basically, if appropriate (the patient is cooperative and capable of following instructions) the patient should inhale as they slowly build up an isometric contraction, hold the breath for the 7–10 second contraction, and release the breath on slowly ceasing the contraction. They should be asked to inhale and exhale fully once more following cessation of all effort as they are instructed to 'let go completely'; during this last exhalation the new barrier is engaged or the barrier is passed as the muscle is stretched (a note 'use appropriate breathing', or some variation on it, will be found in the text describing various MET applications).

Eye movements

Various eye movements are sometimes advocated during contractions and stretches, particularly by Lewit who uses these methods to great effect. The only specific recommendations will be found in regard to muscles such as the scalenes and sternomastoid, where their use is particularly valuable in terms of the gentleness of the contractions they induce (Lewit 1992).

Pulsed muscle energy technique

Pulsed muscle energy technique is based on Ruddy's work and can be substituted for any of the methods described in the text below for treating shortened soft tissue structures, or increasing range of motion in joints (Ruddy 1962). This will be described below.

Co-contraction

There are times when 'co-contraction' is useful, involving contraction of both the agonist and the antagonist. Studies have shown that this approach is particularly useful in treatment of the hamstrings, when both these and the quadriceps are isometrically contracted prior to stretch (Moore et al 1980).

It is seldom necessary to treat all shortened muscles which are identified. For example Lewit and Simons mention that isometric relaxation of the suboccipital muscles will also relax the sternocleidomastoid muscles; treatment of the thoracolumbar muscles induces relaxation of iliopsoas, and vice versa; treatment (MET) of the sternocleidomastoid and scalene muscles relaxes the pectorals. These interactions are worthy of greater study.

A comprehensive outline of all postural muscle assessments and treatments is not within the scope of this text, however, *Muscle Energy Techniques* (Chaitow 1996b) will offer a full range of treatment suggestions for all postural muscles. The assessment and MET treatment guidelines below involve the following selected muscles only:

- Upper trapezius
- Levator scapulae
- Scalenes and sternomastoid
- General suboccipital muscle group.

Assessment for shortness of upper trapezius

Test (a) Lewit simplifies the need to assess for shortness by stating: 'The upper trapezius should be treated if tender and taut'. Since this is an almost universal state in modern life it seems that everyone requires MET application to this muscle. He also notes that a characteristic mounding of the muscle can often be observed when it is very short, producing the effect of 'Gothic shoulders', similar to the architectural supports of a Gothic church tower.

Test (b) Patient is seated and operator stands behind, one hand resting on shoulder of side to be tested. The other hand is placed on the side of the head which is being tested and the

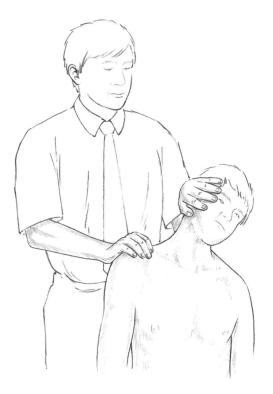

Figure 13.24 Assessment of the relative shortness of the right side upper trapezius. One side is compared with the other (for both the range of unforced motion and the nature of the end-feel of motion) to ascertain the side most in need of MET attention.

head/neck is taken into sidebending away from that side without force whilst the shoulder is stabilised. The same procedure is performed on the other side with the opposite shoulder stabilised.

A comparison is made as to which sidebending manoeuvre produced the greater range and whether the neck can easily reach a 45° angle from the vertical, which it should. If neither side can achieve this degree of sidebend then both trapezius muscles may be short. The relative shortness of one, compared with the other, is evaluated (Fig. 13.24)

Test (c) The patient is seated and the operator stands behind with a hand resting on the shoulder on the side to be assessed. The patient is asked to extend the shoulder, bringing the flexed arm/elbow backwards. If the upper trapezius is very stressed/short on that side it will inappro-

priately activate during this arm movement, and may be assumed to be short.

Test (d) The 'scapulohumeral rhythm test' as described above in the segment covering functional evaluation gives an indication of upper trapezius overactivity (as well as levator scapula) (see Figs. 13.12A and B).

MET treatment of shortened upper trapezius

Method (a) The patient lies supine, head/neck sidebent away from the side to be treated, to or short of the restriction barrier (acute or chronic as appropriate) with the operator stabilising the shoulder with one hand and cupping the ear/mastoid area of the same side of the head with the other.

In order to bring into play all the various fibres of the muscle this stretch needs to be applied with the neck in three different positions of rotation, coupled with the sidebending as described.

- With the neck sidebent and fully rotated the posterior fibres of upper trapezius are involved in any contraction.
- With the neck fully sidebent and half rotated the middle fibres are accessed.
- With the neck fully sidebent and slightly rotated back to the side from which it is sidebent the anterior fibres are being treated (Fig. 13.25).

This manoeuvre can be performed with operator's arms crossed, hands stabilising the mastoid area and shoulder, or not as comfort dictates, and with operator standing at the head or the side, also as comfort dictates.

The patient introduces a resisted effort to take the stabilised shoulder towards the ear (a shrug movement) and the ear towards the shoulder. The double movement (or effort towards movement) is important in order to introduce a contraction of the muscle from both ends. The degree of effort should be mild and no pain should be felt.

After the 10 second (or so) of contraction and complete relaxation of effort the operator gently eases the head/neck into an increased degree of sidebending (back to the barrier if this has been

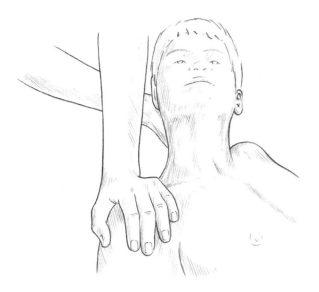

Figure 13.25 MET treatment of right side upper trapezius muscle. The head is in the upright position, with no rotation, in this example, which indicates that the anterior fibres are being treated. Note that stretching in this (or any of the alternative positions which access the middle and posteriour fibres) is achieved following the isometric contraction by means of an easing of the shoulder away from the stabilised head, with no force being applied to the neck and head itself.

reduced before the contraction in a chronic setting, or to the new barrier if it was an acute problem being treated from the resistance barrier) before stretching the shoulder away from the ear whilst stabilising the head, to or through the new barrier of resistance as appropriate. No stretch is introduced from the head end of the muscle as this could stress the neck unduly.

Method (b) Lewit suggests the use of eye movements to facilitate initiation of postisometric relaxation before stretching, an ideal method for acute problems in this region. The patient is supine, while the operator fixes the shoulder and the sidebent (away from the treated side) head and neck at the restriction barrier and asks the patient to look, with the eyes only (i.e. not to turn the head) towards the side away from which the neck is bent. This eye movement is maintained, as is a held breath, while the operator resists the slight isometric contraction that these two factors (eye movement and breath) will have created. On exhalation and complete relaxation the head/neck is taken to a new barrier and the

process repeated. If the shoulder is brought into the equation this is firmly held as it attempts to lightly push into a shrug. After a 10 second push of this sort the muscle will have released somewhat and slack can again be taken out as the head is repositioned, before a repetition of the procedure commences (Lewit 1992).

Levator scapula influences and treatment

Levator scapula, because of its profound influence on the cervical spine (attaching to TPs C1 to C4), is seen to have the potential for disrupting the mechanics of the area. The stretch which is suggested below will influence many of the smaller posterior neck muscles which attach to the cranium.

Assessment and MET treatment for levator scapulae

The assessment position described below is used for treatment, either at the limit of easily reached range of motion, or well short of this, depending upon the degree of chronicity, which will also determine the degree of effort called for (20–30%) and the duration of each contraction (usually 7–10 seconds). Assessment is via the scapulohumeral rhythm test used to assess upper trapezius (see above, Figs. 13.12A and B).

The patient lies supine with the arm of the side to be tested stretched out with the hand and lower arm tucked under the buttocks, palm upwards, to help restrain movement of the shoulder/scapula.

The operator's arm is passed across and beneath the neck to rest on the shoulder of the side to be treated with the forearm supporting the neck. The hand on the shoulder maintains a degree of pressure to prevent the scapula from elevating. The operator's other hand supports the head.

With the forearm, the neck is lifted into full flexion (aided by the other hand) and is turned fully towards sidebending and rotation away from the side to be treated. With the shoulder held caudad by one hand and the head/neck in the position described, levator is held at its elastic barrier.

A gentle springing of the shoulder, caudad, should produce a degree of easy motion. If this is absent, and the 'springing' feels hard or wooden, this confirms that the muscle has shortened (Fig. 13.26).

An isometric contraction may be introduced at this stage (patient is asked to gently 'shrug shoulder' and to take the head and neck 'back to the table' against sustained resistance for 7 seconds). Following this the muscle is taken to its new resting length by means of a slight increase in the flexion, sidebending and rotation of the head/neck to a new barrier.

This is effectively the means of treating tense shortened muscles in FMS, avoiding actual stretching during the acute phases but allowing MET to release hypertonicity.

Assessment of shortness in scalenes

The scalenes are prone to trigger point activity, and are a controversial muscle since they seem to be both postural and phasic, their status being modified by the type(s) of stress to which they are exposed. Janda reports that, 'spasm and/or trigger points are commonly present in the scalenes as also are weakness and/or inhibition' (Janda 1989).

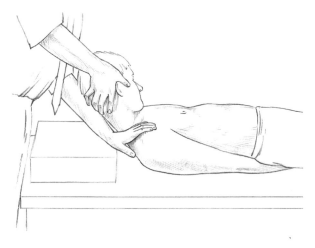

Figure 13.26 MET test and treatment for levator scapula (right side).

There is no easy test for shortness of the scalenes apart from observation, palpation and assessment of trigger point activity/tautness and a functional observation as follows:

• In most people who have marked scalene shortness there is a tendency to over use these (and other upper fixators of the shoulder and neck) as accessory breathing muscles. There may also be a tendency to hyperventilation (and hence for there to possibly be a history of anxiety, phobic behaviour, panic attacks and/or fatigue symptoms). These muscles seem to be excessively tense in many people with chronic fatigue symptoms.
• The observation assessment consists of the operator placing their relaxed hands over the shoulders so that fingertips rest on the clavicles, at which time the seated patient is asked to inhale deeply. If the operator's hands noticeably rise towards the patient's ears during inhalation then there exists inappropriate use of scalenes, which indicates that they are stressed, which also means that by definition they will have become shortened and require stretching.

Alternatively, during the history-taking interview, the patient can be asked to place one hand on the abdomen just above the umbilicus and the other flat against the upper chest. On inhalation the hands are observed, and if the upper one initiates the breathing process, and rises significantly towards the chin, rather than moving forwards, a pattern of upper chest breathing can be assumed and therefore stress, and therefore shortness of the scalenes (and other accessory breathing muscles, notably sternomastoid).

Treatment of short scalenes by MET

Patient lies with head over the end of the table, supported on a cushion which rests on the knees of the seated operator (or the head can be supported by one cupped hand). The head/neck is in slight extension (painless) at this stage.

The head is turned away from the side to be treated. As with treatment of upper trapezius, there are three positions of rotation required, a full rotation producing involvement of the more posterior fibres of the scalenes on the side from which the turn is being made (Fig. 13.27A); a half turn involves the middle fibres (Fig. 13.27B); and a position of only slight turn involves the more anterior fibres (Fig. 13.27 C).

The operator's free hand is placed on the area just below the lateral end of the clavicle of the

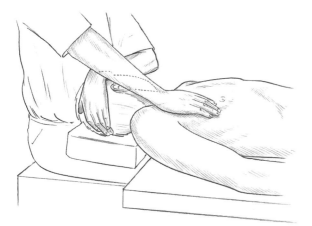

Figure 13.27A   MET for scalenus posticus. On stretching, following the isometric contraction, the neck is allowed to move into slight extension while a mild stretch is introduced by the contact hand which rests on the second rib, below the lateral aspect of the clavicle.

affected side (a side of hand, 'soft', contact is best, resting on the second rib and upper sternal structures).

The patient is instructed, with appropriate breathing cooperation, to lift the forehead a fraction and to attempt to turn the head to the affected side, whilst resistance is applied preventing both movements ('lift and turn'). The effort and therefore the counter-pressure should be modest and painless at all times.

After the 7–10 second contraction the head is allowed to ease into extension and the contact hand on the second rib and upper sternum pushes very gently obliquely away towards the foot on that same side, following the ribs into exhalation where they are held during the period of stretch (up to 30 seconds).

With the head half turned away from the affected side, the hand contact which applies the stretch into the middle fibres of the scalenes is just inferior to the middle aspect of the clavicle; and when the head is in the upright position, for anterior scalene stretch, the hand contact is on the upper sternum itself.

In all other ways the methodology is as described for the first position above.

CAUTION: It is important not to allow heroic degrees of neck extension during any phase of this treatment. There should be some but it

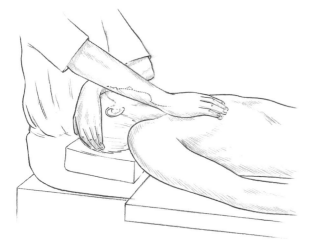

Figure 13.27B   MET treatment for the middle fibres of scalenes. The hand placement (thenar or hypothenar eminence of relaxed hand) is on the second rib below the centre of the clavicle.

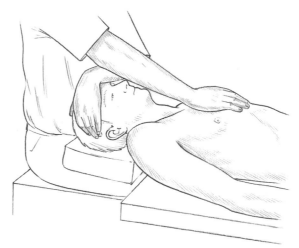

Figure 13.27C   MET treatment of the anterior fibres of the scalenes; hand placement is on the sternum.

should be appropriate to the age and condition of the individual.

A degree of eye movement can assist scalene treatment. If the patient makes the eyes look downwards (towards the feet) and towards the affected side during the isometric contraction she or he will increase the degree of contraction in the muscles. If during the resting phase, when stretch is being introduced the patient looks away from the treated side with eyes focused upwards towards the top of the head, this will enhance the stretch of the muscle.

This whole procedure should be performed several times, in each of the three positions of the head, for each side if necessary.

Assessment for shortness of sternocleidomastoid

As for the scalenes there is no absolute test for shortness but observation of posture (hyperextended neck, chin poked forward) and palpation of the degree of induration, fibrosis and trigger point activity can all alert to probable shortness of sternocleidomastoid (SCM). This is an accessory breathing muscle and, like the scalenes, will be shortened by inappropriate breathing patterns which have become habitual. Observation is an accurate assessment tool. Since SCM is only just observable when normal, if the clavicular insertion is easily visible or any part of the muscle is prominent this can be taken as a clear sign of tightness of the muscle. If the patient's posture involves the head being held forward of the body, often accompanied by cervical lordosis and dorsal kyphosis, weakness of the deep neck flexors and tightness of SCM can be suspected (upper crossed syndrome, see notes earlier in this chapter).

A functional test for shortness is observable by asking the supine patient to very slowly 'raise your head and touch your chin to your chest'. This was described in the functional evaluation methods earlier in this chapter (p. 210, Fig. 13.13).

Recall the importance of the effect on the suboccipital region in general and rectus capitis posterior minor in particular, when SCM is shortened (see Ch. 3 notes on whiplash etc.).

Treatment of shortened sternocleidomastoid using MET

The patient is supine, head over the end of the table, supported by the operator's hand or on cushion on the lap of the seated operator, as in scalene treatment described above.

Whereas in scalene treatment the instruction to the patient was to 'lift and turn' the rotated head/neck against resistance, in treating SCM the instruction is simply to lift the head. When the head is raised there is no need to apply resistance as gravity effectively does this. After 7–10 seconds of this isometric contraction, and held breath, instruct the patient to release the effort (and breathe) and to allow the head/neck to return to a resting position in which some extension of the neck is allowed, while the soft edge of a hand applies oblique pressure/stretch to the sternum to take it away from the head towards the feet. The hand not involved in stretching the sternum away from the head should gently restrain the tendency the head will have to follow this stretch, but should under no circumstances apply pressure to stretch the head/neck while it is in this vulnerable position of slight extension. The degree of extension of the neck should be slight, 10–15° at most. Maintain this stretch for some seconds to achieve release/stretch of hypertonic and fibrotic structures.

General suboccipital muscle release using MET

General (MET enhanced) stretches for the suboccipital muscles, including splenius capitis, semispinalis capitis, rectus capitis posterior major and minor, obliquus capitis inferior and superior.

Treatment(1) Patient is supine, head and neck just beyond the end of the bed supported by the operator's right (in this example) hand with patient's crown of head just touching and lightly supported by operator's abdomen. The operator's left hand cups the chin (avoid larynx) and introduces mild traction

By movement of the operator's body it is possible to introduce controlled flexion to its full extent without force.

A light (10% of strength) attempt is made by the patient to extend the neck against resistance from the operator's hands (or they may merely look upwards as far as possible to initiate light contraction of the extensors of the neck).

After 7–10 seconds of this an increase in flexion is introduced to its fullest pain-free and unforced extent. At the same time the operator can introduce slight downwards (to the floor) pressure on the patient's forehead to increase a stretching flexion of the muscles at the atlanto-occipital junction.

This is held for 10 seconds at least before a slow return to neutral.

Treatment(2) The neck of the supine patient is flexed to its easy barrier of resistance or just short of this and the patient is asked to extend the neck (take it back to the table) using minimal effort on an inhalation, against resistance.

The operator's hands are placed, arms crossed, so that one hand rests on each shoulder, or upper anterior shoulder area, while the patient's head rests on the crossed forearms.

After the contraction, the neck is flexed further to, or through, the barrier of resistance, as appropriate. A further aid during the contraction phase is to have the operator's abdomen in contact with the top of the patient's head, and to use this contact to prevent the patient tilting the head upwards. This allows for an additional isometric contraction and subsequent stretch which involves the short extensor muscles at the base of the skull.

Repetitions of the stretch should be performed until no further gain is possible, or until the chin easily touches the chest on flexion.

No force should be used, or pain produced during this procedure.

Treatment(3) Patient is seated. Operator stands to (left in this example) side with the patient's head supported against the operator's left chest/shoulder area by the left hand and forearm, which embrace the patient's head, palmar surface cupping the right ear and fingers holding the articular and transverse processes of C2.

The operator's right hand stabilises the spinous, articular and transverse processes of C3 and C4.

Utilising this grip, the operator introduces light traction through the long axis of the spine, and introduces flexion of the neck to fully – but without force – take out soft tissue slack, separating the hands to do so.

The patient is asked to look downwards with the eyes and at the same time the operator resists the slight tendency this produce to increase flexion, for 7 seconds or so.

After this – together with the patient's active assistance – a slight increase in flexion is introduced to a new barrier. This is held for a further 10 seconds before a slow return to neutral.

By altering the hold applied by the right hand to a more distal position on the neck, as low as C7–T1, and using the same protocol just described, other attachments can be involved in the flexion stretch.

CAUTION: By carefully, painlessly, and above all without force introducing slight degrees of sidebending and/or rotation, rotational components of these muscles will be lightly stretched.

Ruddy's 'pulsed MET' variation
(Ruddy 1962)

Shortly after the Second World War, osteopathic physician T. J. Ruddy developed a method of rapid pulsating contractions against resistance which he termed 'rapid resistive duction'. It was in part this work which Fred Mitchell Snr DO used as his base for the evolution of MET, along with proprioceptive neuromuscular facilitation (PNF) methodology.

Ruddy's method called for a series of muscle contractions against resistance, at a rate a little faster than the pulse rate. This approach can be applied in all areas where isometric contractions are suitable, and is particularly useful for self-treatment following instruction from a skilled practitioner. It is also particularly useful in acute conditions where a sustained contraction may be painful or difficult to perform – as in FMS.

Ruddy's work is now known as pulsed MET rather than the tongue-twisting 'Ruddy's rapid resistive duction'. Its simplest use involves the dysfunctional tissue/joint being held at its resistance barrier, at which time the patient, ideally (or the operator if the patient cannot adequately cooperate with the instructions) against the resistance offered by the operator, introduces a series of rapid (two per second), very small efforts towards (or sometimes away from) the barrier. The barest initiation of effort is called for with, to use Ruddy's term, 'no wobble and no bounce'.

The use of this 'conditioning' approach involves, in Ruddy's words, contractions which are,'short, rapid and rhythmic, gradually increasing the amplitude and degree of resistance, thus conditioning the proprioceptive system by rapid movements'. This objective could have been designed for the FMS patient where deconditioning is commonly found.

In describing application of this method to the neck (in a case of vertigo), Ruddy gives instruction as to the directions in which the series of resisted efforts should be made. These must include: 'movements . . . in a line of each major direction, forwards, backwards, right forward and right backwards or along an antero-posterior line in four directions along the multiplication 'X' sign, also a half circle, or rotation right and left.'

His suggested timing is to count each series of contractions as follows: 1-1, 1-2; 2-1, 2-2; 3-1, 3-2; 4-1, 4-2 and so on up to 10-2. These 'mini-contractions' are meant to be timed to coincide with each count so that when complete in all the directions available, an effective series of pulsating contractions against the agonists or antagonists will have been achieved.

If reducing joint restriction or elongation of a soft tissue is the objective then, following each series of 20 contractions of this sort, the slack should be taken out, the new barrier engaged, and a further series of contractions should be commenced from this new barrier, possibly in a different direction which can and should be varied according to Ruddy's guidelines, to take account of all the different elements in any restriction.

Despite Ruddy's suggestion that the amplitude of the contractions be increased over time, the effort itself must never exceed the barest beginning of an isometric contraction.

The effects are likely, Ruddy suggests, to include:

- Improved oxygenation
- Enhanced venous and lymphatic circulation through the area being treated.

Furthermore, he believes that the method influences both static and kinetic posture because of the effects on proprioceptive and interoceptive afferent pathways, and that this helps maintain 'dynamic equilibrium', which involves 'a balance in chemical, physical, thermal, electrical and tissue fluid homeostasis'.

Ruddy's work offers a useful means of modifying the use of sustained isometric contractions in MET, which has particular relevance to acute problems.

POSITIONAL RELEASE VARIATIONS (STRAIN/COUNTERSTRAIN)

There are many different methods involving the positioning of an area, or the whole body, in such a way as to evoke a physiological response which helps to resolve musculoskeletal dysfunction. The means whereby the beneficial changes occur seem to involve a combination of neurological and circulatory changes which occur when a distressed area is placed in its most comfortable, its most 'easy', most pain-free, position.

The impetus towards the use of this most basic of treatment methods in a coherent rather than a hit-and-miss manner lies in the work of Lawrence Jones DO, who developed an approach to somatic dysfunction which he termed 'Strain and Counterstrain' (SCS) (Jones 1981).

Walther (1988) describes the moment of discovery in these words:

Jones' initial observation of the efficacy of counterstrain was with a patient who was unresponsive to treatment. The patient had been unable to sleep because of pain. Jones attempted to find a comfortable position for the patient to aid him in sleeping. After twenty minutes of trial and error, a position was finally achieved in which the patient's pain was relieved. Leaving the patient in this position for a short time, Jones was astonished when the patient came out of the position and was able to stand comfortably erect. The relief of pain was lasting and the patient made an uneventful recovery.

The position of 'ease' which Jones found for this patient was an exaggeration of the position in which spasm was holding him, which provided Jones with an insight into the mechanisms involved. Over the years since Jones first made his valuable observation that a position which exaggerated a patient's distortion could provide the opportunity for a release of spasm and hypertonicity, many variations on this basic theme have emerged, some building logically on that first insight with others moving in new directions.

COMMON BASIS

The commonality of all of these approaches is that they move the patient or the affected tissues away from any resistance barriers and towards positions of comfort. The shorthand terms used for these two extremes are 'bind' and 'ease' which anyone who has handled the human body will recognise as extremely apt.

The need for the many variations to be understood should be obvious. Different clinical settings require that a variety of therapeutic approaches be available. Jones's approach requires verbal feedback from the patient as to tenderness in a 'tender' point which is being used as a monitor which the operator is palpating while attempting to find a position of ease. One can imagine a situation in which the use of Jones's 'tender points as a monitor' method would be inappropriate (lost ability to communicate verbally or someone too young to verbalise). In such a case there is a need for a method which allows achievement of the same ends without verbal communication.

This is possible using either 'functional' approaches or 'facilitated positional release' method, involving finding a position of maximum ease by means of palpation alone, assessing for a state of 'ease' in the tissues. As we examine a number of the variations on the same theme of positional release – release by placing the patient or area into 'ease' – the diverse clinical and therapeutic potentials for the use of this approach will become clearer.

It is important to note that if positional release methods are being applied to chronically fibrosed tissue the result would produce a reduction in hypertonicity but cannot produce a reduction in fibrosis. Pain relief or improved mobility may therefore be only temporary in such cases.

1. Exaggeration of distortion (an element of SCS methodology)

Consider the example of an individual bent forward in psoas spasm/'lumbago'. The patient is in considerable discomfort or pain, posturally distorted into flexion together with rotation and sidebending. Any attempt to straighten towards a more physiologically normal posture would be met by increased pain. Engaging the barrier of resistance would therefore not be an ideal first option, in an acute setting such as this.

Moving the area away from the restriction barrier is, however, not usually a problem. The position required to find 'ease' for someone in this state normally involves painlessly increasing the degree of distortion displayed, placing them (in the case of the example given) into some variation based on forward bending, until pain is found to reduce or resolve. After 60–90 seconds in this position of ease, a slow return to neutral would be carried out and commonly in practice the patient will be somewhat or completely relieved of pain and spasm.

2. Replication of position of strain (an element of SCS methodology)

Take as an example someone who is bending to lift a load when an emergency stabilisation is required and strain results (the person slips or the load shifts). The patient could be locked into the same position of 'lumbago-like' distortion as in example 1, above.

If, as SCS suggests, the position of ease equals the position of strain, then the patient needs to go back into flexion in slow motion until tenderness vanishes from the monitor/tender point and/or a sense of 'ease' is perceived in the previously hypertonic shortened tissues. Adding small 'fine-tuning' positioning to the initial position of ease achieved by flexion, usually achieves a maximum reduction in pain. This position is held for 60–90 seconds before slowly returning the patient to neutral, at which time, as in example 1, a partial or total resolution of hypertonicity, spasm and pain should be noted. The position of strain, as described, is probably going to be similar to the position of exaggeration of distortion, as in example 1.

These two elements of SCS are of limited clinical value and are described as examples only, since it is not a frequent occurrence to have patients who can describe precisely in which way their symptoms developed. Nor is obvious spasm such as torticollis or acute anteflexion spasm ('lumbago') the norm and so ways other than 'exaggerated distortion' and 'replication of position of strain' are needed in order to easily be able to identify probable positions of ease.

3. Using Jones's tender points as monitors (Jones 1981)

Over many years of clinical experience Jones compiled lists of specific tender point areas relating to every imaginable strain of most of the joints and muscles of the body. These are his 'proven' (by clinical experience) points. The tender points are usually found in tissues which were in a shortened state at the time of strain, rather than those which were stretched. New points are periodically reported in the osteopathic literature – for example sacral foramen points relating to sacroiliac strains (Ramirez et al 1989).

Jones and his followers have also provided strict guidelines for achieving ease in any tender points which are being palpated (the position of ease usually involving a 'folding' or crowding of the tissues in which the tender point lies). This method involves maintaining pressure on the monitor tender point, or periodically probing it, as a position is achieved in which:

• There is no additional pain in whatever area is symptomatic
• The monitor point pain has reduced by at least 75%.

This is then held for an appropriate length of time (90 seconds according to Jones; however, there are variations suggested for the length of time required in the position of ease as will be explained).

In the example of the person with acute low back pain who is locked in flexion, the tender point will be located on the anterior surface of the abdomen, in the muscle structures which were short at the time of strain (when the patient was in flexion) and the position which removes tenderness from this point will usually require flexion and probably some fine-tuning involving rotation and/or sidebending.

If there is a problem with Jones's formulaic approach it is that while he is frequently correct as to the position of ease recommended for particular points, the mechanics of the particular strain with which the operator is confronted may not coincide with Jones's guidelines. An operator who relies solely on these 'menus' or formulae could find difficulty in handling a situation in which Jones's prescription failed to produce the desired results. Reliance on Jones's menu of points and positions can therefore lead to the operator becoming dependent on them, and it is suggested that a reliance on palpation skills and other variations on Jones's original observations offers a more rounded approach to dealing with strain and pain.

Fortunately Goodheart (and others) have offered less rigid frameworks for using positional release.

4. Goodheart's approach (Goodheart 1984, Walther 1988)

George Goodheart DC (the developer of applied kinesiology) has described an almost universally applicable formula which relies more on the individual features displayed by the patient, and less on rigid formulae as used in Jones's approach.

Goodheart suggests that a suitable tender point be sought in the tissues opposite those 'working' when pain or restriction is noted. If pain/restriction is reported/apparent on any given movement, muscles antagonistic to those operating at the time pain is noted will be those housing the tender point(s). Thus, for example, pain (wherever it is felt) which occurs when the neck is being turned to the left will require that a tender point be located in the muscles which turn the head to the right.

In examples 1 and 2, of a person locked in forward bending with acute pain and spasm, using Goodheart's approach, pain and restriction would be experienced as the person straightened up (moves into extension) from a position of enforced flexion.

This action (straightening up) would usually cause pain in the back but, irrespective of where the pain is noted, a tender point would be sought (and subsequently treated by being taken to a state of ease) in the muscles opposite those working when pain was experienced – i.e. it would lie in the flexor muscles (probably psoas) in this example.

It is important to emphasise this factor, that tender points which are going to be used as 'monitors' during the positioning phase of this approach are not sought in the muscles opposite those where pain is noted, but in the muscles opposite those which are actively moving the patient or area when pain or restriction is noted.

Goodheart has also suggested refinements which are claimed to reduce the amount of time the position of ease needs to be maintained, from 90 seconds (Jones) to 30 seconds.

5. Functional technique (Hoover 1969, Bowles 1981)

Osteopathic functional technique relies on a reduction in palpated tone in stressed (hypertonic/spasm) tissues as the body (or part) is being positioned or fine-tuned in relation to all available directions of movement in a given region. One hand palpates the affected tissues (moulded to them, without invasive pressure). This is described as the 'listening' hand since it assesses changes in tone as the operator's other hand guides the patient or part through a sequence of positions which are aimed at enhancing ease and reducing bind.

A sequence is carried out involving different directions of movement (e.g. flexion/extension,

rotation right and left, sidebending right and left, etc.), with each movement starting at the point of maximum ease revealed by the previous evaluation, or combined point of ease of a number of previous evaluations. In this way one position of ease is 'stacked' on another until all movements have been assessed for ease (Fig. 13.28).

Were the same fictional patient with the low back problem described previously being treated using functional technique, the tense tissues in the low back would be the ones being palpated. Following a sequence of flexion/extension, sidebending and rotating in each direction, translation right and left, translation anterior and posterior, and compression/distraction, so involving all available directions of movement of the area, a position of maximum ease would be arrived at in which (if the position were held for 30–90 seconds) a release of hypertonicity and reduction in pain would result.

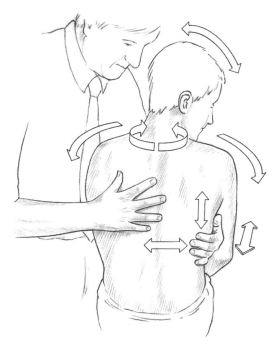

Figure 13.28 Functional palpation (or treatment) of a spinal region/segment during which all possible directions of motion are assessed for their influence on the sense of 'ease and bind' in the palpated tissues. After the first (sequence is irrelevant) position of ease is identified each subsequent assessment commences from the position of ease (or combined positions of ease) identified by the previous assessment(s) in a process known as 'stacking'.

The precise sequence in which the various directions of motion are evaluated is irrelevant, as long as all possibilities are included.

Theoretically (and often in practice) the `position of palpated maximum ease (reduced tone) in the distressed tissues should correspond with the position which would have been found were pain being used as a guide as in either Jones's or Goodheart's approach, or using the more basic 'exaggeration of distortion' or 'replication of position of strain'.

6. Any painful point as a starting place for SCS

All areas which palpate as painful are responding to, or are associated with, some degree of imbalance, dysfunction or reflexive activity which may well involve acute or chronic strain.

Jones identified positions of tender points relating to particular strain positions. It makes just as much sense to work the other way around and to identify where the 'strain' is likely to have occurred in relation to any pain point which has been identified. We might therefore consider that any painful point found during soft tissue evaluation could be treated by positional release, whether we know what strain produced them or not, and whether the problem is acute or chronic.

Experience and simple logic tell us that the response to positional release of a chronically fibrosed area will be less dramatic than from tissues held in simple spasm or hypertonicity. Nevertheless, even in chronic settings, a degree of release can be produced, allowing for easier access to the deeper fibrosis.

This approach, of being able to treat any painful tissue using positional release, is valid whether the pain is being monitored via feedback from the patient (using reducing levels of pain in the palpated point as a guide) or whether the concept of assessing a reduction in tone in the tissues is being used (as above). Again, a lengthy 60–90 seconds are recommended as the time for holding the position of maximum ease, although some (such as Marsh Morrison – see induration technique below) suggest just 20 seconds.

7. Facilitated positional release (FPR) (Schiowitz 1990)

This variation on the theme of functional and SCS methods involves the positioning of the distressed area into the direction of its greatest freedom of movement starting from a position of 'neutral' in terms of the overall body position.

To start with, the seated patient's sagittal posture might be modified to take the body or the part (neck for example) into a more 'neutral' position – a balance between flexion and extension – following which an application of a facilitating force (usually a crowding of the tissues) is introduced. No pain monitor is used but rather a palpating/listening hand is applied (as in functional technique) which senses for changes in ease and bind in distressed tissues as the body/part is carefully positioned and repositioned. The final 'crowding' of the tissues, to encourage a 'slackening' of local tension, is the facilitating aspect of the process according to its theorists. This 'crowding' might involve compression applied through the long axis of a limb perhaps, or directly downwards through the spine via cranially applied pressure, or some such variation. The length of time the position of ease is held is usually suggested at just 5 seconds. It is claimed that altered tissue texture, either surface or deep, can be successfully treated in this way.

8. Induration technique
(Morrison 1969)

Marsh Morrison DC suggested very light palpation, using extremely light touch, as a means of feeling a 'drag' sensation alongside the spine (as lateral as the tips of the transverse processes). Drag relates to increased hydrosis which is a physiological response to increased sympathetic activity and is an invariable factor in skin overlying trigger and other forms of reflexively induced or active myofascial areas. Once drag is noted, pressure into the tissues normally evinces a report of pain.

The operator stands on the side of the prone patient opposite the side in which pain has been discovered in these paraspinal tissues. Once located, tender or painful points (lying no more lateral than the tip of the transverse process) are palpated for the level of their sensitivity to pressure. Once confirmed as painful, the point is held by firm thumb pressure while, with the soft thenar eminence of the other hand, the tip of the spinous process most adjacent to the pain point is very gently eased towards the pain (ounces of pressure only) so crowding and slackening the tissues being palpated, until pain reduces by at least 75%. Direct pressure (lightly applied) towards the pain should lessen the degree of tissue contraction and the sensitivity (Fig. 13.29).

If it does not do so then the angle of 'push' on the spinous process towards the painful spot should be varied slightly so that, somewhere within an arc embracing a half circle, an angle of push towards the pain will be found to abolish the pain totally and will lessen the objective feeling of tension. This position is held for 20 seconds after which the next point is treated.

A full spinal treatment is possible using this extremely gentle approach which incorporates the same principles as SCS and functional technique, the achievement of ease and pain reduction as the treatment focus.

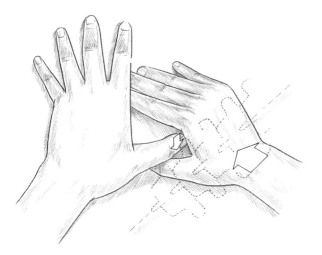

Figure 13.29 Induration technique hand positions. Pressure used on the spinous process is measured in ounces (grams) at most.

9. Integrated neuromuscular inhibition technique (INIT)
(Chaitow 1994)

INIT involves using the position of ease as part of a sequence which commences with the location of a tender/pain/trigger point, followed by application of ischaemic compression (optional – avoided if pain is too intense or the patient too sensitive) followed by the introduction of positional release (as in 6 above). After an appropriate length of time, during which the tissues are held in 'ease', the patient introduces an isometric contraction into the affected tissues for 7–10 seconds, after which these are stretched (or they may be stretched at the same time as the contraction if fibrotic tissue calls for such attention) (Figs. 13.30A, 13.30B, and 13.30C)

INIT method

When a trigger point is being palpated by direct finger or thumb pressure, and when the very tissues in which the trigger point lies are positioned in such a way as to take away the pain (entirely or at least to a great extent), then the most (dis)stressed fibres in which the trigger point is housed are in a position of relative ease.

At this time the trigger point would be under direct inhibitory pressure (mild or perhaps intermittent) and would have been positioned so that the tissues housing it are relaxed (relatively or completely).

Following a period of 20–90 seconds of this position of ease and inhibitory pressure (constant or intermittent), the patient is asked to introduce an isometric contraction into the tissues and to hold this for 7–10 seconds – involving the precise fibres which had been repositioned to obtain the positional release.

The effect of this would be to produce (following the contraction) a reduction in tone in these tissues. The hypertonic or fibrotic tissues could then be gently stretched as in any muscle energy procedure so that the specifically targeted fibres would be stretched.

SCS RULES OF TREATMENT

The following 'rules' are based on clinical experience and should be borne in mind when using positional release (SCS, etc.) methods in treating pain and dysfunction, especially where the patient is fatigued, sensitive and/or distressed:

• Never treat more than 5 'tender' points at any one session, and treat fewer than this in sensitive individuals.

• Forewarn patients that, just as in any other form of bodywork which produces altered function, a period of physiological adaptation is inevitable, and that there will therefore be a 'reaction' on the day(s) following even this extremely light form of treatment. Soreness and stiffness is therefore to be anticipated.

• If there are multiple tender points – as is inevitable in fibromyalgia – select those most proximal and most medial for primary attention – that is those closest to the head and the centre of the body rather than distal and lateral pain points.

• Of these tender points, select those that are most painful for initial attention/treatment.

• If self-treatment of painful and restricted areas is advised – and it should be if at all possible – apprise the patient of these rules (i.e. only a few

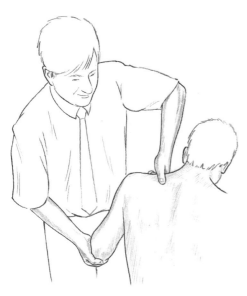

Figure 13.30A First stage of INIT in which a tender/pain/trigger point in supraspinatus is located and ischaemically compressed, either intermittently or persistently.

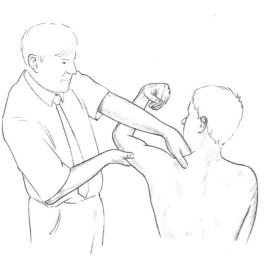

Figure 13.30B The pain is removed from the tender/pain/trigger point by finding a position of ease which is held for at least 20 seconds, following which an isometric contraction is achieved involving the tissues which house the tender/pain/trigger point.

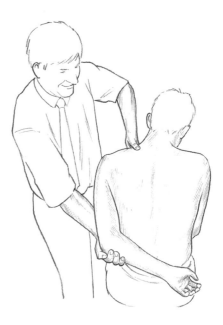

Figure 13.30C Following the holding of the isometric contraction for an appropriate period, the muscle housing the point of local soft tissue dysfunction is stretched. This completes the INIT sequence.

pain points on any day to be given attention, to expect a 'reaction', to select the most painful points and those closest to the head and the centre of the body).

Many manual medicine experts believe that this approach – in which the body tissues are 'allowed' to normalise – is the best way forward since it offers a practical and philosophical alternative to more aggressive interventions which oblige a response (stretching, pressure, etc.).

Positional release can be equated with deep relaxation, therapeutic fasting, the cranial 'still point', neutral (flotation) bathing, wellness massage, etc. – all of which comprise whole-body, non-specific, constitutional interventions.

Learning to apply positional release/SCS

The four keys which allow anyone to efficiently apply positional release/SCS are:

1. An ability to localise soft tissue changes related to particular strain dysfunctions, acute/chronic
2. An ability to sense tissue change, as it moves into a state of ease, comfort, relaxation and reduced resistance
3. The ability to guide the patient as a whole, or the affected body part, towards a state of ease with minimal force
4. The ability to apply minimal palpation force as the changes in the tissues are evaluated.

The guidelines which should therefore be remembered and applied are:

• Locate and palpate the appropriate tender point or area of hypertonicity
• Use minimal force
• Use minimal monitoring pressure
• Achieve maximum ease/comfort/relaxation of tissues
• Produce no additional pain anywhere else.

These elements need to be kept in mind as positional release/SCS methods are learned, and are major points of emphasis in programmes which teach it (Jones 1981).

The general guidelines which Jones gives for relief of the dysfunction with which such tender points are related involves directing the movement of these tissues towards ease, which commonly involves the following elements:

• For tender points on the anterior surface of the body, flexion, sidebending and rotation should be towards the palpated point, followed by fine tuning to reduce sensitivity by at least 70%.
• For tender points on the posterior surface of the body, extension, sidebending and rotation should be away from the palpated point, followed by fine tuning to reduce sensitivity by 70%.
• The closer the tender point is to the midline the less sidebending and rotation should be required and the further from the midline the more sidebending and rotation should be required, in order to effect ease and comfort in the tender point (without producing additional pain).
• The direction towards which sidebending is introduced when trying to find a position of ease often needs to be away from the side of the palpated pain point, especially in relation to tender points found on the posterior aspect of the body, but it may be towards the direction of pain.

SCS cervical flexion restrictions (Fig. 13.31)

Note that SCS is an ideal approach for self-treatment of 'tender' points in fibromyalgia and can safely be taught to patients for home use.

An area of local dysfunction is sought on the anterior surface of the cervical region, using an appropriate form of palpation, such as a 'feather-light', single-finger, stroking touch on the skin areas overlying the tips of the transverse processes. Using this method a feeling of 'drag' is being sought which indicates increased sudo-motor (sympathetic) activity and therefore a likely site of dysfunction, local or reflexively induced (Lewit 1992).

When drag is noted, light compression is introduced to identify and establish a point of sensitivity, a tender point, which in this area represents (based on Jones's findings) a flexion

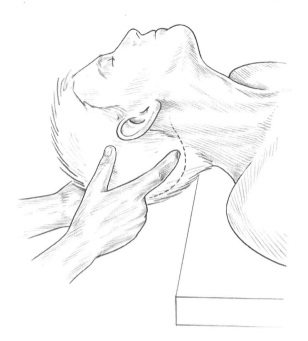

Figure 13.31 First cervical extension strain. The position of ease requires extension of the neck and (usually) rotation away from the side of pain.

strain site. The patient is instructed in the method required for reporting a reduction in pain during the positioning sequence which follows.

The author's approach is to say: 'I want you to score the pain caused by my pressure, before we start moving your head into different positions (in this example) as a '10' and to not speak apart from giving me the present score (out of 10) whenever I ask for it.' The aim is to achieve a reported score of 3 or less before ceasing the positioning process.

The head/neck is then passively taken lightly into flexion until some degree of ease is reported in the tender point (based on the score, or the 'value', reported by the patient) which is either being constantly compressed at this stage (this is author's preference, if discomfort is not too great) (Chaitow 1991) or intermittently probed (which is Jones's preference).

When a reduction of pain by around 50% is achieved, a degree of fine-tuning is commenced in which very small degrees of additional positioning are introduced in order to find the position of maximum ease, at which time the

reported 'score' should be reduced by at least 70%.

At this time the patient may be asked to inhale fully and exhale fully while observing for themselves changes in the palpated pain point, in order to evaluate which phase of the cycle reduces the pain score still more. That phase of the breathing cycle in which they sense the greatest reduction in sensitivity is maintained for a period which is tolerable to the patient (holding the breath in or out or at some point between the two extremes) while the overall position of ease continues to be maintained and the tender/tense area monitored. This position of ease is held for 90 seconds in Jones's methodology, although there exist mechanisms for reducing this.

During the holding of the position of ease the direct compression can be reduced to a mere touching of the point along with a periodic probing to establish that ease has been maintained.

After 90 seconds the neck/head is very slowly returned to the neutral starting position. This slow return to neutral is a vital component of SCS since the neural receptors (muscle spindles) may be provoked into a return to their previously dysfunctional state if a rapid movement is made at the end of the procedure.

The tender point/area may be retested for sensitivity at this time and should be found to be considerably less hypertonic and sensitive.

SCS cervical extension restrictions (Fig. 13.31)

Note that SCS is an ideal approach for self-treatment of 'tender' points in fibromyalgia and can safely be taught to patients for home use.

With the patient in the supine position but with the head clear of the end of the table, fully supported by the operator, areas of localised tenderness are sought by light palpation alongside or over the tips of the spinous processes of the cervical spine.

Having located a tender point, compression is applied to elicit a degree of sensitivity or pain which the patient notes as representing a score of '10'.

The head/neck is then taken into light extension along with sidebending and rotation (usually away from the side of the pain if this is not central) until a reduction of at least 50% is achieved in the reported sensitivity. The pressure on the tender point can be constant or intermittent, with the latter being preferable if sensitivity is great.

Once a reduction in sensitivity is achieved of at least 70%, inhalation and exhalation are monitored by the patient to see which reduces sensitivity even more, and this phase of the cycle is maintained for a comfortable period during which the overall position of ease is maintained. If intermittent pressure on the point is being used, this needs to be applied periodically during the holding period in order to ensure that the position of ease has been maintained.

After 90 seconds a very slow and deliberate return to neutral is performed and the patient is rested for several minutes. The tender point should be repalpated for sensitivity which should have reduced markedly as should any sense of hypertonicity in the surrounding tissues.

Functional release atlanto-occipital region

The operator sits slightly to the side of the head of the supine patient (facing the corner of table). The caudad hand (forearm fully supported by the table) cradles the upper neck so that the atlas is either lightly held between finger and thumb, or rests on the webbing between finger and thumb. The cephalad hand cradles the base of the head with fingers spreading over the crown facing anteriorly.

The caudad hand is a 'listening', diagnostic contact attempting to identify changes taking place in the soft tissues ('ease' and 'bind') with which it is in contact, as the other hand slowly and deliberately moves the head on the atlas in various directions.

As the head is slowly flexed and then extended (slightly in each direction until a sense of tension or 'bind' is noted) variations in tissue response to the movement will be noted by the listening hand. When the most easy, 'softest', most relaxed, preferred position is noted, this is held momentarily (this is the 'first position of ease') at which

time a second range of motion is introduced, possibly sidebending right and then left.

When the second position of ease (the combined first and second position) has been identified, this is used as the starting point for a third range of motions to be assessed, perhaps rotation right and left, or translation ('glide') right and left or anterior/posterior.

By moving from one assessment to another, always commencing the new testing range from the combined position of previous 'ease' positions, the operator is in effect 'stacking' positions of ease on to each other. Eventually, when all options (all directions of motion, in any sequence) have been tried, a point of balanced dynamic neutral will be reached, where the local tissues are at their most relaxed (Bowles 1981).

This position is held for around 90 seconds during which time increased circulation through the tissues as well as neurological resetting (muscle spindle response) creates a sense of 'softening', a sense of warmth and increased relaxation of the tissues.

Following this the neck/head is returned slowly to its starting position and the atlanto-occipital junction will usually display a greater freedom of movement and comfort.

The same principles can be applied to any tissues in the body. The approach will be recognised as essentially the same as that used when skin on fascia was 'slid' to its combined position of ease, in the palpation exercise earlier in this chapter (p. 204). This is an ideal approach in treating FMS, especially if there is any history of trauma to the area or of head/neck tension, and pain is a feature (see whiplash, Ch. 3).

ADDITIONAL SUB-OCCIPITAL TECHNIQUES

Cranial base release

This technique releases the soft tissues where they attach to the cranial base.

The patient is supine and the operator should be seated at the head of the table with arms resting on and supported by the table. The dorsum of the operator's hand rests on the table with fingertips pointing towards the ceiling, acting as a fulcrum on which the patient rests the occiput so that the back of the skull is resting on the palm. The fingertips touch the occiput and the patient allows the head to lie heavily so that the pressure induces tissue release against the fingertips.

As relaxation proceeds and the finger pads sink deeper into the tissues, the arch of the atlas may be palpated and it may be encouraged to disengage from the occiput by application of mild traction cephalad (applied by the middle fingers). This would probably not be for some minutes after commencement of the exercise.

The effect is to relax the muscular attachments in the area being treated. This 'release' of deep structures of the upper neck enhances drainage from the head, and circulation to it, reducing intercranial congestion.

Occipital condyle decompression

The objective of the decompression technique is to separate the occiput from the articular surfaces of the atlas, if they are not freely able to do so.

Upledger & Vredevoogd (1993) report that condylar compression may accompany cranial base and/or lumbosacral compression, and may be related to hyperkinesis in children and headache in adults. The method for achieving decompression is identical with the method for assessing whether or not it is necessary to do so – in other words assessment and treatment are the same.

The cranial base release (above) should be performed first and any muscular influences which might be impeding free motion (upper trapezius, levator scapula, sternomastoid, etc.) should be dealt with using appropriate soft tissue methods as suggested in the section on MET, or by means of positional release techniques.

Method The patient is supine with operator seated at the head of the table. The operator's arms are supported on the table and placed so that the elbows are a little apart. The patient's head rests on the operator's palms. The middle (and perhaps index) finger pads are placed close to the midline and as near the foramen magnum as can comfortably be achieved, without force.

The distal interphalangeal joints of the middle fingers are flexed so that the tips apply a gentle sustained pressure to the occiput which is directed posteriorly and cephalad. If the occiput is free, a sense will be noted of the occiput being able to move freely. If restricted there will be a resistance to the gentle traction applied by the finger pads to the occipital base, in which case this traction is sustained as described until a sense of a free motion (Upledger & Vredevoogd call it a 'glide') is achieved.

At this time the operator's elbows are slowly brought towards each other, the hands pivoting on the hypothenar eminences, so introducing both supination of the hands and a simultaneous separation force to the contact fingers which creates a posterolateral traction on the occiput from these fingers.

The forces being applied should be minimal and sustained until a sense of 'softening' or warmth is noted, ideally on each side of the foramen magnum.

RESPIRATORY FUNCTION ASSESSMENT AND RESPONSES

Seated (Janda 1982)

Test (a) Have the patient place a hand on the upper abdomen and another on the upper chest. Observe the hands as the patient inhales several times. If the upper hand (chest) moves superiorly rather than anteriorly, and moves significantly more than the hand on the abdomen, a first clue is noted as to a dysfunctional pattern of breathing. If this is the case breathing retraining is called for.

Test (b) Stand behind and place both hands gently on upper trapezius area and have the patient inhale – note whether the hands move towards the ceiling significantly. If they do the scalenes are overworked, indicating stress and therefore probable shortening. MET treatment as described above will be appropriate.

Test (c) Stand in front and place the hands on the lower ribs, facing posteriorly, and note whether there is lateral excursion of the hands on inhalation: is there symmetry? If there is asymmetry reevaluate when all the identified restrictions, muscle imbalances, etc. have been worked on.

Stand to the side and observe the spinal contour as the patient fully flexes. Is there evidence of 'flat' areas of the spine (unable to flex fully), especially in the thoracic region, which would imply rib restrictions at those levels? The paraspinal muscles in the 'flat areas' should receive appropriate treatment (MET, NMT, induration technique, etc., and/or possibly spinal joint manipulation).

Supine

Test (d) Observe breathing pattern. Does the abdomen move forwards on inhalation? It should. Or does the upper chest move forwards on inhalation while the abdomen retracts? If it does, breathing retraining is called for as this is a paradoxical pattern. Is there an observable lateral excursion of lower ribs? There should be.

Test (e) Assess for shortness in pectoralis major and latissimus dorsi (arms extended above head). If the patient's arms cannot lie flat on the table, touching along the whole length, there is pectoral shortness; if the elbows deviate laterally significantly there is usually latissimus shortness. If either of these is short, appropriate lengthening procedures should be carried out (MET, etc. – not described in these notes).

Test (f) Observe for chin protrusion on raising of the head (functional test for sternomastoid). If this is positive (chin pokes), SCM is short and MET treatment as described above will be appropriate. (See Fig. 13.13, p. 210)

Test (g) Check psoas using functional assessment previously described (patient supine, arms crossed on chest, knees flexed, attempts to raise shoulders from table slowly; if feet leave table or lower back arches, psoas is implicated). Psoas merges with the diaphragm and requires attention (MET or self-stretching techniques – not described in these notes) if overactive or short, in order to facilitate normal respiration. (See Fig. 13.10, p. 208)

Test (h) Stand at waist level facing the head and place the hands fully extended on each side of the lower rib cage, fingers facing posteriorly along the rib shafts. Test the tissues for their rotational preference, by easing the superficial tissues and the ribs in a rotational manner, right and then left. Do the tissues move more easily when rotated right or left? Whichever it is, hold them lightly in that direction and then test to see whether the tissues in this region prefer to sidebend left or right. Whichever they do, hold them in this direction. A simple functional combined position of ease has been achieved which, if held (90 seconds or so), will effectively 'release' (to an extent) the structures to which the diaphragm attaches.

Side-lying

Test (j) Assess quadratus lumborum by palpation (leg abduction while palpation is carried out as in the functional assessment described earlier in this chapter). Quadratus attaches to the diaphragm as well as the twelfth rib and is often a major player in breathing dysfunction. If it is overactive it will shorten and both re-education and stretching are required (not described in these notes). (See Fig. 13.11, p. 209)

Prone

Test (h) Observe the so-called 'breathing wave' – the movement of spine from sacrum to base of neck on deep inhalation (there should be a continuous wave from the base of the spine to the neck). If movement starts above the sacrum and moves down and up (common), or if regions of the spine move as a 'block', instead of in a sequential wave-like manner, this can be noted as the current representation of the dysfunctional pattern, as it involves spinal movement. As improvement occurs (via bodywork, mobilisation, relaxation, exercise, breathing retraining, etc.), the pattern will be seen gradually to normalise.

Test (i) Palpate and evaluate for trigger point activity in muscles which are shown by previous assessments to be dysfunctional, using NMT and/or other palpation methods. Treat as appropriate using methods previously described (see Ch. 6 and also INIT notes above).

SUMMARY OF SOFT TISSUE APPROACHES TO FMS

1. Identification of local dysfunction, possibly involving:
   — Off-body scan for temperature variations (cold may suggest ischaemia, hot may indicate irritation/inflammation) (p. 202)

— Evaluation of fascial adherence to underlying tissues, indicating deeper dysfunction (Fig. 13.3)
— Assessment of variations in local skin elasticity, where loss of elastic quality indicates hyperalgesic zone and probable deeper dysfunction (e.g. trigger point) or pathology (Fig. 13.5)
— Evaluation of reflexively active areas (triggers, etc.) by means of very light, single-digit palpation seeking phenomenon of 'drag' (Fig. 13.14)
— NMT palpation utilising variable pressure, which 'meets and matches' tissue tonus (p. 209)
— Functional evaluation to assess local tissue response to normal physiological demand (e.g. as in functional tests as described) (Figs. 13.9, 13.10, 13.11, 13.12, 13.13).

2. Short postural muscles:
— Sequential assessment and identification of specific shortened postural muscles, by means of observed and palpated changes, functional evaluation methods, etc. (Box 13.1, p. 200)
— Subsequent treatment of short muscles by means of MET or self-stretching will allow for regaining of strength in antagonist muscles which have become inhibited, after which additional gentle toning exercise may be appropriate (pp. 223–224, Figs 13.25, 13.26).

3. Treatment of local (i.e. trigger points) and whole muscle problems utilising:
— Tissues held at elastic barrier to await physiological release (skin stretch, 'C' bend, 'S' bend, gentle NMT, etc.) (p. 203)
— Use of positional release methods – holding tissues in 'dynamic neutral' (strain/counterstrain, functional technique, induration technique, fascial release methods, etc.) (Fig. 13.7, p. 204)
— Myofascial release methods (not described in this text)
— MET methods for local and whole muscle dysfunction (involving acute, chronic and pulsed [Ruddy's] MET variations as described above) (p. 227)

— Vibrational techniques (rhythmic/rocking/oscillating articulation methods; mechanical or hand vibration)
— Deactivation of myofascial trigger points (if sensitivity allows) utilising INIT (p. 233) (integrated neuromuscular inhibition technique) or other methods (acupuncture, ultrasound, etc.).

4. Whole body approaches such as:
— Wellness massage and/or aromatherapy (pp. 151, 176)
— Hydrotherapy (pp. 175, 178)
— Cranial techniques
— Therapeutic touch
— Lymphatic drainage.

5. Re-education/rehabilitation/self-help approaches:
— Postural (Alexander, etc.)
— Breathing retraining (p. 173)
— Cognitive behavioural modification (Ch. 7)
— Aerobic fitness training (p. 147)
— Yoga-type stretching, T'ai chi
— Deep relaxation methods (autogenics, etc.) (p. 174)
— Pain self-treatment (e.g. self-applied SCS – see Ch. 14).

6. Sound nutrition (Ch. 11 & 12).

CONCLUSION

When people are very ill, as in FMS/CFS where adaptive functions have been stretched to their limits, ANY treatment (however gentle) represents an additional demand for adaptation (i.e. it is yet another stressor). It is therefore essential that treatments and therapeutic interventions are carefully selected and modulated to the patient's current ability to respond, as best as this can be judged (see Fig. 2.4 and Box 2.1, Therapeutic stress).

When symptoms are at their worst, only single changes, or simple interventions, may be appropriate, with time allowed for the body/mind to process and handle these. It may also be worth considering general, whole-body, constitutional, approaches (dietary changes, hydrotherapy, non-specific 'wellness' massage, relaxation methods, etc.) rather than specific interventions, in the initial stages, and during periods when symptoms have flared. Recovery from FMS is slow at best and it is easy to make matters worse by over-enthusiastic and inappropriate interventions. Patience is required by both the health care provider and the patient, avoiding raising false hopes while realistic therapeutic and educational methods are used which do not make matters worse and which offer ease and the best chance of improvement.

REFERENCES

Baldry P 1993 Acupuncture, trigger points and musculoskeletal pain. Churchill Livingstone, London

Barrell J-P 1996 Manual thermal diagnosis. Eastland Press, Seattle

Basmajian J 1974 Muscles alive. Williams and Wilkins, Baltimore

Beal M 1983 Palpatory testing of somatic dysfunction in patients with cardiovascular disease. Journal of the American Osteopathic Association (July)

Bowles C 1981 Functional technique: a modern perspective. Journal of the American Osteopathic Association 80(3): 326–331

Chaitow L 1989 Soft tissue manipulation. Thorsons, London

Chaitow L 1991 Modified 'Strain Counterstrain' in soft tissue manipulation. Healing Arts Press, Rochester, Vermont

Chaitow L 1994 Integrated neuromuscular inhibition technique. British Journal of Osteopathy 13: 17–20

Chaitow L 1996a Modern neuromuscular techniques. Churchill Livingstone, New York

Chaitow L 1996b Muscle energy techniques. Churchill Livingstone, New York

Dickey J 1989 Postoperative osteopathic manipulative management of median sternotomy patients. Journal of the American Osteopathic Association 89(10): 1309–1322

DiGiovanna E (ed) 1991 An osteopathic approach to diagnosis and treatment. Lippincott, Philadelphia

Dvorak J, Dvorak V 1984 Manual medicine: diagnostics. Georg Thiem Verlag Thieme Stratton, Stuttgart

Engel A et al 1986 'Skeletal muscle types' in myology. McGraw Hill, New York

Evjenth O, Hamberg J 1984 Muscle stretching in manual therapy. Alfta Rehab, Oslo

Garland W 1994 Somatic changes in hyperventilating subject. Presentation at Respiratory Function Congress, Paris, 1994

Goodheart G 1984 Applied kinesiology workshop procedure manual 21st edn. Privately published, Detroit

Greenman P 1989 Principles of manual medicine. Williams and Wilkins, Baltimore

Hoover H 1969 Collected papers. Academy of Applied Osteopathy Yearbook 1969

Janda V 1982 Introduction to functional pathology of the motor system. Proceedings of VII Commonwealth and International Conference on Sport. Physiotherapy in Sport 3: 39

Janda V 1983 Muscle function testing. Butterworths, London

Janda V 1989a Differential diagnosis of muscle tone in respect of inhibitory techniques. Presentation Physical Medicine Research Foundation, 21 Sept 1989

Janda V 1989b Muscle function testing. Butterworths, London

Jones L 1981 Strain and counterstrain. Academy of Applied Osteopathy, Colorado Springs

Korr I 1976 Spinal cord as organiser of the disease process. Academy of Applied Osteopathy Yearbook 1976

Korr I 1978 Neurologic mechanisms in manipulative therapy. Plenum Press, New York, p 27

Latey P 1983 Muscular manifesto. Self-published, London

Lewis T 1942. Pain. New York

Lewit K 1986 Muscular patterns in thoraco-lumbar lesions. Manual Medicine 2

Lewit K 1992 Manipulation in rehabilitation of the locomotor system. Butterworths, London

Liebenson C 1990 Muscular relaxation techniques. Journal of Manipulative and Physiological Therapeutics 12(6): 446–454

Liebenson C 1996 Rehabilitation of the spine. Williams and Wilkins, Philadelphia

Lin J-P 1994 Physiological maturation of muscles in childhood. Lancet (June 4): 1386–1389

Melzack R 1983 The challenge of pain. Penguin, London

Mitchell F Snr 1967 Motion discordance. Yearbook of the Academy of Applied Osteopathy, Carmel CA, pp 1–5

Moore M et al 1980 Electromyographic investigation manual of muscle stretching techniques. Medicine and Science in Sports and Exercise 12: 322–329

Morrison M 1969 Lecture notes presentation/seminar. Research Society for Naturopathy, London

Nimmo R 1969 Receptor tonus technique. Lecture notes, London

Ramirez M et al 1989 Low back pain: diagnosis by six newly discovered sacral tender points and treatment with counterstrain technique. Journal of the American Osteopathic Association 89(7): 905–913

Rowlerson A A 1981 Novel myosin. Journal of Muscle Research and Cell Motility 2: 415–438

Ruddy T 1962 Osteopathic rapid rhythmic resistive technicque. Academy of Applied Osteopathy Yearbook, pp 23–31

Schiowitz S 1990 Facilitated positional release. Journal of the American Osteopathic Association 90(2): 145 –156

Selye H 1956 The stress of life. McGraw Hill, New York

Simons D 1987 Myofascial pain due to trigger points. International Rehabilitation Medicine Association Monograph, series 1, Rademaker OH

Travell J, Simon G 1983 Myofascial pain and dysfunction: the trigger point manual. Williams and Wilkins, Baltimore, vol 1

Travell J, Simons D 1986 Myofascial pain and dysfunction, Williams and Wilkins, Baltimore, vol 1

Travell J, Simon G 1991 Myofascial pain and dysfunction: the trigger point manual. Williams and Wilkins, Baltimore, vol 2

Travell J, Simons D 1992 Myofascial pain and dysfunction. Williams and Wilkins, Baltimore, vol 2

Travell J, Simons D 1993 Myofascial pain and dysfunction, Williams and Wilkins, Baltimore, vol 2, 2nd edn

Upledger J, Vredevoogd J 1983 Cranio-Sacral Therapy. Eastland Press, Seattle, WA

Wall P, Melzack R 1989 Textbook of pain. Churchill Livingstone, London

Walther D 1988 Applied kinesiology. Synopsis Systems DC, Pueblo, Colorado

Woo Sl-Y et al 1987 Injury and repair of musculoskeletal soft tissues. American Academy of Orthopedic Surgeons Symposium, Savannah GA

A FIBROMYALGIA PROTOCOL

Where a condition has multiple interacting causes it makes clinical sense to try to reduce the burden of whatever factors are imposing themselves on the defence, immune and repair mechanisms of the body, while at the same time doing all that is possible to enhance those mechanisms without increasing demands on the patient's adaptive capacity and current vitality (Fig. 1.2).

In the author's practice (but not always in the order listed) the aim in treating FMS/CFS is to:

• Get the diagnosis right. Many rheumatic-type problems produce widespread muscular pain (e.g. polymyalgia rheumatica). Laboratory and other tests can identify most no-FMS conditions.

• Identify associated myofascial trigger point activity and treat these using methods chosen from bodywork, injection (xylocaine, etc.), acupuncture, nutrition, hydrotherapy, postural and/or breathing re-education, relaxation methods, etc. (Ch. 6, Box 6.2)

• Assess and treat (or refer elsewhere for attention) associated conditions such as allergy, anxiety, hyperventilation, yeast or viral activity, bowel dysfunction, hypothyroid dysfunction, sleep disturbance, depression, etc. (Ch. 10, 11, 12)

• Introduce (in-house, self-applied or via referral) 'constitutional' health enhancement methods such as:

— breathing retraining (p. 173)
— deep relaxation methods (e.g. autogenic training) (p. 174)
— graduated (aerobic, stretching and toning) exercise programmes (p. 147, Ch. 7 and 9)
— regular (weekly or fortnightly) detoxification (fasting) days (to detoxify as well as boost growth hormone production) (p. 190)
— hydrotherapy, e.g. neutral bath or 'constitutional' progressive cold bathing (depending upon vitality and willingness) (p. 175, 178)
— regular non-specific massage (p. 151)
— acupuncture. (Ch. 6)

• Offer detailed advice as appropriate – including possibly:

— elimination and rotation dietary patterns (p. 168)
— exclusion of nightshade family of foods, sugars, yeast based foods (if appropriate), processed foods, etc.
— inclusion of whole foods (organic if possible), adequate protein, probiotics (p. 157)
— nutritional supplements (antioxidants, magnesium, malic acid, manganese glycinate, methionine, NAC, thiamine, DLPA, 5–HTP, chromium, etc), and/or (p. 153)
— amino acids for growth hormone production (arginine, ornithine) (p. 189)
— specific herbal help to enhance circulation to the brain (e.g. *Ginkgo biloba*) or which have pain reducing properties (e.g. *Boswellia*) or which are relaxing (kava kava, valerian, etc.) or antidepressant effects (hydrastis) or antiviral, immune-enhancing capabilities (*Glycyrrhiza glabra* [licorice], echinacea), etc. (pp. 183–184)
— homeopathic remedies (Rhus Tox 6C) (p. 150).

• Provide appropriate soft tissue treatment (see soft tissue approach summary) plus teaching gentle self-help methods (for daily use), for example:

— 'Strain/counterstrain' (see Ch. 14)

• Advice on regular exercise within tolerance, if possible including cardiovascular training and stretching movements (yoga and/or t'ai chi) (p. 147).

— Suggest medication – under medical supervision only – in appropriate cases, to enhance sleep; antidepressant drugs (very low dosage) may offer short-term benefit (p. 152).

• Encourage patients to join support groups, to read about their condition and health enhancement, to take control of their condition, even if progress is apparently slow (Ch. 7).

• Offer stress or general counselling which may help in the learning of coping skills and lead to stress reduction (Ch. 8 and 12).

The text of this chapter can be adapted and used
for patient education

14

Strain/counterstrain self-treatment for some FMS tender points

The text in this chapter, which describes self-treatment of tender points, can be adapted and used for patient education. The aim is to help patients to learn to use strain/counterstrain methods by focusing on five of the key tender points used in diagnosis of FMS. In doing so, the practical 'how to' principles of SCS self-treatment should become clear and usable in first-aid self-care on any painful area of the body.

USING THE TENDER POINTS

Patient information should include the fact that the diagnosis of FMS depends on there being at least 11 tender points present out of 18 tested using a set amount of pressure. The location of the diagnostic points for FMS should be explained:

1. Either side of the base of the skull where the subocciptal muscles insert
2. Either side of the side of the neck between the fifth and seventh cervical vertebrae (anterior aspects of inter-transverse space)
3. Either side of the body on the midpoint of the muscle which runs from the neck to the shoulder (upper trapezius)
4. Either side of the body, origin of the supraspinatus muscle which runs along the upper border of the shoulder blade
5. Either side, on the upper surface of the rib, where the second rib meets the breast bone, in the pectoral muscle
6. On the outer aspect of either elbow just below the prominence (epicondyle)

7. In the large buttock muscles, either side, on the upper outer aspect in the fold in front of the muscle (gluteus medius)

8. Just behind the large prominence of either hip joint in the muscular insertion of piriformis muscle

9. On either knee in the fatty pad just above the inner aspect of the joint

Plus additional sites sometimes also recommended for testing:

10. Lower portion of the sternomastoid muscle in front on the throat

11. Lateral part of the pectoral muscle at the level of the fourth rib

12. The region of the low lumbar spine around the fourth and fifth lumbar vertebrae.

Because they are almost universally present in FMS, the first five of these sets of points are used in the examples of SCS below. These are described in the first person, speaking to the patient directly, so that the text and pictures can be copied for their use.

1. Suboccipital muscles (Fig. 14.1)

To use SCS on these muscles you should be lying on your side with your head on a low pillow. The points lie at the base of your skull in a hollow just to the side of the centre of the back of the neck.

- Feel for the tender point on the side which is lying on the pillow with the hand on that same side, and press just hard enough to register the pain and score the level of pain this produces as a '10' (where 10 is severe and 0 is no pain at all).
- To take pain away from the pressure you are applying to muscles at the base of the skull, you need to take the head backwards slightly, and usually to lean it and perhaps turn it towards the side of pain.
- First just take the head slightly backwards, very slowly as though you are looking upwards. If the palpated pain changes, give it a score. If it is now below 10 you are on the right lines.
- Play around with slightly more backward bending of the neck, done very slowly, until you find a position which reduces the pain to around a 6 or 7.

- Then allow the head to turn and perhaps lean a little towards the pain side (the side you are lying on) until the score drops some more.
- Keep 'fine-tuning' the position as you slowly reduce the pain score. You should eventually find a position in which it is reduced to 3 or less.
- If the directions of movement of the head described above do not achieve this score reduction, the particular dynamics of your muscular pain might need you to turn the head away from the side of pain, or to find some other slight variation of position to achieve ease; however, the directions given above are the most likely to help you bring the score right down to a 3 or less.
- Once you have found the position of maximum ease (3 or less) just relax in that position. You do not need to maintain pressure on the tender point all the time, just test it from time to time by pressing.
- Remember also that the position which eases the tenderness should not produce any other pain – you should be relatively at ease when resting with the pain point at ease.
- Stay like this for at least 1 minute and then SLOWLY return to a neutral position, turn over and treat the other side in the same way.

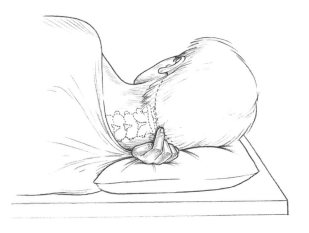

Figure 14.1 Strain/counterstrain self-treatment for suboccipital tender point.

2. Side of neck tender points (Fig. 14.2)

These points lie near the side of the base of the neck directly below the lobe of your ear (between the transverse processes of the fifth and seventh cervical vertebrae).

• You can find the tenderness by running a finger very lightly – skin on skin, no pressure – down the side of your neck starting just below the ear lobe.

• As you run down you should be able to feel the slight 'bump' as you pass over the tips of the transverse processes – the parts of the vertebrae which stick out sideways.

• When you get to the level of your neck which is about level with your chin, start to press in lightly after each 'bump', trying to find an area of tenderness on one side of your neck which, when pressed, allows you to give it a score of '10'.

• Once you have found this, sit or lie and allow your head to bend forwards (use a cushion to support it if you are lying on your back).

• As with the first point treated, you will find that tenderness will be reduced as you take the head forwards. Find the most 'easy' position by experimenting with different amounts of forward bending.

• The tenderness will be reduced even more as you fine tune the position of your head and neck by slowly and slightly sidebending and turning the head either towards or away from the pain side – whichever gives the best results in terms of your 'pain score'.

• When you get the score down to a 3 or less, stay in that position for at least 1 minute and then slowly return to neutral and seek out a tender point at the same level, on the other side of the neck and treat it the same way.

3. Midpoint of upper trapezius muscle (Fig. 14.3)

The trapezius muscle runs from the neck to the shoulder and you can get an easy access to tender points in it by using a slight 'pinching' grip on the muscle using your thumb and index finger of (say) the right hand to gently squeeze the muscle fibres on the left, until something very tender is found.

• If pressure is maintained on this tender point for 3 or 4 seconds it might well start to produce a radiating pain in a distant site, probably the head, in which case the tender point is also a trigger point (the same could be true of any of the tender points you are going to palpate but this one is one of the likeliest and commonest).

• To treat the tenderness you should lie down, using a pillow, on the side opposite that which you are treating.

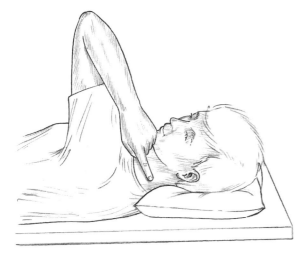

Figure 14.2 Strain/counterstrain self-treatment for lateral cervical tender point.

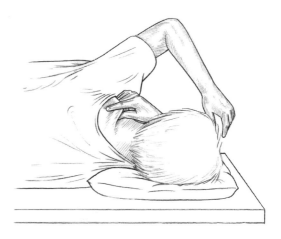

Figure 14.3 Strain/counterstrain self-treatment for tender point in middle fibres of upper trapezius muscle.

- Lightly pinch the point (using the hand on the non-treated side) to produce a score of 10 and try altering the position of the other arm, perhaps taking it up and over your head, to 'slacken' the muscle you are palpating, or altering your neck position by having it sidebend slightly towards the painful side, perhaps by adding an additional cushion.
- Fine tune the arm and head positions until you reduce the score in your pain point (don't pinch it all the time, just now and then, to test whether a new position is easing the sensitivity).
- Once you find your position of maximum ease (score down to 3 or less), stay in that position for not less than 1 minute.
- Slowly return to a neutral position, turn over and seek out a tender point in much the same position on the other side.

4. Origin of the supraspinatus muscle above the shoulder blade
(Fig. 14.4)

Lie on your back, head flat on the floor/bed/surface and, resting your elbow on your chest, ease your hand over your opposite shoulder area to feel with the tips of your fingers for the upper surface (near to the base of your neck) of your other shoulder blade.

- Run your fingers along this upper surface towards the spine until you come to the end of the shoulder blade and there press into the muscles a little, looking for an area of great tenderness (most of us are tender here but in FMS this will usually be very sensitive). You may need to press a little down, or back towards the shoulder or in some other direction until you find what you are looking for and can score the sensitivity as a 10.
- With your upper arm resting at your side (on the affected side), and while a finger of the other hand remains in contact with the tender point, bend the arm on the affected side so that your finger tips rest close to your shoulder.
- Now bring the elbow on the affected side towards the ceiling – very slowly – and let it fall slightly away from the shoulder about half way

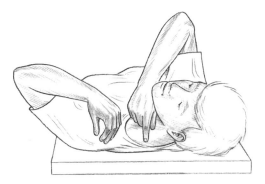

Figure 14.4 Strain/counterstrain self-treatment for supraspinatus tender point.

to the surface on which you are lying. Does this reduce the score?

- It should. Now start to use 'fine tuning' of the arm position in which you rotate the bent arm gently at the shoulder, twisting so that the elbow comes towards the chest and the hand moves away from the shoulder, ever so slightly, until the pain is down to a score of about 3. (The score may also drop if you turn your head towards or away from the treated side slightly.)
- Hold the final 'position of maximum ease' (score 3 or less) for at least 1 minute, and then slowly return to neutral and do the same on the other side.

5. Second rib tender points
(Fig. 14.5)

Sitting in a chair, rest your middle finger on the upper surface of your breast bone, and move it slowly sideways until you touch the end of your collar bone where it joins your breast bone.

- Now run the finger towards your shoulder for not more than 1 inch, along the collar bone and then down towards the chest a half an inch or so, and you should feel first a slight 'valley', after which you will come to the second rib (you cannot easily touch the first rib because it is hidden behind the collar bone).
- Press the upper surface of the second rib firmly and it should be tender, perhaps very tender.
- Search close to here until you find a place where the pressure allows you to score a 10, and

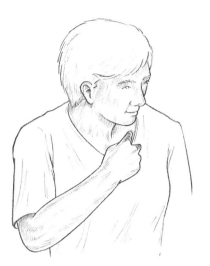

Figure 14.5 Strain/counterstrain self-treatment for second rib tender point.

then begin to take that score down by firstly bending your head and your upper back forwards, slightly (very slightly) towards the side of the pain point, until you feel the pain reduce.

• Find the most 'easy' position of forward and slightly sidebending (the position which reduces the score most) and then see whether slightly tilting the head one way or the other helps to reduce the score even more.

• Try also to take a full deep breath in and then slowly let the breath go, and see which part of your breathing cycle eases the tenderness most.

• Once you have the score down to a 3 or less, add in that most 'easy' phase of the breath (hold the breath at that phase which eases the pain most) for 10–15 seconds.

• Then breathe normally but retain the position of ease for at least 1 minute before slowly returning to neutral and seeking out the tender point on the other side for similar attention.

After trying out these 10 points (five on each side) you can now use SCS to treat any painful point or muscle using these same methods. The relief will be variable, lasting for a short or long period depending on what caused the pain. At least you have with this

technique a practical first-aid measure for reducing pain, often considerably and often for a long period.

Remember the basic rules:

• Find a pain point.
• Score this as 10 while pressing it.
• Move your body, or part of the body, around slowly until the pain is reduced to a 3.
• If the pain is in the front of your body, the movements and positions which ease the pain will usually involve bending forwards and towards the side of the pain.
• If the pain is on the back of your body, the movements which ease the pain will usually involve bending backwards and away from the side of the pain.
• The further a pain point is from the midline, the more sidebending and rotation will usually be needed to ease the pain in the point you are pressing.
• If the pain point is on a leg or arm, then movement of the limb, slowly in various directions, will usually show you which way to go in order to ease the palpated pain.
• Hold the 'position of ease' for 1 minute at least and slowly return to neutral.
That's all there is to SCS – and it works.

As a rule it is movements which 'slacken' the tissues housing the painful point which help reduce the 'score' most.

CAUTION: Do not treat more than 4 or 5 points on any day as the pain may increase for the first day or so after treatment before subsiding: this is because your body has to use the opportunity it has been given when the tender tissues were being held 'at ease' to process and change the tensions and circulation in the area. If you treat too many points you may be asking too much of your repair mechanisms, and may increase pain excessively.

Try these methods on a few points and judge the benefits several days after treating in this way. Are chronic areas less stiff and less painful? If so, treat sensitive areas in this way whenever the pain gets excessive.

RESOURCES

Patient information

Interaction
Journal of Action for ME (3 issues a year)
Action for ME, PO Box 1302
Wells BA5 2WE
UK

Fibromyalgia Network (a quarterly newsletter
for fibromyalgia, fibrositis and CFS support
groups)
PO Box 31750
Tucson, Arizona 85751-1750
USA

The Update
Massachusetts CFIDS Association
808 Main Street
Waltham MA 02154
USA

The CIFDS Chronicle
PO Box 220398
Charlotte NC 28222-0398
USA

Journals for Health Care Professionals

Journal of Musculoskeletal Pain
Haworth Press
10 Alice Street
Binghampton NY 13904
USA

Journal of Bodywork and Movement Therapies
Churchill Livingstone
3 Baxter's Place
Leith Walk
Edinburgh EH1 3AF
UK

Internet connections

USA Fibromyalgia Association
URL:http://www.w2.com/fibro1.html

Fibromyalgia Bibliography
URL:http://www.mabc.bc.ca/biblio/fibro.htm

Fibromyalgia Syndrome Resources
URL:http://prairie.lakes.com/~roseleaf/fibro/
fmswww.html